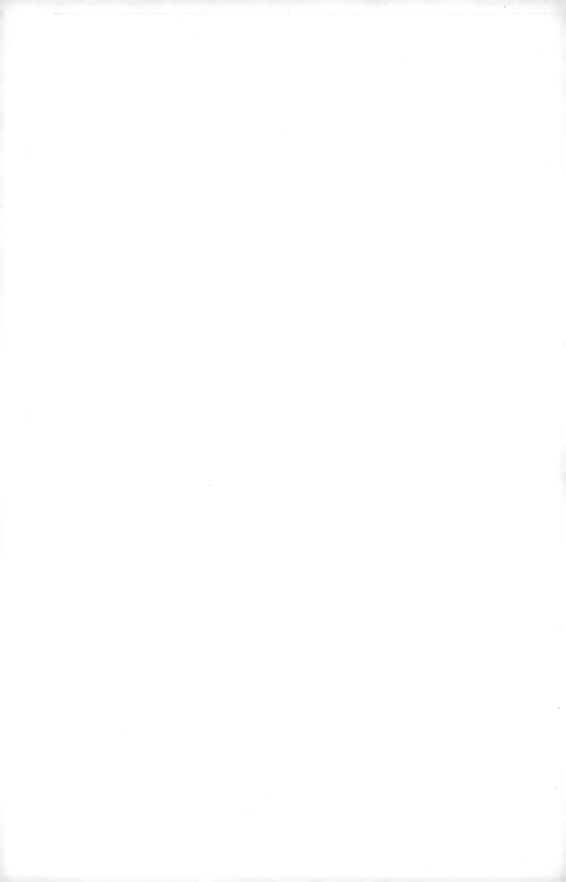

COGNITIVE REHABILITATION

COGNITIVE REHABILITATION

An Integrative Neuropsychological Approach

McKay Moore Sohlberg
Catherine A. Mateer

THE GUILFORD PRESS
New York   London

©2001 The Guilford Press
A Division of Guilford Publications, Inc.
72 Spring Street, New York, NY 10012
www.guilford.com

Printed in the United States of America

This book is printed on acid-free paper.

Last digit is print number: 9 8 7 6 5 4

Library of Congress Cataloging-in-Publication Data
is available from the Publisher.

1-57230-613-0

To Ericka, Tatum, and Emma

About the Authors

McKay Moore Sohlberg, PhD, is a nationally recognized leader in the field of traumatic brain injury rehabilitation. For the past 16 years she has worked as a clinician, researcher, and administrator in the development of programs to assist individuals with brain injury to reintegrate into the community at maximal levels of independence. The types of intervention programs that she has developed and about which she has conducted research have become model programs adopted by rehabilitation centers throughout the United States, Canada, and Europe. Dr. Sohlberg also has a wealth of experience in teaching other professionals and assisting agencies to be more effective in their delivery of community reintegration services to persons with brain injury. She has published numerous articles, chapters, and manuals on managing cognitive impairments following neurogenic insult. Dr. Sohlberg received her master's degree in Speech and Hearing Sciences and her PhD in Educational Psychology at the University of Washington. Currently, she is an associate professor in the Communication Disorders and Sciences program at the University of Oregon.

Catherine A. Mateer, PhD, is a board-certified clinical neuropsychologist with an extensive background in clinical assessment, clinical intervention, and both basic and applied research. She has published over 75 articles and book chapters and two previous books relating to brain organization for language, memory, and praxis, as well as to the assessment and management of acquired disorders of attention, memory, and executive functions in children and adults. Dr. Mateer is known internationally for her pioneering work in the rehabilitation of individuals who have sustained traumatic brain injury. She is also recognized for her basic research on brain and behavior relationships through the use of cortical mapping techniques, electrophysiological studies, and studies of the neuropsychological effects of focal brain lesions and specific neurological disorders. Dr. Mateer received her master's degree in Communication Disorders from the University of Wisconsin, and her PhD in Psychology from the University of Western Ontario. Currently, she is a professor in the Department of Psychology and the Director of the Graduate Program in Clinical Psychology at the University of Victoria in British Columbia, Canada.

Preface

It can no longer be said that cognitive rehabilitation is a "new field." Over the last decade, and since the publication of our first book on cognitive rehabilitation (Sohlberg & Mateer, 1989), substantial growth and development has occurred. The last 2 years have brought the publication of many new texts targeting the rehabilitation of individuals with acquired brain injury. In addition, the research base has broadened, there is greater professional consensus around terminology, the understanding of the theoretical underpinnings of cognitive function has matured, and a wide range of treatment approaches have been articulated. Although there are still many important unanswered questions, the nature of the questions has changed.

The following questions aimed at the rehabilitation field illustrate the complexity of the rehabilitation process from the perspective of cognitive neuropsychology (Shallice, 2000):

- Can the operation of individual damaged subsystems or pathways be improved by retraining on particular input stimuli–output action pairings?
- How easily can a patient acquire and use novel action or thought schemas, which will be required in a rehabilitation procedure?
- Will a newly acquired schema requiring voluntary application eventually lead to effective automatic use?

These and related queries are examples of key issues we attempt to address in this book based on the literature to date. It is exciting to review the insights and possible frameworks for future research. We applaud the efforts of cognitive psychologists as they provide detailed descriptions of cognitive disorders and inform us about the flow of information. We also share their frustrations at the difficulty involved in parsing out cognitive components and evaluating their amenability to change when they are disordered. We are constantly reminded of the need to evaluate and document the result of treatment approaches as they evolve. There is a tendency, however, to erroneously consider cognitive rehabilitation as a singular approach. By analogy, one could not, for example, answer the question "Is surgery effective?" It depends upon the patient, the type of surgical procedure, the surgeon, and the nature of the problem. This text reviews a variety of rehabilitation approaches that run the gamut of behavioral interventions, direct process training, environmental manipulations, and psychotherapy. Their unifying characteristic is their potential effectiveness in helping to alleviate the effects of cognitive problems in persons with acquired deficits.

We also must be vigilant to the larger picture as we use cognitive theory to inform and direct rehabilitation. Cognitive neuropsychology tends to study phenomena at their most minute level (e.g., reading at the word or letter level). What is less understood is the practical impact on a functional level or in context. Cognitive neuropsychology also tends to be tightly organized around a particular process, and, if we are not careful, we might miss the variability associated with related receptive, expressive, and cognitive disorders that may impact treatment. Cognitive modularity is the basis for a number of state-of-the-art theoretical models, and this may be more evident in some systems (e.g., language) than in others (e.g., executive functions). What is heartening is that we are at a point where we can levy such caution.

One of the challenges when writing this book was our desire to reinforce and build upon existing successful rehabilitation techniques while documenting and describing the interventions that have evolved more recently. We fought an occasional urge to jump on the latest rehabilitation bandwagon and abandon careful description of rehabilitation approaches that continue to be effective. For example, attention process training remains a very effective method for managing deficits in attention and concentration in certain clients. The basic techniques are not vastly different from those we described in our earlier text (Sohlberg & Mateer, 1989), although there are more outcome studies suggesting why it may be helpful with some clients and not others, and we have more information about how these processes operate. Thus the chapter on management of attention disorders includes a section that details attention process training in addition to descriptions of other, more contemporary, management approaches. In many ways, however, the field of cognitive rehabilitation has a completely new face.

Perhaps the most important change in the field has been the adoption of a wider lens from which to view rehabilitation. The first text focused on remediation and compensation of damaged cognitive functions. Today, rehabilitation is conducted in a more ecological, contextual framework of service delivery. For example, formerly we acknowledged and studied the impact of head injury on the whole family, but we focused our treatment on the individual. We then began to recognize the importance of educating the family. More recently, we have begun to reap the rehabilitation benefit from collaborating and forming partnerships with families and caregivers.

This recognition of the clinical power inherent in effectively addressing social, emotional, and environmental variables as an integral part of addressing cognitive deficits, plus advances in computer technology and neuroscience necessitated a new volume rather than a second edition of our first text; this volume effectively replaces that text. Chapters covering a broad range of topics including neurobehavioral recovery, management of unawareness, external cognitive aids, collaboration with families, management of social and emotional issues, mild brain injury, and brain injury in children are now included.

In addition to advances in knowledge and experience, changes in service delivery have also profoundly impacted the field of cognitive rehabilitation. Carl Coelho (1997) conceptualized the history of cognitive rehabilitation into several distinct "eras." Our first text was published during the "era of proliferation" for brain injury rehabilitation. In the 1980s, the number of brain injury rehabilitation programs in the United States grew from 10 to over 500. The consumer movement began to flourish with the establishment of the National Head Injury Foundation and the Brain Injury Special Interest Group in the American Congress of Rehabilitation Medicine. In the late 1980s, major government support for research in brain injury was available for the first time and the rehabilitation division of federal education funded five model systems of care. The backdrop against which the current book has been written is vastly different.

We exist now in "an era of consolidation." Health care reform in the United States is a household term. There has been enormous downsizing in programs, shifts toward shorter hospital stays, and less outpatient care, and more severely impaired children are integrated into regular classrooms. Research dollars, however, continue to be available in spite of limited funding to provide clinical services. We are deeply saddened by the restricted access to services for the many people who could benefit from them and we continue to advocate for broader service. One important by-product, however, is that this era has stimulated researchers to develop, utilize, and evaluate the relationship between therapeutic interventions and functional outcome.

To accommodate changes in service delivery, cognitive rehabilitation research must incorporate more participatory action research involving individuals with brain injuries and their families, caregivers, and educators as agents who can deliver cognitive interventions, rather than researchers or rehabilitation professionals. This necessitates learning more about perceptions of the impact of cognitive impairments and using clinical experience to develop intervention and management approaches. The field has moved away from "treatments" and toward "interventions." The goal of these interventions is to expand knowledge about brain injury and its effects, enhance confidence in the ability to self-manage cognitive and behavioral problems, and enable more active discussion between individuals, families, and therapists. This trend has greatly influenced our own research and thinking and is reflected in all of the chapters on specific cognitive abilities, as well as in the addition of chapters reviewing methods to effectively collaborate with families and chapters focusing on methods to work with behavioral and emotional sequelae of brain injury. The primary goals of many of the interventions discussed are client and family education; increased awareness; increased self-regulation of cognitive abilities, behavior, and mood; and a greater sense of self-efficacy with respect to managing the myriad effects of brain injury.

In summary, the overarching goal of this text remains similar to our first book. We attempt to bridge the ever-expanding knowledge of cognitive and behavioral neuroscience with applied rehabilitation so that clinicians can use the text to assist persons with changes in cognitive ability and those who care for them within the real constraints of the environments in which they all function. We strive for a theoretically based yet eminently practical handbook. Occasionally in cognitive neuropsychology and neuroscience circles, our work is criticized as overly applied, confounded by real-world variables, and bordering on unscientific. Occasionally in rehabilitation arenas, it is criticized as too theoretical. We hope this means we are close to building a successful bridge between theory and practice.

REFERENCES

Coelho, C. (1997, October). *Outcomes, efficacy and effectiveness of rehabilitation for cognitive-communicative disorders following traumatic brain injury in adults.* Paper presented at the annual meeting of the Oregon Speech–Language–Hearing Association, Eugene, OR.

Shallice, T. (2000). Cognitive neuropsychology and rehabilitation: Is pessimism justified? *Neuropsychological Rehabilitation, 10*(3), 209–217.

Sohlberg, M. M., & Mateer, C. A. (1989). *Introduction to cognitive rehabilitation.* New York: Guilford Press.

Acknowledgments

This book started out as a process to update our first text. It quickly became clear, however, that the expansion and advancements in neurogenic rehabilitation necessitated a new text. A huge impetus for changes in the field was the efforts of those people most affected by brain injury. Thus, we first acknowledge and thank all persons challenged by brain injury, along with their families, friends, and communities who have contributed so richly to this field. In the 12 years since we wrote the first book, you have become political activists, community advocates, rehabilitation researchers, and authors. You are responsible for many of the advances in cognitive rehabilitation. On a personal note, you do much more than strengthen our professional lives; you deepen our spirits. May we continue to learn from your courage, perseverance, and willingness to educate those around you.

We also thank our past and future students, who are hungry for this information and remain our best critics. You inspire us with your questioning minds and your enthusiasm to form clinical partnerships with persons affected by cognitive disorders. We wish to acknowledge the outstanding editorial assistance from Thomas Boyd, PhD, ABPP. You provide a rare combination of wisdom and heart and serve as a model to all professionals in our field.

Projects such as writing books take large blocks of time, which are only available by taking away time from other responsibilities and enjoyments. McKay thanks Olof for many hours of editorial assistance, his unselfish willingness to take on more domestic tasks, and his continuous support of her passion for this field. You are a soulmate extraordinaire and bring joy to each and every day. She also appreciates her precious daughters, Ericka, Tatum, and Emma, for their support of Mama's "computer days." Your marvelous, unique development in conjunction with your magical sisterly bond has taught her more about cognition and human dynamics than possible through any academic experience. McKay also remains bolstered by loving parents and a greater family spread between two continents—the ultimate safety net.

Katy has experienced major changes in her life since the publication of the previous text, not the least of which was accepting the invitation to move back to Canada, where she completed her doctoral studies many years ago and where she is now involved in developing programs and opportunities for students who will be the clinicians, rehabilitation specialists, and researchers of the future. Many students from the University of Victoria provided valuable assistance with preparation of portions of the text, thoughtful discussion, and valuable reviews of early drafts. Special acknowledgments go to Louise Penkman, Sandra Mish, Nick Bogod, Laura Jansen, Claire Sira, and Jeff Sheer. Lori-Ann, our wonderful clinic manager, provided constant encouragement and helped protect Katy's schedule, enabling her to write. Catherine St. Denis and Pam Duncan are appreciated for their valuable editorial assistance. Katy also thanks her parents and siblings for their constant love and support, and Kim for a life full of more joy, surprise, and adventure than she ever imagined.

Contents

Chapter 8. Management of Dysexecutive Symptoms   230

Chapter 9. The Assessment and Management   269
           of Unawareness

Chapter 10. Communication Issues   306

PART III. INTERVENTIONS FOR BEHAVIORAL, EMOTIONAL, AND PSYCHOSOCIAL CONCERNS

I

FUNDAMENTALS FOR PRACTICING COGNITIVE REHABILITATION

Introduction to
Cognitive Rehabilitation

It has been almost a quarter of a century since the long-term impact of acquired brain injury (ABI), particularly traumatic brain injury (TBI), has been recognized. In that time there has been a surge of interest in understanding the underlying mechanisms of injury, as well as the nature of acquired physical, cognitive, behavioral, and emotional consequences of such injuries. Rehabilitation professionals have met the challenge of working with individuals with acquired brain injury and their families in thoughtful, creative, and dynamic ways. In the United States, at least, these efforts have occurred in the context of major changes in health care delivery and technology.

The term *cognitive rehabilitation* was perhaps always too narrow, and focused too heavily on remediating or compensating for decreased cognitive abilities. The term *rehabilitation of individuals with cognitive impairment* probably better captures the emphasis on injured individuals that has and will always be the target of cognitive rehabilitation. Although some of the fundamental goals of improving and compensating for cognitive abilities continue to be mainstays of rehabilitation efforts with this population, the last 25 years have allowed a richer appreciation for the influence of contextual variables; the personal, emotional, and social impacts of brain injury; and their interactions with cognitive function. All of these factors have been incorporated to an even greater degree into treatment plans and goals. Short- and long-term emotional and social supports are needed for many individuals dealing with persistent sequelae of brain injury.

For decades the field seemed to be trapped in an internal struggle over whether it is better to focus on training processes, skills, or functional abilities, and in what ways and in what contexts that training might be accomplished. Though the struggle is perhaps not entirely over, it is increasingly

3

acknowledged that functional changes must be the goal of treatment, and that there are many ways to go about facilitating those functional changes. If we have learned anything, it is that a cookie-cutter approach will not work. Individuals and families respond differently to different interventions, in different ways, at different times after injury. Premorbid functioning, personality, social support, and environmental demands are but a few of the factors that can profoundly influence outcome. In this variable response to treatment, cognitive rehabilitation is no different from treatment for cancer, diabetes, heart disease, Parkinson's disease, spinal cord injury, psychiatric disorders, or any other injury or disease process for which variable response to different treatments is the norm. Below, we outline some of the major forces that have shaped and continue to shape cognitive rehabilitation.

MAJOR FORCES SHAPING COGNITIVE REHABILITATION

New Perspectives and Findings with Regard to Neuroplasticity

Researchers now know that the brain is a far more plastic organ than was long thought to be the case, and that following injury, it is capable of considerable reorganization that can form the basis of functional recovery. New experimental work has clearly demonstrated changes in regional dendritic arborization that result in increased connections among surviving neurons (Kolb & Gibb, 1999). What are especially important from the point of view of cognitive rehabilitation are the demonstrated relationships among dendritic growth, structured environmental stimulation, and the recovery of lost functions. Our challenge is to understand the principles underlying this recovery and the types of postinjury experience that optimally drive it. This potential to reinstate function in damaged brain region as a consequence of neuroplasticity is discussed in greater length in Chapter 3 of this volume.

Advances in Technology

The exponential growth in new technology has had profound influences on rehabilitation. One way in which these effects can be felt is in the growth and development of powerful information-based tools that can be adapted for individuals with cognitive limitations. Increasingly smaller yet more powerful computers and chip-based technology are putting sophisticated devices for storing and retrieving information at our fingertips. Watches, cell phones, paging systems, and hand-held computer devices can all be linked to other computers and systems to expand ways in which individuals with physical and/or cognitive impairments can interact with the world. Moreover, as the technological revolution continues to advance, costs and size are coming down, and usability and flexibility are going up.

New applications of already existing technology can support sophisticated tracking, orienting, and signaling devices for people with severe memory impairments. The ability to develop skills and knowledge in a functional context is being met in brand new ways through the use of "virtual reality" environments. Individuals with severe physical limitations (even high-spinal-cord injuries) can now interact with and affect their environment through computers signaled by eye movements, or even by keyboards placed on the roof of a person's mouth!

Whole apartments have been adapted and wired to support increased independence in the community. Appliances can be monitored for safety; flexible devices for paging or communicating are available; and adapted equipment allows efficient cooking, bathing, cleaning, gardening, and self-care. These innovations are being fueled not only by technological advances, but by the increased proportion of older adults in our society. Changes are occurring so rapidly that it is difficult to anticipate fully how they will help increase independence even in the next few years.

Emphasis on Empowerment

Over the last few decades, there has been an increased focus on self-sufficiency and self-help. Books, magazines, and opportunities for involvement with groups have promoted a take-charge approach to health, adjustment, and satisfaction. Widespread access to the Internet is arming people with disabilities and their families and caregivers with information, resources, and a wide range of mechanisms for support; as a result, they are beginning to feel less isolated. For example, there is a Web site run for and by individuals with the relatively rare neurological disorder prosopagnosia, which affects a person's ability to recognize even familiar faces. Accessible at http://www.choisser.com/faceblind/, it affords individuals with prosopagnosia the opportunity to gain information and share experiences with others who are "faced" with the same challenges.

A number of empowerment principles should guide rehabilitation efforts. Interventions should have as their ultimate goal an increase in skill or knowledge, a belief, a change in behavior, and/or the use of a compensatory strategy that will increase or improve some aspect of independent function. Interventions sometimes need to balance maximization of safety with risk taking as an individual takes on new skills and challenges. The rehabilitative process should work to reinforce individuals and families by building on their strengths. Individuals and families should be involved in setting goals, but also in selecting, developing, participating in, and evaluating the intervention plan. The role of a therapist in cognitive rehabilitation has been likened to that of a teacher or coach. This is because much of the emphasis in any rehabilitation program is on providing education, fostering awareness, and facilitating goals, rather than on treatment per se, as performed by a doctor or dentist.

Changes in the Health Care Sector in the United States

Rehabilitation professionals and the individuals and families they work with have faced cutbacks similar to, if not more extreme than, those faced by other medical professionals and consumers of health care. This has translated into shorter inpatient stays, reduced outpatient coverage, fewer day treatment programs, and more limited ancillary support services. Every rehabilitation professional has felt the loss of team autonomy in decision making about rehabilitation needs, together with the mandate to reduce costs above all else. The changes have forced rehabilitation professionals to use time as effectively as possible and to focus on short-term, measurable, functional outcomes. Long-term needs are likely to be met by families themselves and other community service agencies, which need to be educated about the effects of brain injury. There is no doubt that families, schools, mental health agencies, and communities have taken up the burden of managing the often lifelong consequences of significant brain injury. Many of the techniques that have been developed and shown to work in increasing independence and promoting self-sufficiency and community involvement, including return to work, are simply now not funded for many people. Restriction of health care dollars to "medical healing" leaves the great majority of clients with brain injuries and their families alone, scrambling to heal functionally, psychologically, and emotionally. It seems ironic that in a time of such unprecedented economic prosperity in the United States, hospitals, rehabilitation programs, outpatient services, and access to psychological support are being cut back or phased out altogether. At the same time, programs in some parts of the world have seen tremendous growth in and commitment to this segment of the population. Let us hope that the pendulum will swing back again.

Focus on Function

Although meaningful changes in an individual's everyday life have always been the goals of rehabilitation, it has been a challenge to articulate and measure appropriate goals and successful outcomes in individuals who have such a broad range of difficulties in many aspects of life. The emphasis on function has, however, encouraged the development of more ecologically based and relevant assessment scales and tools. Individuals affected by brain injury and their families are now much more likely to be involved from the beginning in identifying treatment goals. Indeed, mutual goal setting and involvement of families, friends, and coworkers in the rehabilitation process are now very common.

MANAGEMENT OF ATTENTION, MEMORY, AND EXECUTIVE FUNCTIONS

Although we have broadened the scope of this text to address behavioral issues, issues related to working with families, and a broader range of strategies designed to address emotional and adjustment issues, a strong emphasis on the important role of cognitive impairment remains. It is common in rehabilitation texts to consider the cognitive processes of attention, memory, and executive functions as separate units. Several reasons encourage us to integrate a discussion of the theoretical backdrop for these three cognitive domains. First, these areas are commonly targeted in neurorehabilitation programs. Second, impairments in each of these cognitive processes can have devastating effects on people's day-to-day functioning. Most importantly, the cognitive components involved in attention, memory, and executive functions overlap and interact in complex ways that make it difficult to discuss one process without referring to one of the other domains. The circuitry and structures subserving attention, memory, and executive functions are widely shared and are particularly vulnerable to disruption following acquired brain injury (Finlayson & Garner, 1994; Sohlberg & Mateer, 1989). In particular, these functions are commonly disrupted following injury to anterior frontal and temporal brain systems—areas that are often affected by TBI resulting from acceleration–deceleration forces. Reviews of treatment efficacy have often focused on attention, memory, and executive functions. Coelho, DeRuyter, and Stein (1996), for example, organized a review of treatment efficacy for cognitive–communicative disorders according to these three domains, as did Mateer, Kerns, and Eso (1996) in discussing the management of children with acquired disorders of attention, memory, and executive functions.

It is well established that impairments in attention, memory, and executive functions can profoundly affect an individual's daily functioning. Even mild changes in the ability to attend, process, recall, and act upon information can have significant effects on effectively completing basic everyday tasks. Consider the cognitive skills required for successful meal preparation as an example. The individual must plan a menu, identify needed ingredients, develop a shopping list for required items, and leave sufficient time for shopping and preparing the meal. Then the individual must sequence many food preparation activities in an organized way so that everything is ready at dinner time. Even a mild attention or executive function deficit can render this difficult, ineffective, or even impossible.

Attention, Memory, and Executive Function as Interdependent Processes

Attention, memory, and executive functions are related and interdependent. Their close interdependence stems from both a functional association and their shared neurocircuitry. Various components and subcomponents for each process may be identified, depending upon one's conceptualization of the specific process; however, regardless of one's theoretical framework, a great degree of overlap exists. When attempting to parcel out or define the components of attention, memory, or executive functions, a researcher necessarily borrows from the other two processes. For example, most researchers conceptualize attention as a hierarchy of subcomponents. High in the attention taxonomy are complex attention abilities such as working memory, selective attention, and the ability to shift attention between different tasks (Posner & Petersen, 1990; Sohlberg & Mateer, 1987; Sturm, Willmes, Orgass, & Hartje, 1997). These subcomponents of attention mirror certain abilities one often attributes to executive functions. For example, the ability to make mental shifts and engage in flexible thinking is an accepted subcomponent of executive functions (Lezak, 1993; Stuss & Benson, 1986). Similarly, it is difficult to distinguish between selective attention and mental flexibility.

When one considers the neurocircuitry serving attention, memory, and executive functions, the overlap becomes further evident. For example, a primary function of the prefrontal cortex has been described as the temporal organization, integration, formulation, and execution of novel behavioral sequences that are responsive to both environmental demands and constraints and to internal motivations and drive, such that they contribute to orderly purposive behavior (Mateer, 1999). Obviously, these frontal functions are integrally involved in attention and memory processes, as well as those of executive function.

Functionally, it is difficult to independently evaluate the operations involved in attention, memory, and executive functions. With the exception of laboratory tasks, which may engage very discrete components of one cognitive process, most functional activities involve multiple types of processing. Completing activities that engage the circuitry for one process will necessarily activate other processes. For example, when an individual is using executive function skills to plan and organize the activities involved in meal preparation, the processes of memory and attention will also be required and utilized.

Interdependence between Cognitive Abilities and Other Domains

In the same way that cognitive abilities overlap with each other, cognitive abilities also overlap with, influence, and are influenced by emotional difficulties (e.g., anger, anxiety, depression), behavioral difficulties (e.g., impulsivity, frustration, inappropriateness), and physical problems (e.g., motor impairments, sensory changes, headache, musculoskeletal pain). The artificial distinction among cognition, emotion, and motivation has steadily eroded. However, it is still common in rehabilitation texts to see box diagrams in which cognitive problems are dealt with in cognitive rehabilitation and/or speech therapy; emotional and behavioral problems are dealt with in some sort of affective rehabilitation therapy (e.g., group counseling, individual psychotherapy); and physical problems are dealt with through medical management and by physical and occupational rehabilitation specialists. Although the notions of interdisciplinary or even transdisciplinary treatment attempt to bridge and coordinate the various approaches, there has been very little written or investigated with regard to how to practice this philosophy in patient interactions and not just in a paper trail. In addition, health care practices have in some situations tended to break up rather than to bolster multidisciplinary treatment and teamwork.

Yet working on problems from multiple perspectives is crucial if we are to be successful. It has been suggested, for example, that working on a demanding cognitive task can actually have some effect on the ability of elderly people to maintain balance and equilibrium, potentially contributing to falls (Shumway-Cook, Wollacott, Kerns, & Baldwin, 1997). Combining therapeutic cognitive and motor activities may approximate the demands of everyday life more closely than artificially separating them in separate therapy sessions. The experience of cognitive inefficiency or failure can also give rise to catastrophic emotional reactions, manifested as fear, anxiety, and depression. These can further impede cognitive performance, setting up a cycle of negative self-expectancy on the part of a client, and resulting in conditioned avoidance of activities. Talking about emotional adjustment in the abstract, outside the context of cognitively demanding situations, may not address the underlying triggers for emotional reactions. Every rehabilitation specialist working with cognitively impaired individuals—not just a psychologist or social worker—needs to be alert for, and to have some knowledge and experience in working with, emotional reactions to frustration and loss. Indeed, we argue that dealing with these responses is an integral, not an ancillary, part of effective treatment.

To meet these needs, solid teamwork is essential. Rehabilitation professionals need to approach their task from a broad, long-term perspective, developing information, expertise, and goals with other professionals, clients, and their families. Interventions need to be person-focused rather than discipline-focused (Ponsford, Sloan, & Snow, 1995). This is best accomplished when clinicians are flexible and not overly concerned with role boundaries. Strong interdisciplinary teamwork and communication can reduce stress and provide motivation and encouragement to clinicians, who are often faced with challenging situations and clients. It also allows cross-fertilization of ideas from different perspectives. The interventions discussed in this text can be carried out by different members of the team, depending on the particular structure of the rehabilitation setting, although working as a team will almost always yield better outcomes.

DEVELOPING THEORIES FOR WORKING WITH COGNITIVE IMPAIRMENT

Although we have separate chapters in the book devoted to attention, memory, and executive functions, we are cognizant of the fact that these are highly interactive and interdependent processes. In this section we discuss some of the basic assumptions and models of cognitive processes underlying cognitive rehabilitation.

Basic Assumptions

What theories do clinicians need to understand in order to develop effective interventions with individuals who have acquired cognitive disorders? How can these theories be elaborated and applied to specific assessment and intervention plans? Theories specific to our understanding of particular aspects of cognition are discussed in the chapters dedicated to clinical management. We begin here by identifying some assumptions underlying this book's discussion of cognition and its approach to managing deficits in attention, memory, communication, executive functions, and behavioral and emotional dysregulation, the specifics of which are discussed in the ensuing chapters.

1. *Rehabilitation specialists cannot isolate cognition.* Brain damage affects cognitive, social, behavioral, and emotional functioning. Each of these four domains interacts with the others. It is inappropriate to consider management of difficulties in one domain, such as cognitive function, without attending to the others.

2. *Rehabilitation specialists will need to adopt an eclectic management approach.* Effective management of cognitive disorders requires drawing on a broad range of traditions, including behavioral, sociological, psychological, and neuropsychological disciplines.

3. *Rehabilitation specialists need a way to conceptualize the cognitive areas.* We hold that disorders need to be understood before they can be rehabilitated. Working from a taxonomy or model of a cognitive process helps clinicians to organize assessment and treatment activities and practices.

4. *Rehabilitation specialists need to apply current knowledge from the fields of cognitive psychology and the neurosciences.* There is a rapidly

expanding knowledge base within these fields that should guide our treatment. Having a grasp of the theoretical underpinnings of attention, memory, and executive functions will allow clinicians to develop effective treatments. For example, understanding the notion of preserved priming may provide clues for how best to teach an individual with amnesia to learn to use a compensatory memory system.

5. *Rehabilitation specialists need to form partnerships with clients and their families.* It is important to recognize the clinical power inherent in collaborations that build upon the expert knowledge families have about their own members and functioning. Families provide critical direction for cognitive rehabilitation efforts. Clinicians are unlikely to effect meaningful changes in attention and memory function in the absence of a working relationship with a client's family.

Models of Cognitive Processing

We can now begin to build a theoretical foundation for treatment itself. This involves choosing one or more models, as appropriate, for conceptualizing the various cognitive processes that need to be addressed in the treatment plan. Exploring the nature of attention, memory, and executive functions has been a focus of experimental psychologists for decades. Various theoretical interpretations and conceptual models have been put forth for each of these processes. In their discussion of attention, Kerns and Mateer (1996) describe four different types of models: cognitive processing, factor-analytic, neuroanatomical, and clinical models of attention. We also discuss a fifth type here: functional models.

Cognitive processing models usually examine the target process based on information from a normally functioning population as opposed to clinical samples, using laboratory-based tasks. It is worth mentioning, however, that cognitive psychologists have increasingly looked to clinical samples to inform them about the structure and function of cognition, and cognitive neuroscience is one of the fastest-growing areas of research. Indeed, with the advent of functional neuroimaging, it has become increasingly difficult to study cognitive functions without some consideration of their biological substrate. *Factor-analytic* models consider cognitive processes psychometrically. Constructs for the cognitive process are derived by conducting factor analyses of performance on psychometric tests thought to assess attention, memory, and executive functions. Models for these same cognitive processes have also been generated by identifying each of their *neuroanatomical* substrates. The cognitive processing and factor-analytic models commonly divide a process into a number of distinct components and subcomponents; neuroanatomical models identify the different brain regions that subserve these components.

Each of the models described above draws upon information from normally functioning individuals. With the advent of the field of cognitive rehabilitation, there has been a shift toward incorporating clinical observations from the disordered population into our theoretical models. Clinical models have emerged out of overlapping perspectives from cognitive psychology, neuropsychology, and the detailed analysis of cognitive function in persons with neurological impairment. Similar to factor-analytic models, most clinical models view attention, memory, and executive functions as having a number of dissociable components. Again, these components are based on clinical observations that are matched against components identified by cognitive and experimental psychologists.

A fifth type of modeling that is extremely relevant to cognitive rehabilitation is the use of *functional* descriptions. This involves describing how cognitive processes might be used for the completion of day-to-day tasks. For example, *prospective memory* is the ability to carry out intended actions. It is a very functional memory construct. A task analysis for prospective memory might consist of (1) formation and encoding of the intention and action; (2) a retention interval, during which both the intent to perform an action in the future and the actual task to be performed are held in memory; (3) the performance interval, or the space of time in which the intention is to be recalled; (4) initiation and execution of the intended action; and (5) evaluation and recording of outcome, which prevent the action from being performed again at some later time (Ellis, 1996). Similar models have been developed for everyday problem-solving strategies. Models describing "everyday" attention, memory, and executive functions are increasingly important in guiding our treatment.

As we discuss the theoretical underpinnings of the various cognitive processes in the following chapters, we will be describing cognitive processing theory and identifying the relevant neuroanatomical substrates, but will also be drawing upon clinical and functional models of cognitive functioning. We have used a combination of clinical, cognitive, and functional models in conceptualizing and implementing treatment.

MEASURING EFFICACY AND OUTCOME

Whereas a decade ago we described a vacuum in terms of efficacy work (Sohlberg & Mateer, 1989), there is now a larger literature on the efficacy of rehabilitation. As indicated earlier, research in this area continues to be hampered by methodological problems involving heterogeneity of clients, heterogeneity of treatment approaches and settings, and the fact that almost all of this work goes on in active rehabilitation settings that have clinical service rather than research as their mandate.

Nevertheless, documentation of outcomes is critical to justify the time and resources expended by clients, caregivers, and therapists; to accurately estimate service delivery needs and costs; and to inform the development and delivery of treatment. The aims of outcome documentation should be as follows:

1. To determine whether and which interventions result in functional gains, reduction of handicap, and achievement of goals.
2. To determine whether gains are maintained over time, and, if so, to what degree.
3. To ascertain whether the intervention results in better outcomes than would be expected or observed without provision of rehabilitation, and, if so, how.
4. To obtain the information needed to modify programs to be more effective.

Measurement of treatment efficacy and outcome occurs on many levels. The effectiveness of a specific intervention in one subject or a small group of subjects may be ascertained by the use of single-case designs, which rely heavily on obtaining a stable baseline of performance and then using each subject as his or her own control. For example, the number of times a person initiates conversation in a group can be recorded over 4 or 5 days, and once a baseline level is determined, an intervention can begin (e.g., an educational approach or external prompting) while behavioral data continue to be collected. If the level of initiation increases following initiation of the intervention, it can be inferred that the intervention has made a difference in the behavior. There are a variety of such designs, many of which have been used and reported in rehabilitation to monitor the effects of an intervention and to support its efficacy in published research. For a review of such designs, the reader is referred to Sohlberg and Mateer (1989).

Another technique for measuring individual outcomes in brain-injury rehabilitation is the use of Goal Attainment Scaling (GAS; Malec, 1999; Malec, Smigielski, & DePompolo, 1991). The first step in the GAS process involves identification of general goals, which are then developed into specific goal statements. Once three to six specific goals are satisfactorily negotiated and endorsed by the client, weights are sometimes applied to the goals to indicate the importance of each to the overall treatment plan. The third step is to define the time period after which progress on the goals is assessed. The fourth and fifth steps involve articulating the "expected outcome" in objective, behavioral terms, and specifying other outcome levels. This scaling of goals is typically done on a 5-point scale ranging from −2 to +2, with 0 the "expected" level, −2 "much less than expected," and +2 "much better than expected." The scale can be used to describe such observable, externalized behaviors as the percentage of time a client uses a memory book to record information, as well as internalized behaviors having to do with use of coping skills to manage stress. The sixth step is for the therapist and client together to score the status of the client prior to treatment and at a specified follow-up time. Malec and colleagues propose that GAS is a useful method for measuring progress toward the types of highly individualized goals that characterize rehabilitation.

Although measurement of treatment efficacy at the individual level is important, it is difficult to measure broader outcomes and more global efficacy for rehabilitation in single cases. Case reports and single-case designs, by definition, are unique in some respects; though they are useful, they do not tell us about how the majority of clients would respond. In addition, most individuals receive multiple forms of intervention that are difficult to quantify. There has been a concerted effort to develop and evaluate the efficacy of various tools for quantifying outcome. In 1999 alone, there were entire conferences and journal issues devoted to the issue of evaluating outcome in rehabilitation (e.g., Fleminger & Powell, 1999). Outcome research is now better designed and better supported by health care facilities and granting agencies.

The emphasis on functional assessment and outcome evaluation from a quantitative perspective has been matched by growth in the application of qualitative research methodologies to measurement in rehabilitation. McColl and colleagues (1998), for example, use qualitative techniques to provide an expanded conceptualization of community integration, derived from the perspective of people with brain injuries. For professionals who are frustrated with limitations in the ability to measure change meaningfully and sensitively with psychometric instruments, qualitative techniques often better capture the nature of intervention effects, some of which may not have been anticipated.

Studies of treatment effects on larger numbers of subjects are needed, and several comprehensive reviews of specific program outcomes have been published. Hall and Cope (1995) reviewed 28 studies published between 1984 and 1994 that examined the benefits of TBI rehabilitation. Methods in the various studies included comparing outcomes of patients given rehabilitation versus those not given rehabilitation; outcomes of patients who received different intensities or types of rehabilitation; pre- versus posttreatment abilities in a nonacute population; and outcomes for early versus late initiation of rehabilitation in matched groups. Sample sizes in the studies ranged from 24 to 433. Hall and Cope reported that patients receiving acute rehabilitation had only one-third as long a stay in postacute rehabilitation as those who did not receive such treatment. Outcomes for outpatient and day treatment programs showed a positive benefit in terms of functional outcomes, including long-term involvement in productive activity and return to work. Several studies showed evidence of improvement with rehabilitation treatment after spontaneous recovery had slowed or stopped. Although differences across studies in sample characteristics; in outcomes measured; and in the length, types, and intensity of rehabilitation made firm conclusions difficult, there was generally support for the benefit of rehabilitation.

One of the largest studies of outcomes from a single program was that provided by Ponsford, Olver, Nelms, Curran, and Ponsford (1999), based on their work in at the Bethesda Rehabilitation Centre in Melbourne, Australia. Approximately 120 patients are admitted each year, most still in posttraumatic amnesia. The program offers inpatient rehabilitation (average stay about 48 days) and outpatient or community-based phases, including transitional living resources and a community team (average stay about 4–5 months). Resources are available for supported work trials, integration aides, and ongoing individual support. A total of 1,268 individuals with moderate to severe injury were seen for follow-up between 2 and 10 years after injury. More than 90% had attained independence in mobility and light activities of daily living, but one-third continued to need support in shopping, financial management, and/or home maintenance. Only 45% had returned to previous leisure activities, and more than half were depressed and anxious, with many being socially isolated. Half were working 2 years after injury, but many did not maintain employment. Ponsford and colleagues (1999) stated that the many and varied roles played by persons in our society mean that rehabilitation goals vary greatly from one person to another, and a measure that is meaningful for one individual is not necessarily applicable to another. Changes in the program prompted by the analysis included development of a community-based team, a focus on leisure time, more monitoring and assistance with employment, and a greater emphasis on development of coping strategies to facilitate adjustment.

Controlled studies with large numbers of subjects that either compare different treatments or use a nontreatment control group are still quite limited. An extensive review of published studies (Chesnut et al., 1999) identified 3,098 potential articles, of which 600 were found to apply to the question "Does the application of cognitive rehabilitation improve outcomes for persons who sustain TBI?" In a subsequent analysis, the authors determined that only 32 articles satisfied all of their exclusion and inclusion criteria (Carney et al., 1999). Of these 32, the authors concluded that only 15 reported results of studies that included a control group (either randomized or matched comparison), and of these, only 6 reported results for what they termed "direct" outcome measures (e.g., functional measures of health or employment status) rather than indirect measures (e.g., cognitive status on psychological tests).

Although additional studies are certainly needed, there is a growing consensus about "what works." This consensus has been bolstered by a statement prepared by the National Institutes of Health (NIH) Consensus Development Panel on Rehabilitation of Persons with Traumatic Brain Injury (1998), which addresses the issue of treatment efficacy. Excerpts from that statement are provided below:

The goals of cognitive and behavioral rehabilitation are to enhance the person's capacity to process and interpret information and to improve the person's ability to function in all aspects of family and community life. Restorative training focuses on improving a specific cognitive function, whereas compensatory training focuses on adapting to the presence of a cognitive deficit. Compensatory approaches may have restorative effects at certain times. . . . Despite many descriptions of specific strategies, programs, and interventions, limited data on the effectiveness of cognitive rehabilitation programs are available because of heterogeneity of subjects, interventions, and outcomes studied. Outcome measures present a special problem, since some studies use global "macro"-level measures (e.g., return to work), while others use "intermediate" measures (e.g., improved memory). These studies also have been limited by small sample size, failure to control for spontaneous recovery, and the unspecified effects of social contact. Nevertheless, a number of programs have been described and evaluated.

Cognitive exercises, including computer-assisted strategies, have been used to improve specific neuropsychological processes, predominantly attention, memory, and executive skills. Both randomized controlled studies and case reports have documented the success of these interventions using intermediate outcome measures. . . . Compensatory devices, such as memory books and electronic paging systems, are used both to improve particular cognitive functions and to compensate for specific deficits. Training to use these devices requires structured, sequenced, and repetitive practice. The efficacy of these interventions has been demonstrated.

Psychotherapy, an important component of a comprehensive rehabilitation program, is used to treat depression and loss of self-esteem associated with cognitive dysfunction. Psychotherapy should involve individuals with TBI, their family members, and significant others. Specific goals for this therapy emphasize emotional support, providing explanations of the injury and its effects, helping to achieve self-esteem in the context of realistic self-assessment, reducing denial, and increasing ability to relate to family and society.

The NIH Consensus Statement was further supported by a comprehensive review of cognitive rehabilitation (Cicerone et al., 2000).

There has also been a concerted effort to promote multicenter research on TBI rehabilitation through the Traumatic Brain Injury Model Systems (TBI-MS) network in North America. This group (accessible at http://www.tbims.org) has worked to identify useful outcome measures and to promote large-scale intervention studies. Although such studies will be valuable, it continues to be difficult to organize and interpret studies in a patient population that is so diverse in terms of injury locus, severity, and effects. Even when these variables can be matched or controlled for, individuals still differ widely in terms of their premorbid functioning, emotional and personality makeup, and response to intervention. Small-scale studies, using single-case designs or multiple-baseline designs, continue to provide a valuable contribution to our understanding of what works, as do individual case studies and reports.

Another positive development in the measurement of outcome and treatment efficacy has been the creation of several scales that have proven to be useful in characterizing outcomes following brain injury. Although activities-of-daily-living scales such as the Functional Independence Measure (Granger & Hamilton, 1987), the Disability Rating Scale for Severe Head Trauma (Rappaport, Hall, Hopkins, Belieza, & Cope, 1982), and the Glasgow Outcome Scale (Jennett & Bond, 1975) are widely used in medical settings, their emphasis on self-care and their limited range make them unsuitable for measuring long-term outcome following ABI. Many other measures that tap daily living skills, as well as emotional, social, and vocational outcomes have been developed. These include the Sickness Impact Profile (Bergner, Bobbitt, Carter, & Gibson, 1981), the Katz Adjustment Scale (Katz & Lyerly, 1963), the Neurobehavioral Rating Scale (Levin et al., 1987), the Portland Adaptability Inventory (Lezak, 1987), the Mayo–Portland Adaptability Inventory (Malec & Thompson, 1994), the Supervision Rating Scale (Boake, 1996; Boake & High, 1996), and the Craig Handicap Assessment and Reporting Technique (Whiteneck, Charlifue, Gerhart, Overholser, & Richardson, 1992), to name but a few of the more commonly cited ones. These outcome measures, which are discussed in more detail in Chapter 4, allow clinicians to better address not only daily functioning, but also the ability to fulfill roles in the family, at work, and in social and leisure pursuits.

Outcome and treatment efficacy related to emotional and psychological adjustment has continued to be more difficult to measure. Many of the traditional scales for assessing levels of depression and anxiety are heavily weighted by items that reflect somatic or vegetative symptoms. These include such areas as difficulty with sleep, feelings of fatigue, weakness, and headache, all of which can also be direct consequences of a brain injury. It is important to do an item analysis of responses on such scales, to determine whether one is picking up purely somatic symptoms or a genuine depression. Scales that have relatively few items pertaining to somatic symptomatology may be more sensitive to depression following brain injury (e.g., the Leeds Scales for Self-Assessment of Anxiety and Depression; Snaith, Bridge, & Hamilton, 1976).

The field has also begun to appreciate the importance of such constructs as *awareness of deficit* and *locus of control* in terms of how they affect the participation and rehabilitation progress of individuals affected by brain injury. Individuals who do not accurately perceive how their abilities have changed, who fail to appreciate the impact or consequences of those changes, and/or who feel they have little capacity to change often do not make as much progress as others do in a treatment program (Ben-Yishay & Daniels-Zide, 2000; Prigatano & Ben-Yishay, 1999). Ben-Yishay argues that those who are successful in rehabilitation are those who are self-aware and who have been successful in reconstituting a sense of self. He makes a distinction between clients who learn to *self-examine* and those who *adjust*. Productivity in this model is considered only one important outcome, with life meaning, a sense of peace, social activities, and a capacity for joy and intimacy being equally important and valid constructs and goals

New models for measuring efficacy are unquestionably needed. Despite considerable research supporting various interventions, there is still little consensus about what are specific accepted treatments within the framework of cognitive rehabilitation. The field might profit from adopting criteria that have been used to identify *evidence-based* or *empirically validated* psychological and psychosocial interventions for specific populations (Chambless et al., 1996, 1998; Task Force on Promotion and Dissemination of Psychological Procedures, 1995). In order for a treatment to be deemed empirically valid and either "well-established" or "probably efficacious," the criteria listed in Table 1.1 must be met. With these criteria, specific evidence-based treatments were initially identified for individual outpatient psychotherapy for the treatment of depression and anxiety disorders. This work has now expanded to include couple treatments, interventions for severely mentally ill patients (including family interventions for schizophrenia), interventions for chronic pain conditions, and smoking cessation programs. The designation for behaviorally and psychoeducationally oriented family interventions was based on a demonstrated role for such programs in medication monitoring, case management, prevention of relapse, and other individual treatments. Based on this model, evidence-based treatments could be designated within the realm of cognitive rehabilitation for interventions that improve attentional skills, train the use of compensatory memory or organizational systems, increase awareness, or improve family or social integration.

The Task Force has also taken a two-stage approach to looking at what its members term *efficacy* and *effectiveness* (Chambless et al., 1998, p. 3). They have initially concentrated on *efficacy*, identifying "treatments that are beneficial for patients or clients in well-controlled treatment studies." They go on to state: "Effectiveness studies are of importance as well; these include studies of how well an efficacious treatment can be transported from the research clinic to community and private practice settings." In the field of cognitive rehabilitation, there has often been a huge "burden of proof" attached to intervention studies. Effective training of a memory system, for example, is unlikely in and of itself to get someone living more independently or going back to work; basing a determination of

TABLE 1.1. Criteria for Empirically Validated Treatment
Well-established treatments

I. At least two good between-group design experiments, demonstrating efficacy in one or more of the following ways:
    A. Superior (statistically significantly so) to pill or psychological placebo or to another treatment.
    B. Equivalent to an already established treatment in experiments with adequate sample sizes.

or

II. A large series of single-case design experiments ($n > 9$) demonstrating efficacy. These experiments must have:
    A. Used good experimental designs and
    B. Compared the intervention to another treatment as in IA.

Further criteria for both I and II:
III. Experiments must be conducted with treatment manuals or detailed descriptions.
IV. Characteristics of the client samples must be clearly specified.
V. Effects must have been demonstrated by at least two different investigators or investigating teams.

Probably efficacious treatments

I. Two experiments showing the treatment is superior (statistically significantly so) to a waiting-list control group.

or

II. One or more experiments meeting the Well-Established Treatment criteria IA or IB, III, and IV, but not V.

or

III. A small series of single-case design experiments ($n > 3$) otherwise meeting the Well-Established Treatment criteria.

Note. From "Update on Empirically Validated Therapies II" by D. L. Chambless, M. J. Baker, D. H. Baucom, L. E. Beutler, et al., 1998, *The Clinical Psychologist, 51*, p. 4. Copyright 1998 by the American Psychological Association. Adapted by permission.

efficacy on such an outcome is probably unreasonable. However, effective use of a system may well be one very important element in a set of behaviors, skills, attitudes, and abilities that will increase the likelihood of returning to work. It does not mean that we do not need to understand the best practices for training use of memory systems in cognitively impaired individuals. The same can be said of increasing attention skills, improving initiation, or decreasing anxiety. It is still vitally necessary to establish the efficacy of subsets of skills that together lead to more multidimensional functional outcomes.

In summary, there have been tremendous growth and interest in tools, techniques, and strategies for looking at treatment efficacy and outcome, at both the individual and program levels. Outcome measures are broader and more holistic in their approach. Gains have been made in identifying short- and long-term needs of individuals with brain injuries, and in determining what approaches seem to have an effect. However, this continues to be an area in need of solid interdisciplinary research.

STRATEGIES FOR PROMOTING
MAINTENANCE AND GENERALIZATION

A major and continuing concern with regard to cognitive rehabilitation is whether the abilities or skills targeted in treatment will be maintained and generalized, so as to lead to sustained improvement in targeted aspects of everyday function. Generalization can be measured at multiple levels, including generalization to other similar but untrained treatment activities, to psychometric measures of the process or function addressed, to other abilities that are presumably related to or subserve the process, to structured functional activities, and to spontaneous functional activities. As an example, successful training on a high-level working memory task (e.g., alphabetized sentences) might be expected to result in better performance on other high-level working memory exercises (e.g., number sequencing), to psychometric measures that require working memory (e.g., the Paced Auditory Serial Addition Task), to a structured functional task (e.g., balancing a checkbook), and finally to a spontaneous functional task (e.g., quickly figuring out whether you have enough money for the items in a shopping cart). We have always maintained that therapists should not "expect" generalization, rather that they should "program" for generalization. It has become abundantly clear that spontaneous generalization of skills is improbable if not impossible for many clients with acquired brain injury. However, steps can be taken to facilitate and ensure generalization. Some of the principles to keep in mind with respect to increasing the likelihood of generalization include the following:

- Be explicit in training, but train a variety of target skills and have clients practice these beyond criteria (overlearning).
- Train general strategies and have clients practice these in a variety of natural settings.
- Change the environment to support new skills and behaviors.
- Enlist help and involvement from significant others.
- Promote internal attributions of change.
- Identify barriers to maintenance and plan for high-risk situations.
- Plan for recovery from setbacks, schedule booster sessions, and make long-term maintenance plans.

PRINCIPLES OF COGNITIVE REHABILITATION

Based in part on the efficacy and outcome literature, and in part on our own experience, we have developed the following set of principles for implementing effective rehabilitation with individuals who demonstrate cognitive, behavioral, emotional, and psychosocial difficulties following acquired brain injury.

- Cognitive rehabilitation is informed by medical and neuropsychological diagnosis, but is based on an ever-evolving formulation of the individual client's needs and his or her problems and strengths from physical, cognitive, emotional, and social perspectives.
- Cognitive rehabilitation requires a sound therapeutic alliance among the therapist, client, and family members or other caregivers.
- Cognitive rehabilitation emphasizes collaboration and active participation.
- Cognitive rehabilitation is goal-oriented and, while problem-focused, builds on strengths.
- Cognitive rehabilitation has a primary focus on education, with an emphasis on empowerment, self-control, and self-sufficiency.
- Cognitive rehabilitation sessions are structured, and treatment plans and activities are developed with reference to both assessment results and current performance data.
- Cognitive rehabilitation goals may include improving cognitive and behavioral skills, compensating for cognitive and behavioral limitations, and assisting a client to understand and manage emotional reactions to changes in his or her functioning.
- Cognitive rehabilitation assists clients in achieving a more accurate understanding of their strengths and limitations, and in adjusting to injury-related changes in functioning and in life circumstances.
- Cognitive rehabilitation is eclectic: It uses a variety of techniques and strategies to improve abilities; to teach new and compensatory skills; to facilitate regulation of behavior; and to modify negative or disruptive thoughts, feelings, and emotions.
- Cognitive rehabilitation seeks to understand each client's previous lifestyle, including abilities, goals, values, relationships, values, roles, personality, and behavioral patterns.
- Cognitive rehabilitation is responsive to changing theories and technologies.
- Cognitive rehabilitation professionals recognize and respond to the need to evaluate objectively the effectiveness of interventions.
- Team-based cognitive rehabilitation offers the advantage of seeing a problem or opportunity from a number of related but distinct professional perspectives.

SUMMARY

We have attempted in this chapter to identify some of the major directions, findings, trends, and challenges facing clinicians who work with individuals with cognitive impairment. Although there have been exciting developments in cognitive theory, in knowledge about the effects of brain injury, in neuroscience, and in technology, many challenges remain in our ability to integrate these developments into our conceptualization and implementation of services. Moreover, our ability to do this has been compromised by changes in the delivery and funding of health care and rehabilitation services. There continues to be a pressing need for outcome and efficacy research on multiple levels. We have come away with a broader, more complex perspective on how to approach rehabilitation than the one we articulated over a decade ago (Sohlberg & Mateer, 1989), but many of the principles and beliefs we held then remain relevant and important. Treatment efficacy occurs and must be measured at multiple levels, and every rehabilitation professional has a role to play and a contribution to make in this ever more interesting and exciting endeavor.

REFERENCES

Ben-Yishay, Y., & Daniels-Zide, E. (2000). Examined lives: Outcomes after holistic rehabilitation. *Rehabilitation Psychology, 45,* 112–129.

Bergner, M., Bobbitt, R. A., Carter, W. B., & Gibson, B. G. (1981). The Sickness Impact Profile: Developmental and final revision of a health status measure. *Medical Care, 19,* 787–805.

Boake, C. (1996). Supervision Rating Scale: A measure of functional outcome from brain injury. *Archives of Physical Medicine and Rehabilitation, 77,* 65–72.

Boake, C., & High, W. M. (1996). Functional outcome from traumatic brain injury. *American Journal of Physical Medicine and Rehabilitation, 75,* 1–9.

Carney, N., Chesnut, R. M., Maynard, H., Mann, N. C., Patterson, P., & Helfand, M. (1999). Effect of cognitive rehabilitation on outcomes for persons with traumatic brain injury: A systematic review. *Journal of Head Trauma Rehabilitation, 14,* 277–307.

Chambless, D. L., Baker, M. J., Baucom, D. H., Beutler, L. E., Calhoun, K. S., Crits-Christoph, P., Daiuto, A., DeRubeis, R., Detweiler, J., Haaga, D. A. F., Johnson, S. B., McCurry, S., Mueser, K. T., Pope, K. S., Sanderson, W. C., Shoham, V., Stickle, T., Williams, D. A., & Woody, S. R. (1998). Update on empirically validated therapies II. *The Clinical Psychologist, 51,* 3–16.

Chambless, D. L., Sanderson, W. C., Shoham, V., Bennett Johnson, S., Pope, K. S., Crits-Christoph, P., Baker, M., Johnson, B., Woody, S. R., Sue, S., Beutler, L., Williams, D. A., & McCurry, S. (1996). An update on empirically validated therapies. *The Clinical Psychologist, 49,* 5–18.

Chesnut, R. M., Carney, N., Maynard, H., Mann, N. C., Patterson, P., & Helfand, M. (1999). Summary report: Evidence for the effectiveness of rehabilitation for persons with traumatic brain injury. *Journal of Head Trauma Rehabilitation, 14,* 176–188.

Cicerone, K. D., Dahlberg, C., Kalmar, K., Langenbahn, D. M., Malec, J., Bergquist, T. F., Felicetti, T., Giacino, J. T., Harley, J. P., Harrington, E., Herzog, J., Kneipp, S., Laatsch, L. L., & Morse, P. A. (2000). Evidence-based cognitive rehabilitation: Recommendations for clinical practice. *Archives of Physical Medicine and Rehabilitation, 81,* 1596–1615.

Coelho, C. A., DeRuyter, F., & Stein, M. (1996). Treatment efficacy: Cognitive–communicative disorders resulting from traumatic brain injury in adults. *Journal of Speech and Hearing Research, 39,* S5–S17.

Ellis, J. (1996). Prospective memory or the realization of delayed intentions: A conceptual framework for research. In M. Brandimonte, G. O. Einstein, & M. A. McDaniel (Eds.), *Prospective memory: Theory and applications* (pp. 1–22). Mahwah, NJ: Erlbaum.

Finlayson, M. A., & Garner, S. G. (1994). *Brain injury rehabilitation: Clinical considerations.* Baltimore: Williams & Wilkins.

Fleminger, S., & Powell, J. (Eds.). (1999). Evaluation of outcomes in brain injury rehabilitation [Special issue]. *Neuropsychological Rehabilitation, 9*(3–4).

Granger, C. V., & Hamilton, B. B. (1987). *Uniform data set for medical rehabilitation.* Buffalo, NY: Research Foundation, State University of New York.

Hall, K. M., & Cope, D. N. (1995). The benefit of rehabilitation in traumatic brain injury: A literature review. *Journal of Head Trauma Rehabilitation, 10,* 1–13.

Jennett, B., & Bond, M. (1975). Assessment of outcome after severe brain damage: A practical scale. *Lancet, i,* 480–484.

Katz, M. M., & Lyerly, S. B. (1963). Methods for measuring adjustment and social behaviour in the community: Rationale, description, discriminative validity and scale development. *Psychological Reports, 13,* 503–535.

Kerns, K. A., & Mateer, C. A. (1996). Walking and chewing gum: The impact of attentional capacity on everyday activities. In R. J. Sbordone & C. J. Long (Eds.), *The ecological validity of neuropsychological testing* (pp. 147–169). Delray Beach, FL: GR Press/St. Lucie Press.

Kolb, B., & Gibb, R. (1999). Neuroplasticity and recovery of function after brain injury. In D. T. Stuss, G. Winocur, & I. H. Robertson (Eds.), *Cognitive neurorehabilitation* (pp. 9–25). Cambridge, England: Cambridge University Press.

Levin, H. S., High, W. M., Goethe, K. E., Sisson, R. A., Overall, J. E., Rhoades, H. M., Eisenberg, H. M., Kalinsky, Z., & Gary, H. E. (1987). Neurobehavioral Rating Scale: Assessment of the behavioral sequelae of head injury by the clinician. *Journal of Neurology, Neurosurgery and Psychiatry, 50,* 183–193.

Lezak, M. D. (1987). Relationship between personality disorders, social disturbances, and physical disability following traumatic brain injury. *Journal of Head Trauma Rehabilitation, 2,* 57–69.

Lezak, M. D. (1993). Newer contributions to the neuropsychological assessment of executive functions. *Journal of Head Trauma Rehabilitation, 8,* 24–31.

Malec, J. F. (1999). Goal Attainment Scaling in rehabilitation. *Neuropsychological Rehabilitation, 9,* 253–275.

Malec, J. F., Smigielski, J. S., & DePompolo, R. W. (1991). Goal Attainment Scaling and outcome measurement in postacute brain injury rehabilitation. *Archives of Physical Medicine and Rehabilitation, 72,* 138–143.

Malec, J. F., & Thompson, J. M. (1994). Relationship of the Mayo–Portland Adaptability Inventory to functional outcome and cognitive performance measures. *Journal of Head Trauma Rehabilitation, 9,* 116–124.

Mateer, C. A. (1999). The rehabilitation of executive disorders. In D. T. Stuss, G. Winocur, & I. H. Robertson (Eds.), *Cognitive neurorehabilitation* (pp. 314–332). Cambridge, England: Cambridge University Press.

Mateer, C. A., Kerns, K. A., & Eso, K. L. (1996). Management of attention and memory disorders following traumatic brain injury. *Journal of Learning Disabilities, 29*(6), 618–632.

McColl, M. A., Carlson, P., Johnston, J., Minnes, P., Shue, K., Davies, D., & Karlovits, T. (1998). The definition of community integration: Perspectives of people with brain injuries. *Brain Injury, 12,* 15–30.

National Institutes of Health (NIH) Consensus Development Panel on Rehabilitation of Persons with Traumatic Brain Injury. (1998, October). *Consensus conference: Rehabilitation of persons with traumatic brain injury* [Online]. Available: http://www.odp.od.nih.gov/consensus/.

Ponsford, J., Olver, J., Nelms, R., Curran, C., & Ponsford, M. (1999). Outcome measurement in an inpatient and outpatient traumatic brain injury rehabilitation program. *Neuropsychological Rehabilitation, 9,* 517–534.

Ponsford, J., Sloan, W., & Snow, P. (1995). *Traumatic brain injury: Rehabilitation for everyday adaptive living.* Hove, England: Erlbaum.

Posner, M., & Petersen, S. E. (1990). The attention system of the human brain. *Annual Review of Neuroscience, 13,* 25–42.

Prigatano, G., & Ben-Yishay, Y. (1999). Psychotherapy and psychotherapeutic interventions in brain injury rehabilitation. In M. Rosenthal, E. R. Griffith, J. S. Kreutzer, & B. Pentland (Eds.), *Rehabilitation of the adult and child with traumatic brain injury* (3rd ed., pp. 271–283). Philadelphia: F. A. Davis.

Rappaport, M., Hall, K. M., Hopkins, K., Belieza, T., & Cope, D. N. (1982). Disability Rating Scale for severe head trauma: Coma to community. *Archives of Physical Medicine and Rehabilitation, 63,* 118–123.

Shumway-Cook, A., Wollacott, M., Kerns, K. A., & Baldwin, M. (1997). The effects of two types of cognition tasks on postural stability in older adults with and without a history of falls. *Journal of Gerontology: Medical Sciences, 52A,* M232–M240.

Snaith, R. P., Bridge, G. W., & Hamilton, M. (1976). *The Leeds Scales for Self-Assessment of Anxiety and Depression.* London: Psychological Test Publications.

Sohlberg, M. M., & Mateer, C. A. (1987). Effectiveness of an attention training program. *Journal of Clinical and Experimental Neuropsychology, 19,* 117–130.

Sohlberg, M. M., & Mateer, C. A. (1989). *Introduction to cognitive rehabilitation: theory and practice.* New York: Guilford Press.

Sturm, W., Willmes, K., Orgass, B., & Hartje, W. (1997). Do specific attention deficits need specific training? *Neuropsychological Rehabilitation, 7,* 81–176.

Stuss, D. T., & Benson, D. F. (1986). *The frontal lobes.* New York: Raven Press.

Task Force on Promotion and Dissemination of Psychological Procedures. (1995). Training in and dissemination of empirically validated psychological treatments. *The Clinical Psychologist, 48,* 13–23.

Whiteneck, G. C., Charlifue, S. W., Gerhart, K. A., Overholser, D., & Richardson, G. N. (1992). Quantifying handicap: A new measure of long-term rehabilitation outcomes. *Archives of Physical Medicine and Rehabilitation, 73,* 519–526.

2

Neurological Disorders
Associated with
Cognitive Impairments

It is assumed that individuals reading this book have had some training in basic neuroanatomy and physiology. A basic understanding of normal brain organization and function is essential to appreciating how brain disorders disrupt normal brain function. This chapter describes the pathophysiology, frequent functional impairments, and natural history of the neurological disorders affecting the majority of individuals who are seen for cognitive rehabilitation. These include traumatic brain injury (TBI), stroke, hypoxic–hypotensive injury, encephalitis and other infectious disorders, and brain tumors. Each of these types of neurological disorders is associated with particular patterns of damage to the central nervous system (CNS), and each is associated with different (though often overlapping) syndromes of physical, cognitive, behavioral, and emotional dysfunction. Understanding these differences and their common course facilitates the processes of evaluation, treatment planning, and goal setting for the rehabilitation team.

Each disorder has two stages that contribute to brain injury: (1) the immediate damage to brain tissue resulting from mechanical forces or pathophysiological mechanisms; and (2) secondary brain complications that develop as a consequence of metabolic disturbances or the original neuronal damage. Three primary dimensions to consider in neurological injury are the distribution, the severity, and the type of underlying pathology. Distribution of injury is typically considered as focal, multifocal, or diffuse.

Focal lesions commonly result from cerebrovascular events (hemorrhages or infarcts), neoplasms or tumors, brain abscesses, or in some cases

25

a focal trauma, such as in a penetrating injury (e.g., a gunshot wound). The effect of a focal lesion is directly related to its size, location, and depth. In addition, the type of pathological process involved is important in the effect of the injury, the prognosis, and the natural history. A tumor can often expand to a large size before having a noticeable clinical effect, because it develops over time and neural compensation and reorganization can occur. A lesion of the same size and in the same location may have a devastating effect if it has a sudden onset, as in the case of stroke.

Multifocal lesions can be seen with multiple, distributed occurrences of any of the pathologies described above. Various medical conditions, such as severe cerebrovascular disease and TBI, are commonly characterized by multiple lesion foci. In the case of multifocal injuries, the degree of functional impairment is typically greater when lesions are bilateral than unilateral, and when lesions are caused simultaneously rather than staged or staggered in time.

Diffuse brain injury occurs when the precipitating condition has the potential to affect widely distributed areas of brain tissue. This is true in many cases of TBI involving significant acceleration–deceleration forces; in cases of hypoxic–ischemic injury; and in a variety of metabolic, infectious, and inflammatory disorders. The effect of these injuries depends on the density and nature of the damage to brain structures, and to the specific structures and neural elements involved.

In the following section, the major etiological causes of brain injury are discussed, with specific reference to patterns of recovery and functional outcomes. Later in the chapter, we discuss the major medical diagnostic techniques used for patients with brain injuries.

MECHANISMS OF ACQUIRED BRAIN INJURY

Traumatic Brain Injury

Individuals with TBI have occupied increasing numbers of rehabilitation beds as emergency medical services (including fast-response services) and new medical, surgical, and pharmacological interventions have increased survival rates for ever more severe injuries. The incidence of TBI in the United States is 200 cases per 100,000 persons, or about 500,000 new cases per year, exceeding that of both stroke and epilepsy. Approximately 20% of TBI cases are categorized as moderate to severe injuries, with the remainder classified in the mild range. Although an event resulting in TBI can occur to anyone of any age, men suffer TBI twice as often as women, and individuals in the 15–24 age bracket have the highest incidence of TBI. Motor vehicle accidents are the most common cause of TBI in adolescents and young adults, and almost half of these injuries are believed to be related to alcohol consumption. Falls are the primary cause of TBI in children and older adults. Assaults and firearm injuries are common causes of TBI in some urban areas and in wartime.

Mechanisms

There are multiple sources of damage to the brain in most cases of TBI. First, damage can result from mechanical forces. If the head is struck by, or forcefully contacts, a rigid surface (e.g., a baseball bat, a windshield), there is a translation of forces from the point of contact to the head. This can result in skull fractures and focal damage to the underlying brain tissue. Second, acceleration–deceleration forces occur when the head suddenly stops but the brain continues in the original direction of motion and then rebounds in the opposite direction. Areas of contusion or bruising can occur to brain tissue that collides with the skull. Cortical contusions can be caused by abrasion of tissues and are frequently accompanied by focal areas of bleeding and swelling. A common occurrence in motor vehicle accidents is for an unrestrained passenger in the front seat to hit the windshield with his or her forehead. On impact, as the brain is thrust forward, bruising can occur to brain tissue in the frontal regions. Upon rebounding, areas at the back of the brain may also be contused (see Figure 2.1). Injuries of this sort, occurring on opposite sides of the brain, are called *coup* and *contre-coup* injuries. Injury also commonly occurs as the undersurface of the brain is forcefully shoved over the rough and irregular bony surface at the base of the skull. The orbital and lateral undersurfaces of the frontal and temporal lobes are particularly vulnerable to this sort of injury. Contusions are common causes of focal pathology associated with TBI and are common in motor vehicle accidents and in falls from a height.

Another cause of focal injury occurs with disruption of the vascular system. The acceleration–deceleration forces discussed above can tear small blood vessels of the meninges and brain surface. This can result in bleeding into the space that surrounds the brain (e.g., extradural and subdural hematomas). Accumulations of blood in these spaces can damage or begin to exert pressure on the brain itself. Advances in neuroimaging and its application in emergency medicine have allowed more rapid identification and surgical management of such bleeding. Figure 2.2 shows a CT scan of a brain with a left-sided craniotomy, focal areas of confusion in the left frontal and temporal lobes, and significant brain swelling with a left-to-right shift. Mechanical forces or general swelling can also cause disruptions of the vascular system within the brain itself. Arteries can be torn, resulting in intracerebral hematomas, or can be squeezed, resulting in areas of infarction in which tissue has been deprived of blood perfusion for some time. These pathological processes can result in deep cerebral damage, and the clinical correlates can appear very similar to those of individuals who

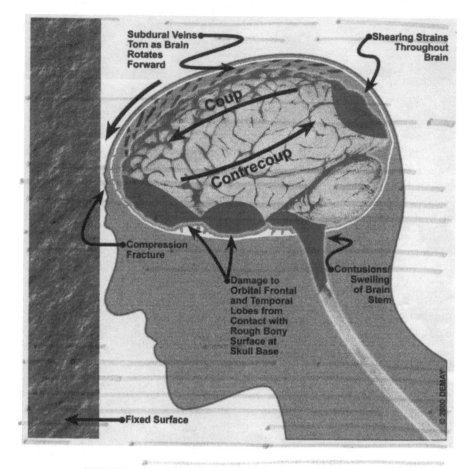

Subdural Veins
Torn as Brain
Rotates
Forward

Shearing Strains
Throughout
Brain

Coup

Contrecoup

Compression
Fracture

Damage to
Orbital Frontal
and Temporal
Lobes from
Contact with
Rough Bony
Surface at
Skull Base

Contusions/
Swelling
of Brain
Stem

© 2000 DEMAY

Fixed Surface

FIGURE 2.1. Brain damage caused by closed head injury.

have suffered strokes. Figure 2.3 shows a gunshot wound to the right temple resulting in bilateral frontal lobe damage.

Acceleration–deceleration forces can also have stretching, deformation, and shearing effects on the neurons. Long fiber tracts coursing throughout the brain are most vulnerable to this kind of injury. Grey matter, consisting mostly of nerve cell bodies in the cortex and subcortical nuclei, is interconnected by massive bundles of axons. Axons, the neuronal processes by which nerve cells communicate, are often of considerable length. These axons are usually covered in myelin, a fatty substance that provides electrical insulation of the fibers and decreases transmission time. The fiber tracts appear as white matter. Imagine you are holding with both hands a bundle of cooked spaghetti strands. Then make a rapid jerking and twisting motion. The broken, stretched, and distorted spaghetti can serve as a metaphor for the kind of injury that can occur in fiber tracts in the brain following exposure to rapid and powerful acceleration–deceleration and rotational forces. Shearing and stretching can result in widespread, though patchy, damage to the axons of nerve cells.

This type of injury has been termed *diffuse axonal injury* (DAI). When an axon is destroyed or significantly damaged, the entire neuron, including the cell body, dies. In addition, other neurons that have depended on the damaged neuron for input may also die. Depending on the amount and location of DAI, large portions of the cerebral hemispheres as well as the brainstem can be damaged. DAI follows a gradient, with least injury in the peripheral cerebral cortex and most injury to the central brain and midbrain. In addition to the physical damage to axons, DAI sets off a cascade of destructive processes, including defective axonal transport and axonal swelling, which can result in the separation of the proximal and distal ends of axons. The process typically occurs within 24 hours of injury, but may continue for some time. The extent of DAI is directly related to the overall severity of TBI and to functional outcome. Trauma related to

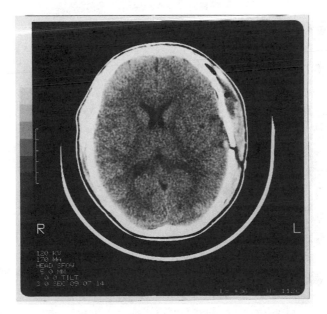

FIGURE 2.2. Traumatic brain injury. CT scan indicates a left-sided craniotomy defect with bone flap in place. There is a small area of pneumocephalus in the left frontal region. Several focal areas of brain contusion are demonstrated in the left frontal and temporal lobes. There is also evidence of some residual edema (swelling) with a shift of the midline structures to the right. This scan was taken 8 days post injury. Surgery was required to relieve intracranial pressure.

(a)

(b)

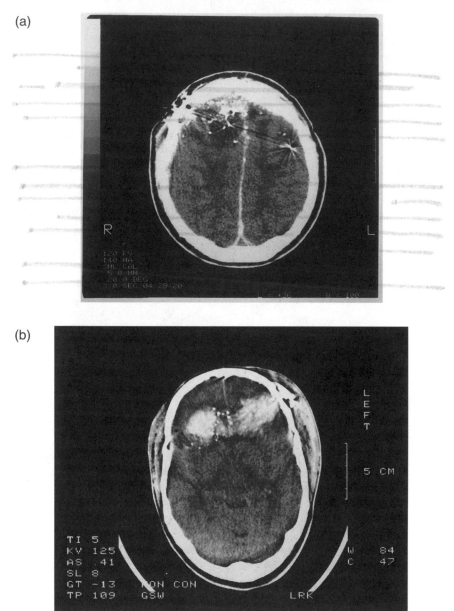

FIGURE 2.3. (a) Penetrating brain wound. CT scan indicates a gunshot wound to the right temple. There is a cranial wound with bone or bullet fragments in the right frontal region and associated bleeding and tissue damage. Brain swelling is indicated by the right to left shift. The bullet crossed the midline of the brain and can be seen lodged in the mid left frontal area. (b) CT scan of another gunshot wound with entry site in the left temple and exit site in the right frontal region. Extensive bleeding and tissue damage are seen around the bullet's path.

DAI is commonly evident in the medial frontal lobes, the corpus callosum, and the superior cerebellar peduncles.

In addition to these primary focal and diffuse injuries, involving contusions, hemorrhages, and DAI, a number of associated secondary phenomena may result in further brain injury. These include surges of excitatory neurotransmitters that create massive neuronal depolarization and that promote the formation of free radicals, which further damage nerve tissues. Diffuse microvascular damage also contributes to edema and brain ischemia. In addition, the rupture of small blood vessels and breakdown of the blood–brain barrier can lead to delayed hemorrhages. These secondary insults compound the damage produced by the primary injury.

Finally, in cases of multiple trauma, injuries to other portions of the body—including crushing chest or airway injuries, choking injuries caused by bleeding into the mouth and larynx, and orthopedic injuries to the face, jaw, ribs, or limbs—can affect normal respiration and thus oxygen supply to the brain. Trauma may also be associated with cardiac or respiratory arrest, resulting in anoxia. Crushing injuries to long bones in the body may result in diffuse showers of fatty emboli, which can clog the lungs and arteries and result in oxygen deprivation and infarction of cerebral tissues. Figure 2.4 shows numerous small, scattered areas of brain affected by fatty emboli. In addition to these cases of injury, there may also be late-developing consequences of TBI in the form of seizure disorders secondary to scar-

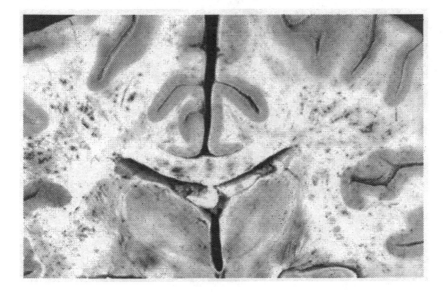

FIGURE 2.4. Small petechial hemorrhages and infarcts secondary to fatty emboli following fracture of the femur.

ring, and/or hydrocephalus secondary to death of brain tissue or blockage of cerebrospinal fluid (CSF).

Although seizures within the acute stage following injury are relatively common, the development of a persistent posttraumatic seizure disorder occurs in only about 4–7% of individuals who have sustained TBI. A seizure disorder is more likely to develop following a severe injury (11.5%), in children as opposed to adults, and following a penetrating injury (35–50%) (Katz & Black, 1999). Focal hemorrhagic lesions of any sort result in a higher risk of seizures (35%). More than half of patients with posttraumatic seizures experience onset within the first year, and 75–80% by the second year. Seizure types can include stereotypical ones lasting a few seconds to minutes, focal motor seizures, complex partial seizures, and generalized seizures (see Yablon, 1993, for a review of this topic). The development of a seizure disorder presents a special challenge to the individual and to the rehabilitation team. Development of such a disorder can limit a person's independence and safety, particularly with respect to such activities as driving, living independently, and engaging in sports. In addition, several of the medications that can be helpful in managing seizures can have a deleterious effect on cognitive functioning. Commonly used anticonvulsants include carbamazepine, gabapentin, phenobarbital, phenytoin, and valproic acid, many of which can affect alertness and arousal, as well as causing additional troublesome side effects.

TBI often involves a large number of these different pathological processes (see Table 2.1 for a summary), resulting in overlapping but quite different constellations of symptoms. Unfortunately, much of the underlying pathology that typically occurs with TBI involves microscopic structures, which cannot be imaged with even the most powerful of the current tech-

---

TABLE 2.1. Mechanisms of TBI

Skull fracture

Primary brain injury
   Cerebral contusion
   Diffuse axonal injury (DAI)

Secondary brain injury
   Intracranial hemorrhage
   Raised intracranial pressure
   Brain swelling
   Respiratory or cardiac failure
   Hypotension
   Ischemic brain damage
   Infection

Delayed complications
   Posttraumatic epilepsy
   Hydrocephalus

---

niques. Hence, although medical/neurological information is important in diagnosis and treatment planning, it must be supplemented by careful evaluation of residual and evolving abilities and disabilities.

Levels of Severity

TBI occurs along a continuum of severity from very mild concussions to catastrophic injuries resulting in death or severe disability. The level of coma in the first 24 hours after injury and the duration of posttraumatic amnesia (PTA) are used to classify injuries as *mild, moderate,* or *severe*. *Coma* is a period of unconsciousness or unawareness following brain damage. The depth of coma in the first few hours after injury is an important early indicator of severity and is commonly measured with an observational instrument called the Glasgow Coma Scale (GCS). This scale uses eye opening, best motor response, and best verbal response to determine the degree of coma and to monitor changes in the level of coma, which may reflect recovery or deterioration of brain function. Scores range from 3 to 15, with scores of 8 or less on the GCS usually indicating severe injury, 9–12 moderate injury, and 13–15 mild injury (Jennett, Snoak, Bond, & Brooks, 1981; Jennett & Teasdale, 1981) (see Table 2.2).

PTA includes the period of coma and extends until the patient's memory for ongoing events becomes reliable, consistent, and accurate. This pe-

TABLE 2.2. Glasgow Coma Scale (GCS)

	Points
Eye opening	
Opens eyes on own	4
Opens eyes on request	3
Opens eyes in response to painful stimuli	2
Does not open eyes	1
Best motor response	
Follows request to move	6
Pushes painful stimulus away	5
Withdraws from painful stimuli	4
Has abnormal (decorticate) flexion	3
Has abnormal (decorticate) extension	2
Makes no motor response	1
Verbal response	
Converses and is oriented	5
Confused speech or disoriented	4
Uses words but doesn't make sense	3
Makes only sounds or incomprehensible words	2
Makes no noise	1

Note. Data from Jennett, Snoak, Bond, and Brooks (1981).

riod may also be associated with disorientation, agitation, and restlessness. One of the common scales used to capture the major features of different levels of functioning with PTA is the Galveston Orientation and Amnesia Test (Levin, O'Donnell, & Grossman, 1979). This questionnaire is used to evaluate whether a patient is oriented to person, place, time, and circumstances. Typically, orientation to person occurs prior to orientation to place and circumstances; orientation to time is often the last to stabilize. The duration of PTA has been found to correlate well with residual physical and cognitive impairments, and also with level of independence and return to work (Dikmen, Machamer, Winn, & Temkin, 1995). TBI severity based on initial GCS score, duration of coma, and length of PTA is indicated in Table 2.3.

Although there are certainly commonalities, there are also many significant differences among patients with different levels of TBI severity in short- and long-term outcomes, as well as in patterns of residual physical, cognitive, emotional, and social functioning. Whereas the majority of individuals who suffer mild traumatic brain injury (MTBI) have relatively uncomplicated recoveries and resume preinjury levels of functioning, the majority of individuals who suffer moderate to severe TBI will have some residual impairments that affect functional activities. Because persistent effects from MTBI represent a special, though certainly important, case, we have chosen to discuss MTBI and the postconcussion syndrome and its management in a separate chapter (Chapter 15). In the following subsection, we describe the common course of recovery and consequences of moderate to severe TBI. In general, the most rapid period of recovery following moderate to severe injury occurs during the first 6 months after injury, with slower yet ongoing recovery up to 2 years following injury. Although spontaneous recovery is much slower beyond that period, many individuals can still benefit from interventions designed to help compensate for deficits even many years after injury.

Patterns of Recovery Following Moderate to Severe TBI

Survivors of moderate to severe TBI, characterized by diffuse pathology caused by DAI and its secondary complications, typically demonstrate a

TABLE 2.3. Classification of Severity of TBI

TBI classification	GCS score	Duration of coma	Length of PTA
Severe	3–8	Over 6 hours	Over 24 hours
Moderate	9–12	Less than 6 hours	1–24 hours
Mild	13–15	20 minutes or less	60 minutes or less

Note. Data from Lezak (1995).

characteristic pattern of improvement. From the point of injury or shortly thereafter, the individual usually suffers a loss of consciousness or significant alteration of awareness. Interventions at this stage are primarily medical, surgical, and/or pharmacological. Other care is palliative, ensuring adequate nutrition, skin care, and minimization of secondary disabilities (e.g., muscle contractures).

Within 4 weeks the majority of survivors spontaneously open their eyes and develop sleep–wake cycles, but do not have any purposeful behavioral responses or apparent understanding of what is going on around them. Only 2% of these patients remain in this state, sometimes termed *vegetative*, for a year or more. The majority of survivors of moderate to severe TBI gradually increase in responsiveness from this point, although their speech, movements, and behaviors remain quite erratic and disorganized. The first signs of this shift are often seen in their tracking of visual stimuli or their orienting to auditory stimuli. These reactions are first seen in the context of automatic or reflexive responses, and gradually appear to come under greater volitional control. The patients may begin to respond to some commands, though they may be mute. This stage is commonly, though not always, associated with agitation and restlessness. Interventions at this stage are usually carried out in subacute treatment units. The environment should be regulated to avoid excessive stimulation, and patients who are easily overstimulated should be treated in quiet, isolated treatment areas. Even after agitation and motor restlessness subside, the patient often demonstrates confusion, disorientation, severe attentional deficits, disinhibition, and significant memory impairment. The inability to demonstrate continuous memory characterizes the period known as posttraumatic amnesia (PTA). Although speech may have recovered substantially, such that an individual is able to respond with apparent understanding, memory and new learning skills may remain very poor.

The next phase is characterized by the restoration of orientation and continuous memory, though significant impairments in memory and new learning may well persist. The length of this very general phase is generally related to the severity of the injury. It is at this stage that most in- and outpatient rehabilitation is focused. At this stage, there is an emphasis on training and resumption/stabilization of self-care activities (e.g., dressing and grooming), and on ambulatory and other motor activities. These often require strengthening, normalizing muscle tone, work on balance and postural control, and restitution of gait patterns. They may also involve compensatory training to use an unimpaired limb, and assistive devices such as a wheelchair or walker. Cognitive deficits can still be very marked at this stage, and efforts are made to stabilize orientation, to facilitate effective communication, to improve attention, and to train the use of compensatory strategies that will help patients deal more effectively with memory difficulties and residual problems with confusion and problem solving. In part due to brain injury and in part due to limited opportunity to engage in previously routine aspects of their lives, many patients at this stage have no or very blunted awareness of the extent or implications of their deficits or functional impairments. Social interaction may improve, but it may be marked by disinhibition and difficulty with pragmatic skills. That is, the person may have trouble starting or stopping conversation, maintaining the topic of conversation, or engaging in normal turn-taking behavior.

Following discharge from inpatient rehabilitation, the great majority of individuals with TBI return home. Depending on the severity of injury and the degree of residual functional impairment, most individuals are able to redevelop some level of independence in self-care. The abilities critical to making decisions in one's own best interest; caring for spouse/partner or children; returning to work or school; and reengaging in former leisure activities, social activities, and other aspects of community integration are often more difficult to recover. Residual problems are often seen in a wide range of cognitive abilities, such as attention and memory; in the organization and carrying out of goal-directed behaviors; in social skills; and in self-regulation of mood, emotion, and behavior. Treatment at this stage is usually more limited.

In the 1980s, prompted by an increased understanding of the long-term impact of TBI on many individuals and their families, there was a proliferation of postacute rehabilitation services aimed at increasing independence, community integration, and long-term social and emotional adjustment to brain injury. However, at least in the United States, with increasing cuts in rehabilitative services, Medicare restrictions, and the introduction of funding based on diagnosis-related groupings, many such services and programs have either closed or been severely cut back. Ethical dilemmas surround the issue of what constitutes medically necessary services versus what constitutes appropriate measures to increase independence and quality of life. Nevertheless, restricted access to such services has undoubtedly put an increased burden on families and on other social service and government agencies, as well as limited potential opportunities for survivors of TBI. When services are available at this stage, the emphasis is usually on accessing community services, increasing emotional adjustment to loss, and assisting with behavioral regulation of common sequelae of TBI (e.g., difficulty with irritability and anger). There is also an emphasis on assisting injured individuals in returning to productive activity in the form of work, school/training, or avocational pursuits.

The Rancho Los Amigos Levels of Cognitive Functioning Scale (Hagen & Malkmus, 1979) was developed to track movement through these various stages following TBI more systematically. It provides a verbal description for many of the typical behaviors seen at each level, and orients rehabilitation staff to behaviors that signify recovery, decline, and/or plateauing of symptoms. Another scale, the Stages of Recovery from Diffuse Axonal Injury Scale (Mills, Cassidy, & Katz, 1997), was originally developed by Alexander (1982) and later modified by Katz (1992). Both scales are useful in identifying and monitoring stages of recovery from TBI; they are presented in Tables 2.4 and 2.5, respectively.

Common Cognitive Impairments

The range and degree of cognitive impairments following TBI can vary greatly, depending on the severity and location of injury. If there has been focal injury to cerebral structures, the individual may demonstrate stroke-like symptoms in the form of aphasias, apraxias, unilateral neglect, or visuospatial dysfunction. Typically, however, these are not prominent features of TBI. The mechanics of the most common form of TBI—acceleration–deceleration injuries—put the ventral and lateral surfaces of the frontal and temporal lobes at highest risk of injury. The most common sequelae of TBI are indeed predicted by what is known about the functions of these areas, and include problems with attention, memory and new learning, planning and problem solving, initiation, impulsivity, self-regulation of mood and emotional reactions, and self-awareness. Attention deficits, initially often very severe in the residual stage, usually involve difficulties in dealing with distraction, shifting mental set, or processing and responding to simultaneously presented stimuli. Long-term memories are typically restored, or remain intact in the first place, but many individuals with TBI continue to have difficulty learning and retaining new information as effectively as before. Working memory, the ability to hold and effectively process information online, is frequently impaired. Some individuals with TBI also continue to demonstrate severe amnesic syndromes, though this is more often the case when there has been an associated period of anoxia or hypoxia.

Various so-called executive functions, thought to be related primarily to frontal lobe structures and function, are also frequently impaired in in-

TABLE 2.4. Rancho Los Amigos Levels of Cognitive Functioning Scale

1	No response
2	Generalized responses
3	Localized responses
4	Confused–agitated
5	Confused–inappropriate
6	Confused–appropriate
7	Automatic–appropriate
8	Purposeful and appropriate

Note. Data from Hagen and Malkmus (1979).

TABLE 2.5. Stages of Recovery from Diffuse Axonal Injury Scale

1. *Coma*
   Unresponsive
   Eyes closed

2. *Vegetative state*
   No cognitive responsiveness
   Gross wakefulness
   Sleep–wake cycles

3. *Minimally conscious state*
   Purposeful wakefulness
   Responds to some commands
   Often mute

4. *Confusional state*
   Recovered speech
   Amnesic (PTA)
   Severe attentional deficits
   Agitated, hypoaroused, and/or labile behavior

5. *Postconfusional, evolving independence*
   Resolution of PTA
   Cognitive improvement
   Achieving independence in daily self-care
   Improving social interaction
   Developing independence at home

6. *Social competence, community reentry*
   Recovering cognitive abilities
   Goal-directed behaviors, social skills, personality
   Developing independence in the community
   Returning to academic or vocational pursuits

Note. From Mills, Cassidy, and Katz (1997, p. 116). Copyright 1997 by Blackwell Scientific Publications. Reprinted by permission.

dividuals with TBI. Individuals with severe frontal injury can appear almost inert and fail to initiate behavior of which they are capable (usually in association with lateral or medial frontal involvement), or can demonstrate excessive behavior and be unable to inhibit inappropriate, repetitious, or dysfunctional/ineffective behaviors. Many individuals with TBI and associated frontal involvement have a wide array of capabilities, but seem unable to initiate, sequence, organize, or monitor their actions in order to reach functional goals. Self-regulation of emotion and behavior is often poor, and problems with irritability and angry outbursts are frequently reported by family members and friends. Social behavior may appear less appropriate—not selfish in the classical sense, but suggesting an unawareness of the needs and feelings of others. Finally, many of these individuals appear to have limited insight into how their abilities and their behavior have changed. This is often a graded impairment, such that awareness of physical limitations is better than awareness of cognitive, social, and behavioral limitations. This gradation of awareness has been identified as a strong predictor of response to rehabilitation and to functional outcomes.

Many of the interventions for cognitive impairment that are discussed in this text were developed in the context of acute and postacute rehabilitation for individuals with TBI. The common cognitive and behavioral syndromes of TBI were not well articulated until the late 1970s and early 1980s, and subsequent work with this population has provided many valuable insights into the nature of cognitive systems and the kinds of interventions for cognitive and behavioral difficulties that may be useful.

Stroke

The terms *stroke* and *cerebrovascular accident* (CVA) are both used to describe brain damage or dysfunction that occurs as a result of some disruption in the vascular supply to or of the brain. Stroke is one of the three major neurological causes of death and disability, together with TBI and dementia. It is the third leading cause of death in the United States. Approximately 25% of stroke patients are less than 65 years of age.

Cerebral Hemorrhage

Intracerebral and subarachnoid hemorrhages account for about 15% of strokes. When a blood vessel weakens, tears, or bursts, blood can leak into the surrounding tissue, damaging its cells. This is considered a *brain hemorrhage* or *bleed*. It can result from several factors, including (1) the breakdown of fragile veins or arteries damaged by atherosclerosis or hypertension; (2) bleeding from abnormally developed vascular tissue (congenital arteriovenous malformations or cavernous hemangiomas); (3) a disorder called *amyloid angiopathy,* which is a degenerative disorder of blood vessels associated with the elderly and is common in dementia of the Alzheimer's type; or (4) impaired blood clotting due to congenital impairments such as hemophilia, acquired disorders such as chronic liver disease, or medications such as warfarin or aspirin. The common results of cerebral hemorrhage are focal damage in the area of bleeding, as well as damage to "downstream" tissue and structures that lose their blood supply when the flow is disturbed. The most common sites of ruptured aneurysms are at the junctions of vessels, particularly of the posterior communicating and anterior cerebral arteries, and at the origin of the middle cerebral artery. Patients with intracerebral hemorrhage have a high acute mortality (30%), which is related to intraventricular bleeding and overall size of hemorrhage (Jorgenson, Nakayama, Raaschoy, & Olsen, 1995).

Cerebral Infarction

When a blood vessel is blocked—for example, by a blood clot (*thrombosis*) or atherosclerotic plaque—tissue that is deprived of blood as a result of the blockage quickly suffers damage. The inadequate blood flow is termed *ischemia*, and brain tissue damaged in the area of ischemia is considered to be an *infarction*. Approximately 85% of strokes are infarctions. Mortality (approximately 15%) is usually related to the size of the infarct, though striking cognitive and behavioral abnormalities can be seen with even very small infarcts, depending on their location (Allen, 1984). Recurrent stroke and myocardial infarction are often associated risk factors in this group of patients. The three primary causes of infarction include (1) complete or partial blockage of an artery due to arteriosclerosis; (2) blockage of an artery by a cerebral *embolus* (a blood clot or atherosclerotic plaque); and (3) *lipohyalinosis,* or specific degeneration of small blood vessels, resulting in lacunar infarcts.

Diagnostic procedures with regard to stroke etiology and location have improved dramatically with the advent of better neuroimaging techniques, which enhance treatment options and provide more accurate estimates of mortality and recurrence. Unfortunately, however, the clinical diagnosis of stroke subtype offers little predictive power in terms of functional outcome. Rather, anatomical location, lesion size, and individual factors related to age, general health, and prior neurological events or underlying neurological disease contribute to functional prognosis. In the following subsections, the typical and primary consequences of strokes involving different vascular distributions are presented.

CVA Involving the Middle Cerebral Artery

The artery most commonly involved in CVA is the middle cerebral artery of either hemisphere. This originates in the neck, and its branches perfuse most of the lateral surface of the frontal, temporal, and parietal lobes. The reader will recall from basic neuroanatomy that a *homunculus,* or "map" of the body, is laid out on either side of the central or longitudinal sulcus that divides the frontal and parietal cortices. In front of the sulcus, in the posterior part of the frontal lobe, is a body "map" related to motor functions for structures on the opposite side of the body. Large areas involved in movement of the lips, tongue, and fingers occupy the lower portion of the map, while structures that have less fine motor control capabilities (such as the arms and legs) occupy the more superior regions actually crossing over the top of the brain and moving down the mesial surface between the hemispheres. A similar "map," but one sensitive to sensory inputs from the opposite side of the body, lies just behind the central sulcus in the anterior portion of the parietal lobe. Figure 2.5 are CT scans depicting a bleed in the right temporal lobe.

The most common physical effects of stroke reflect disruption of these areas; they include difficulties with ambulation, upper-extremity paralysis or paresis, tactile sensory impairments in the contralateral limb, and visual defects involving the contralateral visual field. Common cognitive impairments associated with left middle cerebral artery CVA include aphasia, oral and limb apraxia, and verbal learning impairments, whereas the most common deficits following right middle cerebral artery CVA include visuospatial impairments, nonverbal learning impairments, impaired awareness of deficits, impairments in the pragmatic aspects of communication, and impaired attention. Aphasic syndromes have been reported following lesions involving many structures, including the internal capsule, the

(a)

(b)

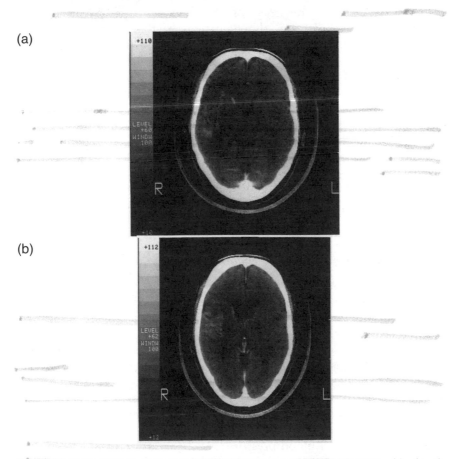

FIGURE 2.5a and b. Cerebrovascular accident (CVA). CT scan indicating a bleed in the right temporal lobe.

lenticulostriate area, the thalamus, and the basal ganglia. It has been difficult to specify the roles that subcortical structures may play, however; brain regions are highly interconnected, and a lesion in a subcortical area will result in reducing the afferent and efferent inputs from that area to many other subcortical and cortical areas with which it was connected. Also problematic in patients who have had strokes are changes in mood, particularly depression, which is seen in approximately 36% of cases. The frequency is equal for left- and right-sided strokes, although there appears to be a higher proportion of severe depression in patients with left-sided strokes, particularly those with deep frontal lesions (Starkstein, Robinson, & Price, 1988).

CVA Involving the Posterior Cerebral Artery

Strokes involving the territory of the posterior cerebral artery are thought to be relatively rare, though it may be that the symptoms that result from strokes in this region do not typically involve motor and sensory losses, and thus may not bring individuals to medical attention. The posterior cerebral arteries supply blood to the occipital lobes and to the medial and inferior parts of the temporal lobes. Branches also supply the thalamus. Strokes in this area result in memory impairments and in a variety of thalamic stroke syndromes. Bilateral thalamic strokes are most devastating and result in severely impaired attention and memory, confabulation, lack of spontaneity, apathy, flat affect, and eye movement disturbances. They may also result in a thalamic pain syndrome. Persistent, severe amnesia has been reported after bilateral anterothalamic infarcts and bilateral medial temporal gyri (involving the hippocampus and related structures).

CVA Involving the Anterior Communicating Artery

The anterior communicating artery is a small artery crossing the midline at the base of the brain, and forming the anterior portion of the circle of Willis. It is called *communicating* because it physically connects the anterior cerebral arteries. From the circle of Willis, these arteries each extend forward and upward, supplying the mesial, inner surface of the frontal lobes, including the cingulate and supplementary motor cortex. The anterior communicating artery is a common site for *aneurysms*—balloon-like structures that develop when vessel walls are weak or develop abnormally. Although the abnormality in vascular structure is probably lifelong, aneurysms may increase in size and vulnerability with age, cerebrovascular disease, and/or increased blood pressure. Bleeds involving aneurysms in this territory commonly result in a syndrome characterized by confabulation, disinhibition, unconcern, severe anterograde and retrograde amnesia, executive function impairments, and limited awareness. The affected structures include the mesial surfaces of the frontal lobes and the basal forebrain.

Stroke rehabilitation has a long history, though refinements continue to be made. This text will not review approaches to the treatment of primary aphasias and apraxias, as a discussion of these issues would be beyond the scope of this book. However, it is important to note that many of the approaches to treatment of attention, memory, and executive function disorders that initially were reported primarily in the context of rehabilitation for individuals with TBI have now been used for patients with strokes. Stroke rehabilitation and recovery has also been positively impacted by the dramatic new role of "clot busting" agents (e.g., tPA) in the emergent treatment of stroke. For a more comprehensive review of stroke and stroke syndromes in the context of rehabilitation, we refer readers to Mills and colleagues (1997).

Hypoxic–Hypotensive Brain Injury

Cerebral hypoxia (or *cerebral anoxia*; the two terms are often used interchangeably) refers to a condition in which there is some deprivation of oxygen to the brain. *Cerebral hypotension* refers to a condition in which the cerebral perfusion of the brain is inadequate, due to insufficient blood pressure or flow to maintain brain oxygenation (insufficient blood flow, as noted above, is also called *ischemia*). These two conditions are often associated. Hypoxic and/or hypotensive injuries can occur whenever conditions are such that the individual does not have normal cardiac or respiratory function. The outcome of these injuries tends to be bimodal. There is rapid recovery in most cases of mild anoxic–hypotensive brain injury. In contrast, in severe cases, following coma of similar duration, the prognosis for patients with anoxic–hypotensive injury is much worse than for patients with TBI.

Four different types of anoxia or hypoxia have been identified (Mills et al., 1997):

Anoxic anoxia. This type of anoxia is due to an inadequate oxygen supply, and can result from asphyxiation, near-drowning, crushing chest injuries, or respiratory arrest from other sources.

Anemic anoxia. This type of anoxia is due to inadequate oxygen-carrying capacity of the blood, such as in conditions of massive blood loss, severe anemia, or carbon monoxide poisoning.

Stagnant hypoxia. This is due to a critical reduction of cerebral blood flow or pressure, such as in cardiac arrest, shock, prolonged cardiac arrhythmia, strangulation, or myocardial infarction.

Toxic hypoxia. This is due to toxins or metabolites that may interfere with oxygen utilization, such as in cyanide poisoning or hypo-glycemia.

Although brain damage will be generalized with prolonged hypoxic–hypotensive episodes, certain areas of the brain are particularly susceptible to hypoxic–ischemic injury. The occipitoparietal cortex and the cerebellum demonstrate selective vulnerability, giving rise to problems with agnosia and motor control. The hippocampus is also highly susceptible to ischemic injury. As a consequence, significant impairments in memory, including full-blown amnesic syndromes, are common in such injuries. The most common form of memory disorder is an anterograde memory disorder similar to Korsakoff's syndrome, most likely caused by anoxic–ischemic damage to the hippocampus (Cummings, Tomiyasu, Read, & Benson, 1984; Kuwert et al., 1993; Zola-Morgan, Squire, & Amaral, 1986). Other areas known to be vulnerable to anoxia include the basal ganglia and the thalamus. Many incidents of hypoxia, such as a near-drowning episode, are unique events characterized by a specific set of parameters. This makes it difficult to generalize about the effects of a hypoxic episode. Somewhat more specificity is available for specific etiologies of hypoxia. Roine, Kajaste, and Kaste (1993), for example, followed 155 survivors of cardiac arrest. Despite good performance on a variety of neuropsychological measures for the group as a whole, from 30% to 35% of these patients demonstrated moderate to severe memory impairment, dyscalculia, or visuoconstructive impairment at 12 months.

Anoxia is often followed by a period of coma. Prognosis is better with coma durations of less than 24–48 hours; if coma lasts longer than this, mortality is high, and a chance of meaningful recovery is extremely low. After a patient emerges from coma, there is often a period of confusion and disorientation, similar to that seen after TBI or frontal system dysfunction; this is followed by gradual recovery of orientation, but a persisting and often severe memory impairment. Unfortunately, it is not uncommon to see a delayed decline in functioning following anoxic–hypotensive brain injury, probably related to extensive demyelination of deep cerebral white matter. This is associated with the emergence of movement disorders, including rigidity, tremor, dystonia, chorea, tics, and myoclonus, related to basal ganglia damage.

Only scattered reports in the literature have addressed the rehabilitation of patients with anoxic–hypotensive brain damage. Most reports suggest that the underlying memory disorder, often the most pronounced cognitive residual effect, is modest and occurs over a much longer period of time than recovery from most brain injury events. However, depending on the integrity of other cognitive functions, these individuals can learn and use effective compensatory memory strategies. Behavioral syndromes that follow some of these injuries, including apathy, inertia, and impulsivity, are extremely difficult to treat, although behavioral strategies and pharmacological interventions may be helpful.

Encephalitis and Other Infectious Disorders

Various infectious disorders constitute another cause of brain damage. Infectious agents may involve the meninges covering the brain (*meningitis*), the brain tissue itself (*encephalitis*), or both (*meningoencephalitis*). The most common causes of brain infection are viral, with a few exceptions. Abscesses, for example, are usually bacterial, and may occur in either brain tissue or the meninges. Although some slow viral infections have been identified, and there are some chronic degenerative diseases of viral origin, most patients seen in rehabilitation units with this type of pathology have had some kind of acute viral infection or a postinfectious encephalomyelitis.

The herpes simplex virus is one of the most common infectious agents. It can affect individuals of all ages and accounts for 5–10% of acute encephalitis cases in North America. There are also several epidemic, seasonal, and geographically related viruses. Epidemic and seasonal viruses are often transmitted from infected vertebrate carriers (e.g., horses, rodents, or birds) to humans by mosquitoes, and are most common in the late summer and fall.

The effects of most viral infections of the brain are difficult to predict. There may be widespread destruction of neurons in many locations throughout the brain, or damage may be limited to small microscopic foci. In contrast, the clinical picture associated with the herpes simplex virus is quite distinctive. This virus is thought to move up from the trigeminal ganglion and to spread along fibers innervating the meninges of the anterior and middle cranial fossa. As a result of this pattern, there is usually extensive damage to the inferior and medial temporal lobes, to the basal and orbital portions of the frontal lobes, and to the insular cortex.

Fever and evidence of meningeal involvement characterize the acute phase of viral encephalitis. Depending on the nature, severity, and course of the infection, the individual may present with a range of symptoms from headache and stiff neck to either generalized neurological signs (such as seizures, confusion, delirium, or coma) or more specific neurological signs (such as aphasia, mutism, motor disorders, or nystagmus). A week or two after onset, patients who survive the infection begin to regain consciousness, after which specific neurological impairments may become evident. Although there is no distinct clinical syndrome attached with most viral infections, it is not uncommon to see global cognitive, motor, and behavioral problems. The herpes simplex virus is typically associated with a more characteristic clinical profile—one that is directly related to limbic and corticolimbic damage involving the temporal and frontal systems. Lesions affecting the medial temporal structures, including the hippocampus, result in anterograde episodic amnesia and new learning deficits, whereas lesions extending into anterior temporal association areas and the insula result in retrograde amnesia and semantic memory loss. Involvement of the basal forebrain results in a behavioral syndrome that looks very much like that seen after CVA involving the anterior communicating artery—specifically, confabulation, executive function impairments, source memory errors, and both memory encoding and retrieval deficits. Mood disorders, including euphoria, mania, aggression, and irritability, affect over half of patients who have had the herpes simplex virus. Inability to speak or swallow has been described in some cases with bilateral frontal opercular involvement.

One follow-up study by Hokkanen and colleagues (1996) indicated full recovery in 44% of patients with non-herpes simplex infections, but in only 12% of patients with herpes simplex encephalitis. In this same sample, 46% of surviving patients with the herpes simplex virus returned to work, whereas 89% of patients with infections of other types returned to work. However, it should be noted that the antiviral agent acyclovir has recently improved the outlook of those contracting herpes simplex encephalitis. In addition to the type of virus, presence and depth of coma, distribution of neuropathology, and age all contribute to outcome.

Rehabilitation is largely driven by a client's presentation of symptoms and postinfection stage. Careful evaluation of memory functions in all their manifestations (anterograde, retrograde, encoding, retrieval, episodic, and semantic) is crucial in this population. With such an assessment, appropriate compensatory approaches to address the specific areas of memory difficulty can be implemented. Strategies for working with attentional, executive function, and behavioral difficulties are also useful with this population.

Cerebral Tumors

Brain tumors are abnormal growths of tissue found inside the skull. The word *tumor* is used to describe both abnormal growths that are new (*neoplasms*) and those present at birth (*congenital tumors*). Tumors are usually classed as *benign* (or noncancerous) if the cells that make up the growth are similar to other normal cells, grow relatively slowly, and are confined to one location. Tumors are usually named for the type of cells involved. For example, a *glioma* involves glial cells (support cells to neurons); an *astrocytoma* involves astrocytes; and a *meningioma* involves the meninges, or covering of the brain. Thus meningiomas often grow inward from the surface, not necessarily invading brain tissue but putting increasing pressure on it. Figure 2.6 depicts a right frontal tumor in MRI scans.

Tumors are called *malignant* (or cancerous) when the cells are very different from normal cells, grow relatively quickly, and can spread easily

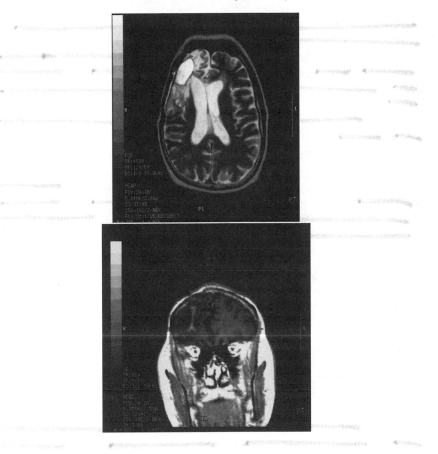

FIGURE 2.6. MRIs demonstrate extensive mass lesion involving the right frontal horn and right lateral ventricle with prominent mass effects (in sagittal and coronal views).

to other locations. Because the brain is housed within the rigid, bony quarters of the skull, any abnormal growth, even a nonmalignant one, can place pressure on sensitive tissues and impair function. Also, tumors located near vital brain structures can seriously threaten critical life support systems. A benign tumor growing next to an important blood vessel in the brain does not have to grow very large before it can block blood flow. Or, if a benign tumor is found deep inside the brain, surgery to remove it may be very risky because of the chances of damaging vital brain centers. On the other hand, a tumor located near the brain's surface can often be removed surgically.

Brain tumors can cause a bewildering array of symptoms, depending on their size, type, and location. Certain symptoms are quite specific because they result from damage to particular brain areas. Other, more general symptoms are triggered by increased pressure within the skull as the growing tumor encroaches on the brain's limited space or blocks the flow of CSF. Some of the more common symptoms of a brain tumor include headaches, seizures, nausea and vomiting, motor problems, balance problems, vision or hearing problems, and both behavioral and cognitive symptoms.

The three most commonly used treatments for brain tumors are surgery, radiation, and chemotherapy. New and often safer surgical techniques, including microsurgery, stereotaxic procedures, laser surgery, and the use of ultrasonic aspirators, are allowing many more tumors to be treated without extensive damage to other brain structures. If a tumor is malignant, doctors often recommend additional treatment, including radiation and/or chemotherapy. In radiation therapy, the tumor is bombarded with beams of energy that kill tumor cells; however, the radiation may also cause damage to healthy brain tissue. Some research has shown, for example, that radiation often has a deleterious impact on memory.

Other Neurological Disorders Associated with Cognitive Disturbance

Many other neurological conditions can give rise to cognitive impairments. Although individuals with these disorders are less commonly seen in an inpatient or outpatient rehabilitation setting, they are frequently seen in the context of specialty medical or neurological clinics. Many of them may benefit from the interventions and compensatory strategies discussed in this text. Individuals with multiple sclerosis or other demyelinating diseases, primary seizure disorders, toxic encephalopathies, Parkinson's disease, and many other neurological conditions frequently have associated cognitive impairments that contribute to disability. Individual case studies have demonstrated that patients with cognitive and behavioral impairment resulting from a wide variety of etiologies can benefit from systematic evaluation of their abilities and assistance in managing cognitive impairments. There is no expectation that cognitive interventions will affect the neurological course of a progressive disease, such as dementia. However, early interventions in the form of family education and the implementation of systems for compensating for memory and other cognitive difficulties are often appropriate and may foster better functioning in an individual's home environment for a longer time than would be the case without such interventions.

With increasing knowledge regarding some of the classical psychiatric syndromes, the specific brain systems responsible for certain cognitive syndromes have been identified. Schizophrenia, for example, is well known to be associated with abnormalities of frontal lobe function, and cognitive impairments in attention and executive function are often what contribute most importantly to functional deficits on a day-to-day basis. Clinicians have begun to evaluate the effectiveness of some interventions, originally designed for individuals with acquired neurological deficits, for individuals with primarily psychiatric diagnoses.

REVIEW OF MEDICAL DIAGNOSTIC TECHNIQUES

Specialized tests and neuroradiological procedures are used to determine the location of lesions within the CNS, to provide information regarding the etiology of the disease process, and to estimate the progression of a patient's disease or the patient's response to therapy. The following review is intended to provide rehabilitation professionals with a basic understanding of medical diagnostic techniques commonly used for patients with neurological injury or disease.

Lumbar Puncture

Lumbar puncture involves the insertion of a needle between the third and fourth lumbar vertebrae into the subarachnoid space. This procedure may be performed for a variety of reasons: (1) to obtain a sample of CSF to aid in the diagnosis of conditions such as meningitis, encephalitis, subarachnoid hemorrhage, multiple sclerosis, and neoplasms; (2) to measure intracranial pressure; (3) to instill medications such as antibiotics or chemotherapeutic agents; (4) to instill contrast material for neuroimaging; and (5) to determine the presence of a spinal block (Guberman, 1994).

Roentgenography (X-Rays)

Plain skull X-rays to evaluate the bones of the skull and sinuses are typically done during preliminary investigation of a patient with TBI. X-rays of the skull are considered mandatory for patients with TBI who present with a loss of consciousness or amnesia; neurological symptoms or signs; blood or CSF leakage from the nose or ear; or scalp laceration, bruising, or swelling suggestive of a penetrating injury (Briggs, 1984). Skull fractures are often associated with intracranial hematoma and with the risk of infection. In addition to identifying fractures, skull X-rays are also useful in determining the presence of calcified tumors or blood vessels, foreign bodies, tumors involving the skull, and evidence of raised intracranial pressure (DeGroot & Chusid, 1991).

Pneumoencephalography (Air Encephalogram)

Pneumoencephalography is occasionally used to assess patients with epilepsy, cerebral atrophy, congenital brain lesions, and posttraumatic cerebral disorders. This technique involves replacing measured quantities of CSF with air or another gas by means of lumbar puncture. X-rays of the brain are then performed and may reveal blockages in the ventricles, displacements in their positions, enlargements (as in hydrocephalus), and atrophy due to dementia. Whereas pneumoencephalography was previously quite commonly used, this procedure is now only rarely used due to its aversive side effects (e.g., severe headache, nausea, and vomiting), and because it is hazardous when used with patients with elevated CSF pressure. We now rely on other, less invasive imaging techniques.

Angiogram

Angiograms are used primarily in cases in which a vessel abnormality (such as occlusion, malformation, or aneurysm) is suspected. It can also be used to determine whether the position of the vessels in relation to other intracranial structures is normal or pathologically changed. Angiograms are performed by injecting a contrast medium or dye into the major cerebral blood vessels and conducting a series of X-rays following each injection. They clearly reveal occlusions, abnormalities (e.g., AUMs), or swelling in the vessels, as well as displacements of vessels or ventricles, which may indicate the presence of a tumor. The use of angiograms in assessing vascular disease has decreased with the advent of computed tomography (CT; see below), but they are still important for some procedures and may be used as an adjunct during surgical interventions.

In the last 20 years there have been extraordinary developments in neurological diagnostic procedures, and especially in techniques for imaging—imaging not only of brain anatomy, but of brain function. There was great excitement when *static* images based on the new imaging techniques revealed a level of anatomical detail never before imagined for a living brain. There has been even more excitement (and a flurry of research activity) with respect to the *dynamic* images that display functional characteristics of not only the living, but also the sensing, thinking, and behaving brain. Below, we review two techniques for imaging brain structure (CT and magnetic resonance imagery [MRI]), followed by four techniques for imaging brain function (positron emission tomography [PET], single-photon emission computed tomography [SPECT], functional MFI [fMRI], and electrophysiological studies).

Computed Tomography

Since its introduction in 1973, CT has revolutionized neurological diagnosis. CT scanning is noninvasive, fast, safe, and painless. Its use has decreased the need for invasive neuroradiological procedures (e.g., pneu-moencephalography, angiography) and has contributed significantly to the understanding of a variety of neurological conditions (Guberman, 1994). CT scanning relies on the principle that tissues of differing electron density differentially absorb X-rays. In CT, an X-ray source is rotated around the head and passes thin beams of radiation though the body, while the detec-tors are arrayed to detect nonabsorbed X-rays on the opposite side. A com-puter then applies a mathematical algorithm to create slices from multiple linear X-ray projections. Images of brain slices between 2 and 12 millime-ters in thickness are generated, and a computer then reconstructs a three-dimensional image representing structures within the planes. Contrast media may be used to improve the spatial and density resolution of the im-ages. In particular, imaging of the major blood vessels is improved through the use of contrast materials.

CT allows direct visualization of intracranial soft tissues, as well as bone, ventricles, cisterns and subarachnoid spaces, orbits, sinuses, and ves-sels. It has become the preferred method of investigation to diagnose con-genital abnormalities of the brain, the presence of abnormal calcifications, demyelinating diseases, brain edema, hydrocephalus, many types of tumors and cysts, hemorrhages, and cerebrovascular disease.

In patients presenting with TBI, CT scanning is considered crucial in cases in which a skull fracture is present, the GCS score is below 15 for 24 hours or more, seizures have occurred, and/or a focal neurological deficit has been found (Servadei et al., 1988; Teasdale, 1990). Repeat CT scans are sometimes necessary, given that some epidural hematomas or intra-cranial mass lesions become evident 2 or more days after injury.

Magnetic Resonance Imaging

The use of MRI scanning over the past 15 years has led to further refine-ment and resolution in identifying brain structure and pathology. This pro-cedure utilizes computer processing of radiofrequency-induced excitations of protons aligned in a strong magnetic field. With MRI, three-dimensional reconstructed images of the brain and surrounding skull can be produced.

Because it provides so much more detailed imaging of anatomical structures than CT, MRI is the primary method of examination for intracranial tumors, cerebrovascular insults, multi-infarct disease, multiple sclerosis, and the brain degeneration and atrophy associated with degener-ative disorders. A major benefit of MRI over CT is that small lesions in the brainstem and other deeper structures can be seen. In addition, unlike CT scanning, which may not pick up stroke-related changes for days, MRI can demonstrate an ischemic cerebral infarct only a few hours following the clinical incident. MRI has also become the method of choice when investi-gators are looking for areas of scarring or gliosis associated with seizure disorders. Finally, with MRI, the flow of blood within medium-sized and larger arteries and veins can be evaluated directly, without the need for potentially dangerous intravenous injections of a contrast agent. The main disadvantages of MRI are the longer imaging times; its incompatibility with many life support systems, given the need to expose the patient to a strong magnetic field; and the lack of availability in many centers. In addition, patients often complain that the procedure is noisy and confining.

Positron Emission Tomography and Single-Photon Emission Computed Tomography

PET and SPECT are techniques that image cerebral blood flow, brain metabolism, and other chemical processes within the brain while the subject is engaged in different activities. These techniques are therefore considered dynamic rather than static in nature, since they reveal information about the nature and localization of brain activity as the subject is engaged in various forms of motor, sensory, or cognitive stimulation or behavior. PET utilizes positron emissions from radioactive isotopes of oxygen, carbon, nitrogen, and fluorine. Patients inhale or are injected with a radioactivity-labeled form of glucose, and emissions from the various compounds listed above are measured with a gamma-ray detector system as they are utilized during different functional activities. Brain areas that are highly active utilize more glucose, and thus radioactivity will be more concentrated there. A major application of PET technology is the assessment of metabolic activity and neurotransmitter function in different brain regions in various forms of neural pathology. PET has also been used widely in research to specify brain areas activated in normal subjects when they are performing motor, language, or sensory tasks.

SPECT is based on principles similar to those of PET, but because of its lower cost, it is more widely used clinically. SPECT utilizes conventional nuclear medicine instrumentation. The gamma rays emitted following injection of radiotracers are detected by specialized receptors placed externally on the scalp. An increased proportion of the tracer material, which readily crosses the blood–brain barrier, is evident in areas of increased blood flow. A cross-sectional image is reconstructed that reveals the relative activity of different cerebral areas. SPECT is used primarily to identify epileptogenic foci and locate brain lesions. Recently three-dimensional SPECT images have become possible, promising even greater spatial specificity.

A dynamic imaging study is more likely than a static study to identify areas of brain dysfunction, in part because there can be functional damage to areas distant from the actual lesioned area as a result of reduced or faulty input and output from the damaged area. For example, Nedd and colleagues (1993) compared SPECT and CT scan results in 16 patients with mild to moderate TBI. SPECT showed differences in cerebral blood flow significantly more often than CT revealed structural lesions (87.5% vs. 37.5%). Even in patients whose scans in both modalities demonstrated abnormalities, the area of involvement was larger on SPECT scans than on CT scans. This is consistent with the notion that regions adjacent to a lesion site have reduced levels of functioning. Jacobs, Put, Ingels, and Bossuy (1994) reported that SPECT alterations correlated well with both overall severity of trauma and with the number and degree of subjective postacute symptoms in individuals with mild to moderate TBI.

Because PET and SPECT are not widely available, these methods are currently used more for research than for clinical purposes. Other limitations of these procedures include their lack of detailed resolution and their high cost. Furthermore, as with any new technology, it will take additional time and study to determine their reliability and utility. Although they may be very sensitive to brain activity, it may be difficult to reliably discriminate normal and abnormal brain functioning. It is also difficult to determine whether an area of increased activity is directly related to a functional task, is related to some unknown background activity, or is related to excitatory or inhibitory processes.

Functional Magnetic Resonance Imaging

Although initial MRI technology displayed exquisite images of the brain, the scans did not provide any information about how structures were actually functioning. However, more recent and advanced fMRI applications, including magnetic resonance spectroscopy, diffusion-weighted MRI, and magnetic resonance angiography, have begun to supply some exquisite information with regard to functional brain activity and dynamic changes in function following brain injury. These fMRI techniques are generally based on the fact that the flow of blood through the tissues of the body varies with the level of metabolism and functional activity in those tissues. The functional activity of an area of tissue is closely tied to its oxygen uptake. Oxygen is supplied to tissues by the blood stream and a rise in oxygen demand is met by an increased flow of oxygenated blood. Cerebral metabolism and blood flow are thus increased during the normal activation of regions of the cerebral cortex involved in the performance of specific tasks. Thus it is possible to localize brain functions by studying regional variations in blood flow through the use of fMRI.

Both PET and SPECT have significant research and clinical limitations because they require use of radioactive isotopes. Thus the cost is high, access is limited, and there is some risk associated with radioactive substances. In addition, it is inadvisable to repeat either procedure with any frequency. In contrast, fMRI entails much less risk and can be used repeatedly. It has already largely taken over the role in functional brain imaging originally anticipated for PET. It has been widely used as a dynamic indicator of functional brain activity, not only in patient populations, but also in control subjects. Dynamic functional imaging of control subjects is providing important insights into the nature of brain organization for many cognitive capacities.

Of interest to readers of this book, both PET and fMRI have begun to be used in the investigation of changes in the location and degree of brain activity that occur over the course of recovery from brain injury or following a course of therapeutic intervention. For example, Weiller and colleagues (1995) investigated possible reorganization within language networks in patients with aphasia secondary to damage to the left posterior perisylvian region (Wernicke's area). Patients and control subjects were studied during tasks that involved generating verbs and repeating pseudowords. Controls demonstrated left posterior temporal activity during both tasks, and left inferior prefrontal activity during the verb generation task, but only minimal activation of homologous areas in the right hemisphere. Patients lacked left posterior activation, but showed increased left inferior prefrontal activation and substantially more activity than controls in homologous anterior and posterior regions of the right hemisphere. Results suggested that recovery of language functions after posterior left-hemisphere lesions is made possible by changes in the left anterior portion of the language network, as well as by recruitment of homologous right-hemisphere regions that play only rudimentary roles during normal language functions. Another interesting example was reported by Buckner, Corbetta, Schatz, Raichle, and Peterson (1996), who studied a patient with a left inferior frontal infarct and residual aphasia. PET scans were done during a word stem completion task that the patient could perform well. Compared to controls, who demonstrated increased blood flow to the inferior frontal cortex, the patient demonstrated activation of a homologous region of the right prefrontal cortex. This suggests either recruitment of a new area or reorganization of the language network to rely more heavily on the right-hemisphere structures.

Electrophysiological Studies

Electrophysiological studies include routine electroencephalography (EEG) and evoked potential studies. These methods complement imaging techniques by providing a noninvasive measure of physiological brain function. EEG provides a sampling of electrical activity of the cortex through small electrodes posted on specific areas of the skull. Fluctuations in electrical activity are recorded by the electrodes and are amplified and displayed on a polygraph. EEG is generally considered a nonspecific indicator of cerebral function; any pathophysiological insult to the CNS can result in alterations in electrophysiology. Although standard EEG is considered a crude measure of the brain's electrical activity, it remains crucial in the diagnosis of epilepsy, as seizure disorders are associated with recognizable EEG abnormalities.

The measurement of sensory evoked potentials is commonly used to assess the intactness of the visual, auditory, and somatosensory pathways, particularly in patients who remain unresponsive for a long time or who are unable to communicate. Very-low-voltage potentials evoked by visual, auditory, or somatosensory stimuli may be recorded by externally placed electrodes. The latencies and amplitudes of the various evoked potential components are measured, and comparisons are made between right- and left-sided stimulation and with normative data. It is possible to determine the integrity of specific sensory pathways and to determine at what level, if any, information is failing to be processed. In minimally responsive patients, this can provide some information about the functioning of brainstem, midbrain, thalamic, and cortical sensory networks.

Although standard clinical EEG analysis rarely indicates any significant abnormality in individuals with mild TBI, finer-grained analysis of brain electrical activity through spectral or quantitative analyses of the EEG signal have sometimes suggested underlying abnormalities in these individuals. This technology is variously termed *computerized EEG, quantitative EEG (qEEG), or brain mapping.* It purports to demonstrate EEG abnormalities that cannot readily be detected by observation of the EEG trace, but that emerge when it is subjected to mathematical analyses. Tebano and colleagues (1988), for example, found a significant increase in the mean power of slow alpha, a reduction of fast alpha, and a reduction of fast beta in 18 patients who had sustained minor head injuries 3–10 days earlier, in comparison to age- and sex-matched controls. These changes could not be identified in a standard EEG reading. This work suggested changes in brain function in the early stages following MTBI, consistent with many other reports of cognitive inefficiency during this period. However, qEEG remains quite controversial in terms of its clinical utility and remains primarily a research tool at this time.

In the last decade, many experimental and even some clinical investigations have utilized devices that can obtain recordings from a much larger number of channels. These studies have provided much more detailed information about the sources and topography of brain electrical activity during a wide variety of cognitive and linguistic activities (see Posner & Raichle, 1994, for a detailed discussion of these techniques). Finally, changes in EEG activity and in the P300 evoked potential response have been used as indicators of possible change in brain electrical activity following cognitive interventions (Baribeau, Ethier, & Braun, 1989). Penkman (2000), for example, reported decreased latency of the P300 only after attention training, and not after an equal amount of supportive counseling.

As indicated in the prior sections, there have been major advances in the capacity to image not only brain structure, but also function in the living brain. These advances have greatly influenced the ability to diagnose neurological disease and to initiate timely and effective surgical and other medical interventions. It is important to remember, however, that imaging techniques are still relatively insensitive to subtle changes in brain structure and/or to microscopic or neuropharmacological changes in brain function. In addition, many apparent "abnormalities" can be identified in persons without any apparent neurological impairment, suggesting a range of normality in brain structure and substantial individual differences in this domain.

SUMMARY

Important tools of the rehabilitation specialist include an understanding of brain systems, an appreciation of how cognitive systems are organized, and a working knowledge of the common cognitive and behavioral profiles associated with various neurological diseases and disorders. Prognosis, treatment planning, and the selection and timing of intervention strategies will be most accurate and effective if these variables are considered in the context of each and every case. Although every person who is seen for rehabilitation is unique and presents with a specified set of premorbid characteristics and injury/illness-related variables, an appreciation of neurological syndromes is a valuable asset in providing the most effective rehabilitation. Knowledge about contemporary techniques for medical diagnosis is helpful in reviewing medical records, understanding the nature and extent of brain injury, and providing information about which functional systems have been affected. In the future, these techniques are likely to play an even greater role in treatment planning and in identifying treatment-related changes in brain functioning.

REFERENCES

Alexander, M. P. (1982). Traumatic brain injury. In D. F. Benson & D. Blumer (Eds.), *Psychiatric aspects of neurologic disease* (pp. 251–278). New York: McGraw-Hill.

Allen, C. M. C. (1984). Predicting the outcome of acute stroke: A prognostic score. *Journal of Neurology, Neurosurgery and Psychiatry, 47*, 475–480.

Baribeau, J., Ethier, M., & Braun, C. (1989). A neurophysiological assessment of selective attention before and after cognitive remediation in patients with severe closed head injury. *Journal of Neurological Rehabilitation, 3*, 71–92.

Briggs, M. (1984). Guidelines for initial management after head injury in adults. *British Medical Journal, 288*, 983–985.

Buckner, R. L., Corbetta, M., Schatz, J., Raichle, M. E., & Peterson, S. E. (1996). Preserved speech abilities and compensation following prefrontal damage. *Proceedings of the National Academy of Sciences USA, 93*, 1249–1253.

Cummings, J. L., Tomiyasu, U., Read, S., & Benson, F. D. (1984). Amnesia with hippocampal lesions after cardiopulmonary arrest. *Neurology, 34*, 679–681.

DeGroot, J., & Chusid, J. G. (1991). *Correlative neuroanatomy* (21st ed.). Norwalk, CT: Appleton & Lange.

Dikmen, S. S., Machamer, J. E., Winn, H. R., & Temkin, N. R. (1995). Neuropsychological outcome at 1-year post head injury. *Neuropsychology, 9*, 80–90.

Guberman, A. (1994). *An introduction to clinical neurology: Pathophysiology, diagnosis and treatment*. Boston: Little, Brown.

Hagen, C., & Malkmus, D. (1979). *Intervention strategies for language disorders secondary to head trauma*. Atlanta: American Speech–Language–Hearing Association.

Hokkanen, L., Poutiainen, E., Valaane, L., Salonen, O., Livanainen, M., & Launes, J. (1996). Cognitive impairment after acute encephalitis: Comparison of herpes simplex and other aetiologies. *Journal of Neurology, Neurosurgery and Psychiatry, 61*, 478–484.

Jacobs, A., Put, E., Ingels, M., & Bossuy, A. (1994). Prospective valuation of technetium-99m-HMPAO SPECT in mild to moderate traumatic brain injury. *Journal of Nuclear Medicine, 35*, 942–947.

Jennett, B., Snoak, J., Bond, M., & Brooks, N. (1981). Disability after severe head injury: Observations on the use of the Glasgow Outcome Scale. *Journal of Neurology, Neurosurgery and Psychiatry, 44*, 285–293.

Jennett, B., & Teasdale, G. (1981). *Management of head injuries*. Philadelphia: F. A. Davis.

Jorgenson, H. S., Nakayama, H., Raaschoy, H. O., & Olsen, T. S. (1995). Intracerebral hemorrhage versus infarction: Stroke severity, risk factors and prognosis. *Annals of Neurology, 38*, 45–50.

Katz, D. I. (1992). Neuropathology and neurobehavioral recovery from closed head injury. *Journal of Head Trauma Rehabilitation, 7*, 1–15.

Katz, D. I., & Black, S. E. (1999). Neurological and neuroradiological evaluation. In M. Rosenthal, E. R. Griffith, J. S. Kreutzer, & B. Pentland (Eds.), *Rehabilitation of the adult and child with traumatic brain injury* (3rd ed., pp. 89–116). Philadelphia: F. A. Davis.

Kuwert, T., Homberg, V., Steinmetz, H., Unverhau, S., Langen, K. J., Herzog, H., & Feinendegen, L. E. (1993). Posthypoxic amnesia: Regional cerebral glucose consumption measured by positron emission tomography. *Journal of Neurological Science, 118*, 10–16.

Levin, H. S., O'Donnell, V. M., & Grossman, R. G. (1979). The Galveston Orientation and Amnesia Test: A practical scale to assess cognition after head injury. *Journal of Nervous and Mental Disease, 167*, 675–684.

Lezak, M. D. (1995). *Neuropsychological assessment* (3rd ed.). New York: Oxford University Press.

Mills, V. M., Cassidy, J. W., & Katz, D. I. (1997). *Neurologic rehabilitation: A guide to diagnosis, prognosis, and treatment planning*. Malden, MA: Blackwell Scientific.

Nedd, K., Sfakianakis, G., Ganz, W., Uricchio, B., Vernberg, D., Villanueva, P., Jabir,

A. M., Vartlett, J., & Keena, J. (1993). TcHMPAO SPECT of the brain in mild to moderate traumatic brain injury patients compared with CT: A prospective study. *Brain Injury, 7*, 469–479.

Penkman, L. (2000). *Rehabilitation of attention deficits in traumatic brain injury.* Unpublished doctoral dissertation, University of Victoria, Victoria, British Columbia, Canada.

Posner, M. I., & Raichle, M. E. (1994). *Images of mind.* New York: Scientific American Books.

Roine, R., Kajaste, S., & Kaste, M. (1993). Neuropsychological sequelae of cardiac arrest. *Journal of the American Medical Association, 269*, 237–242.

Servadei, F., Piazza, G., Seracchioli, A., Acciarri, N., Pozzati, E., & Gaist, G. (1988). Extradural haematomas: Analysis of the changing characteristics of patients admitted from 1980–1986: Diagnostic and therapeutic implications in 158 cases. *Brain Injury, 2*, 87–100.

Starkstein, S. E., Robinson, R. G., & Price, T. R. (1988). Comparison of patients with and without poststroke major depression matched for size and location of lesion. *Archives of General Psychiatry, 45*, 247–252.

Teasdale, G. M., Murray, G., Anderson, E., Mendelow, A. D., MacMillen, R., Jennett, B., & Brookes, M. (1990). Risks of acute traumatic intracranial haematoma in children and adults: Implications for managing head injuries. *British Medical Journal, 300*, 363—367.

Tebano, M. T., Cameroni, M., Gallozzi, G., Loizzo, A., Palazzino, G., Pezzini, G., & Ricci, G. F. (1988). EEG spectral analysis after minor head injury in man. *Electroencephalography and Clinical Neurophysiology, 70*, 185–189.

Weiller, C., Isensee, C., Rijntjes, M., Huber, W., Muller, S., Bier, D., Dutschka, K., Woods, R. P., Noth, J., & Diener, H. C. (1995). Recovery from Wernicke's aphasia: A positron emission tomography study. *Annals of Neurology, 37*, 723–732.

Yablon, S. A. (1993). Posttraumatic seizures. *Archives of Physical Medicine and Rehabilitation, 74*, 983–1001.

Zola-Morgan, S., Squire, L. R., & Amaral, D. G. (1986). Human amnesia and the medial temporal region: Enduring memory impairment following a bilateral lesion limited to field CA1 of the hippocampus. *Journal of Neuroscience, 6*, 2950–2967.

3

Variables Contributing to Neurological and Neurobehavioral Recovery

There is no doubt that individuals who sustain damage to the brain demonstrate changes in functioning over time. For the most part, in nondegenerative disorders, changes appear to reflect recovery of abilities and function. Orientation, speech, language abilities, and memory often show marked improvement in the days, weeks, and months following injury. However, sometimes changes that actually serve to *decrease* function occur in the period following injury. A key example of this is the development of spasticity following damage to motor neurons in the central nervous system (CNS). This spasticity, not present immediately after injury, can severely limit the recovery of mobility and other motor functions. The goal of rehabilitation is to foster and guide natural recovery processes; to decrease the development of maladaptive patterns; and to implement physical, pharmacological, cognitive, and behavioral interventions that will increase the rate and level of functional recovery.

A number of general principles related to recovery have emerged from the study of individuals who have sustained various forms and degrees of brain injury. Although every injury and every injured individual are unique, it is useful to appreciate the various factors that appear to influence recovery after neurological injury. An understanding of these factors is necessary if rehabilitation methods are to be refined and improved. Some of the more important influences on recovery are as follows:

1. Demographic variables.
2. Factors related to the injury itself.

59

3. Psychological factors, especially awareness and readiness to engage in and benefit from rehabilitation.
4. Mechanisms underlying neuroplasticity and synaptic reorganization.
5. Factors related to training programs and interventions.

DEMOGRAPHIC VARIABLES

Age at Injury

It has been postulated that individuals at both ends of the age spectrum (i.e., children and older adults) demonstrate greater effects of brain injury than do young adults. In the case of children, there is concern that damage occurring to a developing system may not appear particularly severe at an early age, but that the children will show increasing lags in development and unexpected deficits as they get older. In the case of older adults, there is concern that acquired brain injury occurs in the context of an already aging and somewhat compromised brain, such that it is more difficult to cope with and compensate for the acquired deficits. We discuss these concepts in more depth below.

Infants and Children

Neurons undergo massive changes in their form and connectivity during normal development and aging. The mammalian brain follows a general pattern of development involving several stages, including cell birth (mitosis), cell migration, cell differentiation, dendritic and axonal growth, synaptogenesis, and cell and synaptic death. In humans, nerve cell migration to appropriate targets in the CNS is generally complete by about 1 month after birth. As neurons reach their final destination, they begin to develop axons and dendrites that will form synapses. Dendritic growth is most intense at about 8 months of age, and the infant achieves maximum synaptic density by about 1 year. After this, waves of pruning, in which synapses are deleted, occur. The number and appearance of dendrites and synapses have been shown, in another mammalion species (i.e., rats), to be directly related to the complexity and quality of their environment and experiences and the time frame during which these experiences are provided.

A very early theory, known as the *Kennard principle* (Kennard, 1940), held that recovery from neurological insult is more complete if lesions are sustained early in life. The original work supporting this theory was based on studies of motor cortex lesions, which showed that animals with early lesions showed better recovery than animals lesioned in adulthood.

In contrast to Kennard, Hebb (1949) postulated that brain injury early in life can, under some circumstances, result in more severe behavior-

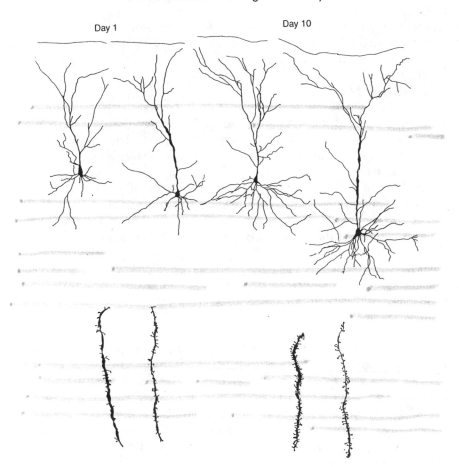

FIGURE 3.1. *Top:* Drawings of representative neurons in the parietal cortex of adult rats with medial frontal lesion made on day 1 and day 10 after birth. Neurons show far more extensive dendritic arborization after a lesion made later in development. *Bottom:* Segments of the terminal dendrites from cells from the same brains illustrated above, showing a clear difference in the density of dendritic spines. From Kolb and Gibb (1999). Copyright 1999 by Cambridge University Press. Reprinted by permission.

al disruption than similar damage later in life. Although he was able to demonstrate this phenomenon behaviorally in experimental animals, more recent work has provided additional neuroanatomical support for the finding. For example, rats with very early lesions to the medial frontal lobe—that is, in the first 4 days of life as opposed to the 7th to 10th days of life—demonstrated dismal behavioral outcomes, as well as a marked atrophy of dendritic arbors and a decrease in spine density in the parietal lobe. These differences in dendritic growth and density of dendritic spines are illustrated in Figure 3.1. Rats with early lesions were not capable of learning and performed poorly on many behavioral tests. This is reminiscent of the retardation sometimes seen after injuries in humans in the third trimester of pregnancy, and such children have also been shown to have a decrease in the density of dendritic spines.

Human infants have also been shown to be particularly susceptible to damage from subdural hematoma, often showing a massive loss of brain tissue, which is associated with severe disability (Duhaime, Bilaniuk, & Zimmerman, 1993). Infants with bilateral diffuse hemispheric hypodensity appear to have a uniformly poor outcome, and remain blind, nonverbal,and nonambulatory, even many years after injury. Even with less severe injuries, early bilateral or diffuse insults in childhood associated with later seizure disorders were found to be associated with lower intellectual levels and verbal abilities than were unilateral insults also associated with seizure disorders (Mateer & Dodrill, 1993). Thus, although the "earlier is better" theory may hold true for focal lesions incurred in childhood, recovery from prenatal injury, early diffuse injury, or early injury to particular brain regions may have very profound and long-lasting effects on many aspects of adaptive behavior.

Indeed, there are many examples of early-acquired injury associated with seriously disordered development and long-term disability (e.g., cerebral palsy, meningitis). Early injury can significantly affect the acquisition and development of many motor, linguistic, cognitive, and social skills. In contrast, injuries sustained after acquisition of a skill may be associated with substantial recovery of abilities, as cortical networks for skills have already been established. Children with focal deficits secondary to trauma may show gratifying improvement in the months after injury, whereas infants with only a focal weakness of the extremities may show more disability with maturation as spasticity and differential growth occur.

It is also important to consider what is meant by *recovery*. Even in situations in which recovery appears to be strong, more careful and detailed observation of function can reveal substantial deficits. For example, after early left hemispherectomy or early lesions to left-hemisphere language areas, substantial language abilities can develop. However, careful examination often reveals residual limitations in grammatical and syntactic functions that presumably cannot be fully supported by remaining areas of the brain (Dennis & Whitaker, 1977). Similarly, there is evidence that early injury to the frontal lobes can have long-term and devastating effects on the development of a wide variety of social skills and executive functions (Eslinger & Damasio, 1985). Some of these difficulties may not be evident until a child reaches an age at which these abilities are expected to develop. In a recent paper, Anderson, Damasio, Tranel, and Damasio (in press) reported on two adults with significant cognitive, behavioral, social, and emotional difficulties, both of whom had sustained early focal frontal injuries evident on scans taken later in life. Although the injuries were recognized at the time as significant events, as children these individuals appeared to have made a full recovery in the acute stage. Thus, although it is true that younger brains certainly have more potential for plasticity, critical lesions can result in permanent deficits.

Young Adults

As a group, younger adults consistently show better levels of recovery than do older individuals. This is true not only when young and old individuals are compared, but also when relatively closely spaced age groups are studied. Teuber (1975), for example, examined the rates of recovery for a variety of different functions in soldiers who had received penetrating brain injuries. He found that 17- to 20-year-olds made better recoveries than 21- to 25-year-olds, who had better recoveries than did individuals aged 26 and over. This pattern held true for motor deficits, somatosensory deficits, visual field defects, and aphasia. Strikingly, these age-related effects held up even when the former soldiers were followed up 40 years later (Corkin, 1989).

Age effects can also be seen in long-term adaptation to brain injury, in that recovery of function following injury may show partial reversal as an individual ages. In the Corkin (1989) follow-up study, individuals who had sustained brain injuries 30 years previously showed a greater decline in performance than did individuals who did not have a history of brain injury. Indeed, some studies have suggested that the incidence of prior brain injury is higher in the population of elderly adults who develop dementia.

Older Adults

Although traumatic brain injury (TBI) is most common among young adult males aged 16–25 (Willer, Abasch, & Dahmer, 1990), older adults are also a high-risk group (Fields & Coffey, 1994), but falls rather than motor vehicle accidents are the major cause of injury. Studies of normal aging indicate age-associated declines in attention, memory, and executive processes (Craik, Anderson, Kerr, & Li, 1995). As such, the impact of injury on an older individual may be expected to vary with age-related maintenance or decline of cognitive abilities. In addition, age-related neuronal cell shrinkage is most pronounced in the frontal region (Hachinski, Potter, & Merskey, 1987)—the same brain region that is most vulnerable to traumatic damage following head injury. Over the course of normal aging, the frontal lobes show greater volume reduction, neuronal loss, and blood flow reduction than do the parietal, occipital, or temporal regions of the brain. Consistent with these findings, cognitive processes supported by the frontal lobes show earlier and greater declines than cognitive processes supported by other brain regions (Albert, 1994).

A study by Mazzuchi and colleagues (1992), examined the performance of patients aged 50–75 years, with TBI of varying severity, up to 3 years after injury. Subjects showed a high level of cognitive impairment, and those with mild TBI (MTBI) were no more likely to have a better outcome than those with severe injury. Richards (2000) examined the separate and combined effects of MTBI on neuropsychological performance in healthy young individuals, young patients with MTBI, healthy elderly individuals, and elderly patients with MTBI. Both age and MTBI negatively affected performance in the elderly group, and the deficits in performance were due to additive rather than interactive effects; that is, each factor produced independent decrements. It may be that there is a protective factor of reserve capacity that is vulnerable to depletion with age. The concept of *brain reserve capacity* hypothesizes that there is a pool of available brain capacity that provides protection from clinical symptoms but is vulnerable to depletion via deleterious organismic and extrinsic events. Alternatively, aging and MTBI may exert differential effects on brain structure and function, which would also be consistent with an additive versus interactive effect of these two factors. TBI & aging = additive effect

Overall, the data suggest that older individuals are more vulnerable to the effects of brain injury. On the other hand, from a rehabilitation perspective, older adults often have a more stable lifestyle, better coping skills, more support, and fewer life demands than younger individuals—all factors that can have a positive impact on rehabilitation outcomes. And, while there is evidence of better recovery of some basic functions in younger versus older adults, there is no reason to believe that older individuals are not able to learn to compensate for residual deficits just as well as younger individuals. Indeed, there has been considerable interest in how individuals learn to compensate for the cognitive declines associated with normal aging (Dixon & Backman, 1995). Although expectations for recovery of underlying processes may be more limited with an older patient, many older individuals have been shown to develop very effective compensatory skills and are often better able to adapt to some of the changes associated with neurological injury or disease than younger individuals.

Premorbid Intelligence and Educational Levels

Preinjury intelligence and educational levels are significant predictors of degree of function recovery following closed head injury (Brooks & McKinlay, 1987; Grafman, 1986). The hypothesis put forward to account for these findings is that the level of impairment is related to the amount of preinjury learning that has taken place. The varied cognitive requirements associated with educational activities may contribute to increased connectivity of neural networks. Indeed, Jacobs, Schall, and Scheibel (1993) found a relationship between the extent of dendritic arborization in Wernicke's area and an individual's level of education. Cortical neurons from the brains of deceased people with a university education had more dendritic arbors than those of people with a high school education. These people, in turn, had more dendritic material than those with less than high school education. It has been suggested that the volume of nodes of connectivity is associated with a richer understanding of, and multiple associations among, concepts. Practice of skills during the course of education may also result in more automatization of computational or cognitive skills. However, it may be that individuals that are more capable continue in school for a longer period, and there is certainly some indication that intellectual ability may be at least in part genetically determined. Undoubtedly, both innate ability and exposure to and involvement in various experiences contribute to functional capacities and to brain physiology. Other factors must also be considered in the recovery of brighter or more educated individuals: They are more likely to have better or more practiced premorbid learning abilities, and potentially more motivation for participation in rehabilitation, more family support, and/or more access to rehabilitation services.

Gender

There has not been a great deal of research concerning possible gender effects on recovery of function. The potential influences on recovery include the fact that some brain structures differ in shape and size in males and females, and that these differences result in both inter- and intrahemispheric gender differences. In addition, potential recovery mechanisms (e.g., dendritic branching and synaptic contacts) appear to be influenced by fluctuations in gonadal hormones such as estrogen. The most compelling data with regard to gender differences in response to neurological injury have been drawn from patients who have sustained strokes. Kimura (1983) examined the incidence of aphasia and apraxia in 224 patients with single left-hemisphere lesions. Aphasia was more frequent in males. In addition, women had speech and apraxic disorders more often from damage to the anterior part of the left hemisphere than from damage to the posterior region, whereas this was not true for the men. Overall, women appeared to have better recovery after left-hemisphere lesions than men, though this may have been due to the higher probability of a posterior rather than an anterior stroke.

There is also some indication that circulating gender-related hormones can have an effect on recovery mechanisms following brain injury. For example, female rats given frontal cortex lesions when progesterone levels were high compared to estrogen levels showed significantly less functional impairment than did female rats lesioned when their progesterone levels were low relative to their estrogen levels (Attella, Nattinville, & Stein, 1987). This suggested that certain hormones might confer a protective effect under conditions of neurological injury. In another study, Roof, Duvdevani, and Stein (1993) found that following bilateral contusion of the medial frontal cortex while under deep anesthesia, male rats had much more cerebral edema than did female rats, and female rats with very high levels of progesterone (pseudopregnancy) had almost no cerebral edema. Interestingly, Basso, Capitani, and Morashini (1983) reported that female patients with injury to the frontal cortex showed less impairment on cognitive tasks than did males with the same locus of injury. The logical extensions of this work are possible applications for prevention and treatment of injury. Tantalizing findings related to this are the results of a study by Roof, Duvdevani, Braswell, and Stein (1992). Both female and male rats treated with progesterone following bilateral medial frontal contusions showed a dramatic decline in postinjury edema, compared to untreated rats. Differences were also noted in cognitive recovery (Roof, Duvdevani, Braswell, & Stein, 1994). Progesterone has been shown to have a variety of effects at the neuronal level; these include enhancement of neuritic outgrowth, the formation of new myelin sheaths, and the regulation of gamma-aminobutyric acid receptors, which can influence the cascade of excitatory and excitotoxic activity that occurs after brain injury. Detailed discussion of these issues is not possible here, but it seems clear that sex hormones and hormonal cycling play an important role in an organism's response to injury (see Stein, Roof, & Fulop, 1999, for a recent review of this research).

Cultural Background

Differences in cultural background include not just language differences, but also differences in group identity, beliefs, and values (Dana, 1993), all of which influence the use of services, the presentation of symptoms, the assessment techniques used, and all other aspects of treatment. The literature suggests that multicultural clients are more likely to end treatment prematurely, due to frustration, misunderstanding, role ambiguities, and differences in the priorities of treatment (Sue & Zane, 1987). Individual identity or self-concept includes culturally mediated norms about assertiveness, aggression, the expression of emotion, and individual goal attainment versus sacrificing for the greater good. Cultural factors may influence what a person believes about illness and its meaning, including the fundamental nature and cause of physical and cognitive losses (Raskin, 2000). Whereas personal independence is highly valued in Western culture, it is not necessarily a goal in other cultures, which have different beliefs about (1) a person's degree of responsibility and control over health and (2) the role of family in dealing with illness. There is also a need to develop culturally relevant and appropriate treatment materials and activities. Involvement of therapists in the community of the same culture, especially for aspects of psychosocial counseling and willingness to work with traditional culture-specific healers or healing techniques, can be beneficial.

Premorbid or Current Drug and Alcohol Abuse

As a group, individuals with TBI have a higher rate of drug and alcohol abuse prior to injury; indeed, in many cases substance use is a contributory factor in their injury. Although some individuals continue to abuse substances after their injury, there is no indication that substance use increases, and a number of studies have reported decrease in substance abuse after injury (Stroup, 1999). In addition to low socioeconomic status and an unstable work history, alcohol use after injury is predictive of poor vocational outcome (Dikmen et al., 1994; Stroup, 1999). Alcohol use may further impair brain function, interrupt neurological recovery mechanisms, impede motivation, or simply limit vocational options. The problem is compounded by the low success rates for dealing with substance abuse in the population in general, and by the lack of programs designed to meet the needs of patients with dual diagnoses of brain injury and substance abuse.

INJURY-RELATED VARIABLES

Time since Injury

The rate of recovery is typically fastest in the early stages after brain injury, and usually decreases over time following injury. In moderate to severe injury, recovery is most rapid during the first 6 months, with slower but significant recovery occurring over the next 2 years. After this, spontaneous recovery is slower, although accommodations and compensations may be developed and implemented at any time after injury. There is also some evidence that underlying motor and cognitive skills, such as attention, can improve with structured interventions even years after injury. After mild injuries, recovery rates are even faster, with resolution of symptoms by 3–6 months in 70% of those injured, and 85% asymptomatic by 12 months after injury (see Chapter 15 of this volume for more details and references in regard to MTBI).

The mechanism for these differences in rate of recovery is thought to be that immediately after injury, areas that are not actually damaged are deprived of neuronal input from and to the damaged area. This deprivation alters the functioning of undamaged areas and results in a large area of functional lesion. Von Monakow (1914) introduced the term *diaschisis,* which he used to describe depression of activity in remote, nondamaged brain sites that are functionally connected to lesioned areas. As these nonlesioned areas become reconnected with other areas, or adjust to their lack of input from the lesioned areas, they begin to resume functioning. A significant amount of early recovery from what initially appear to be very severe functional impairments has been hypothesized to be due to recovery from diaschisis. The other reason for more rapid early recovery is that there is likely to be resolution of nonspecific factors, such as edema, during this period.

Injury Extent and Severity

The rate and extent of recovery vary with the severity of injury, such that those individuals with relatively mild injuries typically recover very quickly, while individuals with more severe injuries typically recover more slowly. Dikmen, Machamer, Winn, and Temkin (1995) demonstrated impressive "dose–response" curves indicating a close relationship between the severity of TBI and the expected recovery curve. Recovery also tends to occur more rapidly after focal pathology than after diffuse pathology, although this is often related to overall size of injury. However, some small focal lesions can have a significant and long-term impact if they affect a critical brain area for which the function cannot be compensated.

Although diaschisis undoubtedly plays a role in recovery, some types or degrees of brain damage may cause neural circuits to be so depleted or so disconnected that no amount of synaptic reorganization will ever allow reconnection. And indeed, some neuropsychological disorders—including aphasia, amnesia, agnosia, neglect, and others—can in some cases remain remarkably stable over many decades. It may be necessary for a certain amount of functionally related circuitry to be undamaged for reconnections to take place or be meaningful. Kolb (1995) has argued that whereas small lesions can result in restitution of function and quite faithful recovery of the original behavior, recovery from large lesions is based more on compensation and behavioral adaptation. Careful examination of the behaviors that appear to have recovered may reveal that they are being carried out in a different (and often less efficient) manner.

There is also some indication that the effects of an injury can be exacerbated if there has been a prior injury. A classic example is the "punch-drunk" phenomenon (*dementia pugilistica*)—a form of severe cognitive impairment that can be seen in individuals who, in the course of years of boxing, suffer repeated blows to the head and multiple concussive episodes. There are very few actual data to support the hypothesis of exponential effects of multiple brain injuries, particularly following a single episode of brain injury. However, it follows from the brain reserve capacity theory described earlier that the brain becomes increasingly less able to re-organize and compensate for damage once this has already occurred.

Recovery of Different Functions at Different Rates

Recovery of relatively simple, highly familiar, overlearned tasks typically occurs at a faster rate than recovery of more complex or novel activities. This makes sense if one thinks of complex tasks not only involving multiple underlying and interconnected skills, but also requiring more conscious and flexible control. Consistent with this notion, functions of the frontal lobe involved in effortful attention, flexible planning, organizing, and problem solving are often among the most persistent impairments after even diffuse brain injury. Differential recovery may also relate to the extent of lesion. For example, the trajectories for recovery from Wernicke's and Broca's aphasias are very similar—both showing gradual though usually incomplete improvement—while the trajectory for recovery from global aphasia is very depressed in comparison (Kertesz, Harlock, & Coates, 1979). In addition, recovery from aphasia after TBI often shows quick and dramatic recovery, perhaps because there has been less severe focal injury to primary language systems.

PSYCHOLOGICAL FACTORS

The process of rehabilitation should not constitute doing something for or to someone; it should involve an interactive partnership. In the best of circumstances, rehabilitation is a consensual and cooperative enterprise engaged in by the client, his or her family or support system, and the therapist. Ideally, the entire process is grounded in respect, trust, and commitment. The therapist needs to attend to the level of readiness and coping capacity of the family, as well as the client; there is evidence that the success of the intervention process with patients is intricately related to the working relationship therapists have with family members. Many factors can interfere with the rehabilitative partnership—some of them related to effects of the injury; some related to premorbid personality features of the client, the family, and/or the therapist; and some related to problems in negotiating the therapeutic relationship and treatment plan. The importance of developing and fostering therapeutic rapport cannot be overemphasized, and we discuss this at greater length in several other chapters (which include principles and strategies for working with families, as well as ways of working with emotional distress). Depression and anxiety, in particular, are very common sequelae of TBI and other acquired brain injuries. Although problems in these areas often result from cognitive impairments and losses, they can further erode cognitive efficiency; can decrease motivation; and can contribute to hopelessness, despair, and isolation. In the long run, these negative emotions and resultant behavior patterns have tremendous potential to limit personal and social adjustment and community reintegration.

Of the many difficulties that professionals face in the rehabilitation of individuals with brain injuries, lack of awareness of deficit can be one of the more significant obstacles. Clients who lack awareness may not acknowledge changes in their functioning, and, not recognizing the need for any treatment, are often resistant to rehabilitation activities. Impaired self-awareness is often associated with poor self-monitoring and poor self-regulatory behavior (Fleming, Strong & Ashton, 1996). Lack of awareness can lead to difficulties in many aspects of rehabilitation, including successful engagement in and completion of treatment regimens, maintenance of deficit-reducing compensatory aids, and inappropriate vocational choices (Allen & Ruff, 1990; Lam, McMahon, Priddy, & Gehred-Schulz, 1988; Melamed, Grosswasser, & Stern, 1992). Chapter 9 reviews strategies for assessing and managing problems with awareness.

Other clients, though reasonably aware of their impairments, are resistant to the rehabilitation process. The system of rehabilitation can be viewed by such clients as coercive and/or manipulative, sometimes with good reason. Anger, resistance, and refusals to participate in rehabilitation can pose real obstacles to progress. Readiness to engage in and benefit from rehabilitation is facilitated by open communication and involvement of a patient and family in mutual goal setting and in selecting and implementing treatment approaches and plans. As discussed in more detail below, experience-dependent plastic reorganization appears to require that attention be paid to the activity or experience. It is important to effectively engage the patient (and family members) in the therapeutic process. Client-centered movements focused on patients' rights and their ability to choose treatment fit well with the notion of a therapeutic relationship in which the views and wishes of all parties are respected.

In the early stages after injury or following very severe injuries, patients themselves may not be capable of entering into the process. Behaviorally based interventions can be extremely effective at this point in modifying the environment and other influences on such clients, and thereby allowing more effective regulation of behavior (see Chapter 11). As awareness and self-regulation of behavior increase, therapists have a responsibility to work toward creating an effective context for rehabilitation that provides structure, motivation, support, and honesty. Management of depression and anxiety through pharmacotherapy and supportive psychotherapy can also be a valuable adjunct to rehabilitation efforts. Throughout this text, there are many specific suggestions for ways to manage clients' emotional responses to cognitive deficits, to changes in function, and to the process of therapy itself. Chapter 12 specifically addresses working with individuals who are experiencing emotional consequences as a result of their injuries.

NEUROPLASTICITY AND SYNAPTIC REORGANIZATION

Neuroscience and, indeed, observation of human behavior leave little doubt that the brain must be fundamentally altered by experience. The notion of *neuroplasticity*—the brain's capacity to change and alter its structure and function—is particularly relevant to rehabilitation and an understanding of recovery processes, both natural and induced. Several mechanisms underlying neuroplasticity have important implications for rehabilitation (see Table 3.1). One of these mechanisms, diaschisis, has been discussed above in connection with time since injury. In this section, we explore some of the evidence with regard to other mechanisms involved in recovery of function and neuroplasticity that may contribute to a stronger theoretical basis for rehabilitation efforts. We then consider the issue of *bottom-up* versus *top-down* processes in rehabilitation, and conclude the section with a brief summary of future directions and guiding principles.

Functional Reorganization

Luria (1973), following in the tradition of Kurt Goldstein, proposed a compensatory process known as *functional reorganization*, by which neural circuits that survive after injury reorganize to accomplish a given behavior in a different way. Luria's emphasis was on compensation as a mechanism of recovery rather than restitution of impaired neuropsychological processes. Traditionally, rehabilitation has focused on assisting pa-

TABLE 3.1. Mechanisms Underlying Neuroplasticity after Brain Injury

Mechanism	Description
Diaschisis	There is a (sometimes temporary) loss of function in areas remote from a lesioned area, but neuronally connected to it.
Functional reorganization	Recruitment of quite different or remote neural circuits allows a given behavior to occur, though perhaps in a different manner.
Modification of synaptic connectivity	Surviving neurons develop new dendrites (or dendritic branches) to receive information from another neuron in the circuit or from a more distant circuit.
Influences on neural circuitry	Structured sensory input can increase connectivity of partially disconnected neural circuits; training in self-awareness can decrease circuit activation, if a decrease is desired.
Impact of interhemispheric competition	Damage to one side of the brain alters the natural balance of functioning, such that the undamaged hemisphere inhibits preserved or recovering functions in the damaged one.

tients to learn to compensate for impaired function, while attempting to maximize functioning of impaired systems. An individual with a hemiparetic limb, for example, is provided with training and practice in using the unimpaired limb for functional activities, while efforts to strengthen and increase range of motion in the impaired limb are also undertaken. Although this approach seems perfectly reasonable, there have been few data or theories underlying its implementation, or direction as to the most effective timing of various interventions. Whereas compensation was long held to be the principal basis of recovery, recent advances in knowledge about the plasticity of the adult CNS require new models for rehabilitation practices that incorporate the best ways to facilitate both compensation and restitution.

Although functional reorganization may seem to be a highly desirable mechanism for behavioral recovery, there is some evidence that it may sometimes actually inhibit the potential for restitution of damaged circuits. In a striking example of this, LeVere and LeVere (1982) demonstrated that rats with visual cortex lesions would ignore visual cues and respond only to nonvisual cues in a learning paradigm. However, if the nonvisual cues were made irrelevant, it became clear that the rats could still use visual cues, though at a less efficient level than previously. The authors concluded that residual spared functioning in the damaged visual system was suppressed, masked, or dominated by functioning of the nonvisual neural system. They argued that reliance on compensatory systems not only can decrease activation in partially lesioned circuits, but can actively inhibit such activation by means of inhibitory processes. It is currently difficult to determine whether a compensatory adjustment is a useful short-term mechanism, or whether it has the potential to actually inhibit restitutive function.

Modification of Synaptic Connectivity

There is clear evidence that learning and experience cause physical changes in the adult brain. The same neural mechanisms that support normal learning are activated in individuals with brain damage, and undoubtedly contribute to recovery of function. Most of the evidence for these neural mechanisms comes from animal work, since detailed microscopic investigation of neural structures is not possible in a living person. Animal studies have investigated neurological changes, such as dendritic sprouting in the cortex following lesions to various areas and in relation to various forms of pre- and postlesion experience (Kolb & Gibb, 1999).

Modification of synaptic activity through dendritic branching and, to a lesser extent, axonal sprouting is an ongoing process present in all adults on a continuous basis. A neuron that has lost input from a damaged neuron can develop new dendrites or dendritic spines to receive information from another neuron in the same circuit, or even from another, more distant circuit. This synaptic plasticity is apparent in both recovery processes and normal learning. Importantly, it is directly related to, and indeed dependent on, experience. Without inputs that drive the system, these new connections do not form. An important implication of this for rehabilitation is that variations in an injured person's experience affect the kind and degree of input to damaged circuitry and thus will influence recovery.

Hebb (1949) hypothesized that strengthening of synaptic connections occurs when pre- and postsynaptic neurons are activated at the same time. This simultaneous activation can occur when each of them is connected to another circuit, which, when activated, causes simultaneous activations in the disconnected neurons. This principle has been summed up as "Cells that fire together, wire together." This firing, of course, depends on the basic viability of the neurons and may be a mechanism that operates most effectively, in the case of a damaged brain, at the margins of a lesion. Current work suggests that plasticity indeed appears to be a property of the synapse, as this is where reorganization and changes in neural connectivity take place.

In rehabilitation, there is a tendency to think of compensation only in the behavioral sense, but it should be thought of in a neurological sense as well. That is, the new behavior that provides compensation for the old engages quite different neurophysiological systems in the performance of the task. Take, for example, experiments in which monkeys trained on a finger dexterity task were given lesions in areas of sensory cortex normally utilized in doing this task. With training, the monkeys were able to reacquire the skill, and there was evidence that this was associated with redistribution of sensory inputs to nondamaged areas of sensory cortex (Xerri, Merzenich, Peterson, & Jenkins, 1998). In humans with tumors in the cortical sensory area for the hand, contralateral hand movements were linked to blood flow increases in the adjacent areas of the motor cortex, but also in the premotor cortex or the parietal somatosensory cortex (Seitz et al., 1995). Such findings lend support to the notion of restitutive reconnection and reorganization in related circuitry, as well as compensatory reorganization in quite different or more remote neural circuits.

Although much of the research supporting more expanded notions of neuronal plasticity comes from animal studies, there is certainly work suggesting that similar mechanisms are functioning in the recovery of humans. For example, it is widely acknowledged that almost all patients with aphasia demonstrate some degree of spontaneous recovery (Wertz, 1996). The neuronal process underlying recovery from aphasia has, however, remained largely unknown. Recently, data have been emerging to allow some of the theories that have been put forward about the underlying basis of recovery to be tested. Some positron emission tomography (PET) studies, for example, have supported the role of the left hemisphere's preserved language zones in the recovery process. In addition, and as originally proposed by Wernicke, the restitution of language after stroke may be mediated through compensation by analogous brain regions in the contralateral, undamaged hemisphere (Gainotti, 1993).

Mimura and colleagues (1998) conducted prospective and retrospective studies of recovery from aphasia following infarction of the left middle cerebral artery, using single-photon emission computed tomography (SPECT). Average cerebral blood flow in the left hemisphere did not differ between good- and poor-recovery groups; however, the good-recovery group demonstrated higher cerebral blood flow in the right frontal and thalamic regions and in the left frontal region. Mimura and colleagues hypothesized that language recovery within the first year was most closely linked to recovery in the dominant hemisphere, and that increased perfusion of areas adjacent to the lesion was crucial for early recovery. However, they suggested that subsequent and long-term language recovery appeared more related to slow and compensatory functions in the contralateral hemisphere, and specifically in homotopic frontal and thalamic areas. In another blood flow study (Musso et al., 1999), training-induced improvements in language comprehension were correlated with increased blood flow in the posterior part of the right superior temporal gyrus and the left precuneus. This was one of the first studies to look specifically at brain-related change during the course of treatment, and it again suggested a role in recovery for both adjacent regions in the damaged hemisphere and homologous regions in the opposite hemisphere.

Influences on Neural Circuitry

A critical question for rehabilitation is this: What can be done to foster reconnectivity of partially disconnected neural circuitry? This is of particular importance, since loss of stimulation, even in an undamaged brain, results in declining connectivity in a circuit. (A good example of this is the trouble one has dredging up those French verb tenses so well studied in high school, but not very available on the trip to Paris 15 years later.) One model for providing increased facilitation involves providing additional structured input to circuits. For example, rats given visual cortex transplants only benefited from the transplants when the circuits were "driven" through opportunities for relevant perceptual motor learning (Mayer, Brown, Dunnett, & Robbins, 1992). Similarly, Nudo, Wise, SiFuentes, and Milliken (1996) found that following lesions to the hand area in monkeys, hand movement representations in initially undamaged areas adjacent to the lesion were lost. Exercise and training of hand use prevented this loss of representation in adjacent tissue; in fact, it resulted in larger areas of hand representation, even well beyond the initial area of representation. These findings suggest that the structured sensory input and structured activity, akin to rehabilitative training, guided synaptic reorganization and functional hand recovery in these monkeys.

Another series of studies focusing on the rehabilitation of unilateral left neglect is illustrative with regard to the issue of how to influence neuronal circuitry. *Neglect* is a visuospatial attentional disorder leading to impaired perception of and diminished responses to stimuli presented in one side of space, more commonly the left. Robertson and North (1992, 1993) examined the therapeutic effects of left-arm activation in patients with left-sided neglect. Moving the left fingers in left side of visual space reduced neglect in comparison to verbal instruction; in contrast, right-finger movements or movements in right hemispace did not reduce neglect. One hypothesis for this effect was that the production of voluntary movements with the left hand activated or enhanced somatosensory circuits that, in turn, produced enhancement of sensations in the left half of personal space. In a follow-up study designed to capitalize on this phenomenon in rehabilitation, Robertson, Hogg, and McMillan (1998) induced movement of the left limb by using a "neglect alert device," which emitted random sounds that the patient had to prevent or terminate by pressing a switch with the left hand. Daily ratings of mobility difficulty arising from neglect showed improvements following implementation of the intervention.

In some situations, it may be desirable to decrease the activation of circuits. For example, it has been suggested that fluent aphasic speech may actually increase the likelihood of reinforcing dysfunctional connections. When awareness of impaired speech is low, as is common in individuals with fluent aphasia, it may be beneficial to provide external cues or supports to reduce talking. Training in self-awareness of impaired speech may be the most appropriate target for rehabilitation. In this example, treatment is directed at the attentional and self-awareness systems of the brain. It may be that these more generic or "umbrella" functions can be used to exert more modulatory influence on functions subserved by more focally organized primary motor and sensory areas. As in the case of a client with a posterior lesion resulting in jargon aphasia, presumably intact frontal systems may be effectively recruited for improved self-monitoring.

The Impact of Interhemispheric Competition

Another consideration in understanding neuroplasticity in the context of recovery is the somewhat competitive relationship that exists between the hemispheres (Kinsbourne, 1993). This relationship becomes important in that, after damage to one hemisphere, there is some evidence that its natural inhibitory influence on the other is lost or reduced. It has been proposed that damaged circuits in the brain can suffer further loss of function because of inhibitory competition from undamaged circuits. There is evidence that the undamaged hemisphere of the brain in a group of patients who had suffered unilateral strokes showed higher levels of regional blood flow than did that hemisphere of the brain in control subjects (Buckner, Corbetta, Schatz, Raichle, & Petersen, 1996; Grady & Kapur, 1999; Weiller, Chollet, Friston, Wise, & Frackowiak, 1992) (see Figure 3.2). Although such increased activity may contribute to some of the compensatory gains, it may also be exerting an inhibitory affect on the damaged hemisphere that reduces the potential recovery of its damaged circuits. Indeed, sometimes paradoxical improvements in performance occur after a second lesion on the opposite side of the brain. In one client we worked with, who had marked left-sided neglect following a right-hemisphere stroke, there was a resolution of the neglect following a left-hemisphere stroke several months later. Perhaps this occurred because the new lesion reduced the activity of left-sided neural networks that were excessively inhibiting the originally damaged right-hemisphere circuitry.

Recovery of function may in part be determined by the extent to which the inhibition of damaged circuits can be reduced, either by activating circuits in the damaged hemisphere itself, or by reducing activation in the undamaged hemisphere. Robertson and North (1992, 1993) provided an example of this from their studies of limb activation to reduce unilateral neglect. Left-sided spatial neglect was reduced by the simultaneous activation of the left limb in left hemispace, presumably because this activated right-hemisphere sensorimotor circuits. However, the beneficial effects of left-limb activation on neglect were eliminated if the right limb was simultaneously moved. The authors hypothesized that whereas left-limb activity

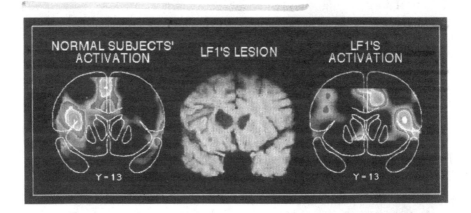

FIGURE 3.2. *Left:* Functional magnetic resonance imaging (fMRI) showing primary left temporal lobe activation during speaking in a normal subject. *Middle:* Scan showing a lesion in the left temporal lobe resulting from stroke. *Right:* Primary activation in the homologous right temporal lobe during speaking in this patient after a period of recovery from the stroke. From Buckner, Corbetta, Schatz, Raichle, and Petersen (1996). Copyright 1999 by Cambridge University Press. Reprinted by permission.

activated circuitry in the right hemisphere, bilateral movements activated competitor circuits in the undamaged left hemisphere at the same time, thereby extinguishing any competitive advantage provided by the unilateral movement. Perhaps application of motor rehabilitation strategies that emphasize the need for bilateral activation of limbs may actually hinder recovery if such activity enhances circuits that competitively inhibit the impaired networks. In addition to interhemispheric inhibition, there may also be sources of inhibition operating within the same hemisphere (see Classen et al., 1997).

Bottom-Up versus Top-Down Processes in Rehabilitation

Robertson and Murre (1999) have proposed a distinction between *bottom-up* and *top-down* processes in rehabilitation (see Table 3.2). *Bottom-up processes refer to the provision of perceptual, motor, or other externally generated or cued inputs to the lesioned network.* One example of this comes from a rehabilitation study focusing on motor recovery. Therapy consisting of highly repetitive hand and finger movements using the impaired arm resulted in greater improvement in hand and finger function than did standard hand and finger exercises involving a range of movements during training (Butefisch, Hummelsheim, Denzler, & Mauritz, 1995). The authors argued that repetitive training more consistently activated the same sets of neurons in the damaged network, allowing faster and more efficient synaptic reconnectivity.

It has also been demonstrated that individuals with partial upper-limb hemiplegia demonstrated improved function in this limb with a treatment program that discouraged use of the unaffected limb and encouraged concentrated, vigorous, and repetitive use of the affected limb (Taub, Uswatte, & Pidikiti, 1999). Even years after injury, improvements lasting up to 2

TABLE 3.2. Examples of Bottom-Up versus Top-Down Training Approaches

Bottom-up approaches provide patterned input to lesioned or dysfunctional networks.
- Repetitive movement or practice
- Structured sensory stimulation
- Constraint-induced therapy
- Training in phonemic or acoustic discriminations
- Provision of external cues to maintain attention

Top-down approaches "stimulate" higher systems (e.g., frontal executive systems) to modify/regulate processing in other systems.
- Improvement of attention skills
- Training in metacognitive and self-monitoring strategies

Note. Data from Robertson and Murre (1999).

years were observed following just 2 weeks of practice with the hemiplegic limb, even in patients for whom spontaneous recovery had appeared quite good.

Recently, there has been substantial interest in an approach to treating children with developmental speech and language disorders that uses what could be considered a bottom-up approach. Tallal, Merzenich, and colleagues (Merzenich et al., 1996; Tallal et al., 1996) propose that speech recognition, and in particular phoneme recognition, can be improved by providing repeated opportunities to make temporal discriminations between very similar auditory stimuli. The training materials consist of acoustically modified stimuli that encourage a child to discriminate successive approximations to temporal differences in the acoustic signal, which are similar in length to those critical for speech perception. These authors have suggested that the repeated (bottom-up) stimulation actually causes plastic reorganization of circuitry involved in temporal segmentation and discrimination.

Robertson, Manly, Andrade, Baddeley, and Yiend (1997) have provided another example of bottom-up input in patients with TBI. The Sustained Attention to Response Task (SART) requires that subjects press a key each time a number appears on the screen, except for one particular target number to which no response should be made. Not pressing these rare targets requires considerable attention to the task at hand and monitoring of responses. Patients with TBI and with right-hemisphere strokes have substantial difficulty on the SART. However, if an external auditory cue is presented occasionally during the task, errors are significantly reduced. Robertson and colleagues have argued that this suggests a bottom-up alerting effect, which improves attention on this task.

There is also some suggestion that certain types of stimulation may foster a dysfunctional connectivity. Sturm, Willmes, Orgass, and Hartje (1997) provided attention training to patients who had sustained strokes. Individuals received training in basic attentional processes (vigilance and selective attention) and in higher-level attention control functions (divided attention). Subjects who first received training in basic processes improved on both those processes and higher-level control functions. In contrast, subjects who received training on higher-level tasks first did not show gains on either the basic or the higher-level processes, and in some cases even demonstrated a decline in their function. Sturm and colleagues argued for the importance of providing hierarchically sequenced training, and cautioned against training higher-level skills before lower-level skills are stabilized.

Top-down processes are based on experimental findings indicating that "higher" brain centers, such as the frontal lobes and thalamus, play a part in determining what sensory information is selected for further processing. Attentional circuits in the frontal lobe are considered to be important in such gating of sensory information. As an example, blood flow to the primary sensory cortex decreases in areas where stimulation is not expected (Drevets et al., 1995). Meyer and colleagues (1991) conducted a study in which vibrotactile stimulation was applied to the fingertips. In subjects who paid attention to the vibration, there was 13% more activation in the hand sensory area than there was when subjects received the same stimulation but did not attend to it. These studies suggest that attention and expectancy, both of which are internally generated processes, enhance brain activation in response to sensory input. Robertson and Murre (1999) argue that synaptic activity, which forms the basis for plastic changes in the brain, is modulated in a top-down fashion by such frontal attentional circuits.

According to this line of thinking, recovery of function should be at least in part related to the integrity of frontal attentional brain systems. Robertson and Murre (1999) have hypothesized that if top-down input from frontal circuits can foster connectivity in the nondamaged brain, then such input should also foster reconnection and repair in the damaged brain. And, indeed, there is considerable evidence that frontal attentional functioning is a strong predictor of recovery of function following brain damage. There are data to suggest that sustained attention is strongly related to right-hemisphere functioning, particularly right frontal functioning (Coull, Frith, Frackowiak, & Grasby, 1996). The ability to sustain attention to a tone-counting task was a significant predictor of long-term left-hand motor recovery and everyday life function following stroke (Robertson et al., 1997). Following TBI, return to work, even several years after the injury, was significantly predicted by postinjury attentional function (Brooks & McKinlay, 1987). Indeed, a number of studies have found that functional recovery from stroke (Hier, Mondlock, & Caplan, 1983) and closed head injury (Bayless, Varney, & Roberts, 1989; Butler, Anderson, Furst, Namerow, & Satz, 1989; Mattson & Levin, 1990; Melamed, Stern, Rahmani, Grosswasser, & Najenson, 1985; Najenson, Grosswasser, Mendelson, & Hackett, 1980; Vilkki et al., 1994; Wilson et al., 1993) is predicted by frontal executive function. These findings are also compatible with animal studies showing that activity-dependent reorganization in sensory and motor maps requires active attention to the relevant stimuli, and that passive stimulation while attention is deployed elsewhere does not result in plastic reorganization of the stimulated circuits.

An obvious implication of these findings is that impaired attention may hinder neuroplastic changes during recovery, and that efforts to improve attention may have widespread positive impact on recovery of a variety of functions, not just attention per se. As an example, one study found that activation of sustained attention resulted in significant improvements in unilateral neglect (Robertson et al., 1997). In another study, we (Mateer & Sohlberg, 1988; Mateer, Sohlberg, & Youngman, 1990) showed that improvements in attention following attention training were associated with improvements in learning and recall abilities in a series of patients with brain injury. Overall, the evidence suggests that frontal lobe damage and attentional deficits are very strong predictors of recovery of a wide variety of functions, and that efforts to increase attention during the rehabilitation process are beneficial.

Neuroplasticity: Future Directions and Guiding Principles

It is clear from this cursory review that research into neuroplasticity and the various influences on how the brain responds to injury is rapidly expanding. We expect that in the next decade, major advances will be made in understanding the natural processes involved, as well as in manipulating them. There is great interest in developing pharmacological interventions that will alter the various biochemical changes occurring after injury, so that damaging effects will be reduced. Various forms of neural implants or cell grafting that will stimulate growth of cells or cell connections will undoubtedly become more widely used. Although this technique was originally studied in the context of degenerative disorders like Parkinson's disease, it will surely become more widely applied, particularly as stem cells—the basic cells from which the CNS (like all other organs) is derived—become more readily available. Increasingly, we will also see an important contribution from the exciting research on gene therapy (e.g., gene transfer and gene splicing) and pharmacogenetic treatments (see Dickinson-Anson, Aubert, & Gage, 1999, for a review).

What are the implications of work in neuroplasticity and recovery for rehabilitation practice? Several principles can be derived from these areas of basic and clinical research, and these should guide our thinking and our development of intervention strategies:

- The brain is a dynamic organ, capable of extensive neurological reorganization over the lifetime of the individual and following injury.
- Motor, sensory, and cognitive abilities can and usually do improve over time, although recovery is generally prolonged and the sequelae of brain injury usually persist to some degree.
- Structural changes in the brain, particularly in dendritic fields and synapses, underlie behavioral changes. There are many influences on synaptic connectivity.
- Enhanced recovery of neurobehavioral function is associated with environmental stimulation and the structuring of experience in both the normal and the damaged brain.
- There is a role for both restitutive and compensatory approaches in rehabilitation.

- Functional reorganization typically involves recruitment of areas adjacent to the lesion and in homologous areas of the contralateral hemisphere.
- Behavioral outcomes reflect a complex interplay of bottom-up and top-down processes and of intra- and interhemispheric influences.

FACTORS RELATED TO TRAINING PROGRAMS AND INTERVENTIONS

Recovery will depend in part on the nature, quality, and quantity of postinjury experience. It is therefore important to consider how and when to implement rehabilitation programs, maximizing their effectiveness while keeping in mind practical and financial constraints. Clinicians, hospital administrators, insurers, and researchers have struggled with the issue of whether to provide intensive services early, or to provide less intensive but more prolonged treatment. Certainly clients have different needs at different stages of recovery. There are undoubtedly neurophysiological mechanisms underlying recovery that are more effective or can be more easily manipulated/recruited at different stages after injury. Unfortunately, information about these mechanisms is not currently available. In addition, constraints related to availability of resources and readiness for treatment must be considered.

The following recommendations are particularly important in the early stages of recovery from neurological injury:

- Make sure the patient is rested. There is some work suggesting that rapid-eye-movement (REM) sleep and/or sleep cycle disorganization may be necessary for consolidation of learning. Thus drugs that interfere with sleep, or poor sleep in general, may affect cerebral plasticity and may retard recovery (Ficca, Lombardo, Rossi, & Salzarulo, 2000).
- Make informed use of pharmacological interventions. A combination of pharmacological and behavioral interventions may be helpful in facilitating arousal. However, caution is in order: Some commonly used drugs reduce the potential for plastic changes to the brain, whereas others may enhance them. Diazepam, for example, which is frequently used for controlling agitation, has been shown to impair plastic recovery in animals (Stein, Brailowsky, & Will, 1995). The use of drugs such as this should be minimized during rehabilitation.
- Make use of natural windows of increased arousal and responsiveness. Patients will respond best to interventions when they are alert and able to attend, however briefly, to the task at hand. Brief, intermittent periods of intervention are likely to be more effective when patients are minimally or inconsistently aroused.
- Monitor and control the attentional load on the patient. Over-

stimulation can lead to both the inability to process information effectively and the reduced awareness of errors. Increase attentional load gradually and systematically, using strategies designed to support and improve sustained, selective, and divided attention. Provide structured, systematic stimulation in a hierarchical manner to ensure success and stabilize skills.

- Many behaviors can be elicited by an effective cue, be it verbal, tactile, or visual. Make use of graded cueing, moving from motor or verbal prompts and assists to more subtle or partial cues.
- Distributed practice for short periods is likely to be more effective than massed practice conducted in a single session. This is consistent with learning theory and clinical observations.

As patients become better able to participate actively in the rehabilitation process, a number of other principles become important:

- Use shaping and behavioral chaining strategies based on learning principles. Partial behaviors can be shaped gradually, and components of behavior can be linked and scaffolded to develop and support more complex behavior sequences.
- Emphasis on modifying antecedents as well as consequences in behaviorally oriented training are particularly relevant to individuals with brain injury.
- Many individuals with brain damage are ineffective learners. Once the nature of a patient's learning and memory deficit is understood, teaching strategies that are most effective for that particular individual can be used. Errorless learning techniques (which are discussed at length in Chapter 6), for example, can be very effective for enabling individuals with severe memory impairments to learn new information.
- Success breeds success, as well as self-esteem and satisfaction. Maximize the likelihood of a correct response, rather than focusing on correction of incorrect responses.
- Work for speed and efficiency of processing and responding while minimizing error rates.
- Make use of mental rehearsal and attentional focus to provide more top-down control. Overt self-talk can be used for self-regulation of many behaviors and skills.
- Recognize which deficits do and do not respond to stimulation-based treatments. For example, attentional skills often respond to repetition and practice, whereas episodic memory skills are less likely to increase with explicit practice. These latter skills are much more effectively dealt with through compensatory approaches.
- In order for a patient to demonstrate improvements in daily life in a variety of settings and over time, it is important to become familiar with and utilize effective generalization strategies.

SUMMARY

Many different factors influence recovery from damage to the brain. Some of these, such as demographic factors, are fixed and not subject to manipulation. We can, however, use information about such factors to make informed predictions about a client's natural course of recovery. Factors related to the injury itself are also not typically under the control of rehabilitation specialists, though medical science is certainly making inroads in decreasing the secondary damage caused by stroke and trauma, primarily through innovative pharmacological interventions. Although our understanding of brain plasticity and of the mechanisms underlying it is still quite primitive, what is emerging provides substantial evidence for a greater degree of plasticity in the adult brain than was previously believed. We are beginning to understand something about the nature of neural reorganization and dynamic synaptic connectivity, and about what influences and drives these natural forces. A consideration of these mechanisms is providing direction for the development of exciting new theoretically based, rehabilitative strategies. At the same time, these new discoveries highlight the complexity of the overall challenge of rehabilitation. Implications for best clinical practice are confusing at times, but this reflects where the field is in the process of assimilating and applying new information. Although a greater understanding of the biological underpinnings of recovery is exciting and vital to the field, it is important to keep in mind many of the principles of rehabilitation practice that we know facilitate the recovery process. Consider, for example, the important role that mood and motivation play in rehabilitation, and the importance of building a therapeutic relationship that will maximize a patient's engagement in the rehabilitative process. This chapter has attempted to illustrate the breadth of operative mechanisms in recovery, from the molecular to the psychosocial. We feel that such a broad consideration of issues is important, and that the increasingly interdisciplinary field of rehabilitation research is very promising and exciting.

REFERENCES

Albert, M. S. (1994). Age related changes in cognitive function. In M. L. Albert & J. E. Knoefel (Eds.), *Clinical neurology of aging* (pp. 314–328). New York: Oxford University Press.

Allen, C. C., & Ruff, R. M. (1990). Self-rating versus neuropsychological performance of moderate versus severe head-injured patients. *Brain Injury, 4,* 7–17.

Anderson, S. W., Damasio, H., Tranel, D., & Damasio, A. R. (in press). Severe long term sequelae of prefrontal cortex damage acquired in early childhood. *Developmental Psychology.*

Attella, M. J., Nattinville, A., & Stein, D. G. (1987). Hormonal state affects recovery from frontal cortex lesions in adult female rats. *Behavioral and Neural Biology, 48*, 352–367.

Basso, A., Capitani, E., & Morashini, S. (1983). Sex differences in recovery from aphasia. *Cortex, 18*, 469–475.

Bayless, J. D., Varney, N. R., & Roberts, R. J. (1989). Tinker Toy Test performance and vocational outcome in patients with closed-head injuries. *Journal of Clinical and Experimental Neuropsychology, 11*, 913–917.

Buckner, R. L., Corbetta, M., Schatz, J., Raichle, M. E., & Petersen, S. E. (1996). Preserved speech abilities and compensation following prefrontal damage. *Proceedings of the National Academy of Science USA, 93*, 1249–1253.

Brooks, D. N., & McKinlay, W. (1987). Return to work within the first seven years of severe head injury. *Brain Injury, 1*, 5–15.

Butefisch, C., Hummelsheim, H., Denzler, P., & Mauritz, K. H. (1995). Repetitive training of isolated movements improves the outcome of motor rehabilitation of the centrally paretic hand. *Journal of the Neurological Sciences, 130*, 59–68.

Butler, R. W., Anderson, L., Furst, C. J., Namerow, N. S., & Satz, P. (1989). Behavioral assessment in neuropsychological rehabilitation: A method for measuring vocational-related skills. *The Clinical Neuropsychologist, 3*, 235–243.

Classen, J., Schnitzler, A., Binkofski, F., Werhahn, K. J., Kim, Y. S., Kessler, K. R., & Benecke, R. (1997). The motor syndrome associated with exaggeration inhibition within the primary motor cortex. *Brain, 120*, 605–619.

Corkin, S. (1989). Penetrating head injury in young adulthood exacerbates cognitive decline in later years. *Journal of Neuroscience, 9*, 3876–3883.

Coull, J. T., Frith, C. D., Frackowiak, R. S. J., & Grasby, P. M. (1996). A fronto-parietal network for rapid visual information processing: A PET study of sustained attention and working memory. *Neuropsychologia, 34*, 1085–1095.

Craik, F. I. M., Anderson, N. D., Kerr, S. A., & Li, K. Z. (1995). Memory changes in normal aging. In A. D. Baddeley, B. A. Wilson, & F. N. Watts (Eds.), *Handbook of memory disorders* (pp. 211–242). Chichester, England: Wiley.

Dana, R. (1993). *Multicultural assessment perspectives for professional psychology.* Boston: Allyn & Bacon.

Dennis, M., & Whitaker, H. A. (1977). Hemispheric equipotentiality and language acquisition. In S. J. Segalowitz & F. A. Gruber (Eds.), *Language development and neurological theory* (pp. 93–106). New York: Academic Press.

Dickinson-Anson, H., Aubert, I., & Gage, F. H. (1999). Intracerebral transplantation and regeneration: Practical implications. In D. T. Stuss, G. Winocur, & I. Robertson (Eds.), *Cognitive neurorehabilitation* (pp. 26–46). Cambridge, England: Cambridge University Press.

Dikmen, S. S., Machamer, J. E., Winn, H. R., & Temkin, N. R. (1995). Neuropsychological outcome at 1-year post head injury. *Neuropsychology, 9*, 98–90.

Dikmen, S. S., Temkin, N. R., Machamer, J. E., Hlubkov, A. L., Fraser, R. T., & Winn, R. (1994). Employment following traumatic brain injuries. *Archives of Neurology, 51*, 177–186.

Dixon, R. A., & Backman, L. (1995). *Compensating for psychological deficits and declines: Managing losses and promoting gains.* Mahwah, NJ: Erlbaum.

Drevets, W. C., Burton, H., Videen, T. O., Snyder, A. Z., Simpson, J. R., Jr., & Raichle, M. E. (1995). Blood flow changes in human somatosensory cortex during anticipated stimulation. *Nature, 373*, 249–252.

Duhaime, A. C., Bilaniuk, L., & Zimmerman, R. (1993). The "big glack brain": Radiographic changes after severe inflicted head injury in infancy. *Journal of Neurotrauma*, 10(Suppl. 1), S59.

Eslinger, P. J., & Damasio, A. R. (1985). Severe disturbance of higher cognition after bilateral frontal lobe ablation: Patient E. V. R. *Neurology, 35*, 1731–1741.

Ficca, G., Lombardo, P., Rossi, L., & Salzarulo, P. (2000). Morning recall of verbal material depends on prior sleep organization. *Behavioral Brain Research, 112*, 159–163.

Fields, R. B., & Coffey, M. D. (1994). Traumatic brain injury. In C. Coffey & J. Cummings (Eds.), *The American textbook of geriatric neuropsychiatry* (pp. 479–508). Washington, DC: American Psychiatric Press.

Fleming, J. M., Strong, J., & Ashton, R. (1996). Self-awareness of deficits in adults with traumatic brain injury: How best to measure? *Brain Injury, 10*, 1–15.

Gainotti, G. (1993). The riddle of the right hemisphere's contribution to the recovery of language. *European Journal of Disorders of Communication, 28,* 227–246.

Grady, C. L., & Kapur, S. (1999). The use of neuroimaging in neurorehabilitative research. In D. T. Stuss, G. Winocur, & I. H. Robertson (Eds.), *Cognitive neurorehabilitation* (pp. 47–58). Cambridge, England: Cambridge University Press.

Grafman, J. (1986). The relationship of brain tissue loss volume and lesion location to cognitive deficit. *Journal of Neuroscience, 6*, 301–307.

Hachinski, V. C., Potter, P., & Merskey, H. (1987). Leuko-araiosis. *Archives of Neurology, 44*, 21–23.

Hebb, D. O. (1949). *The organization of behavior: A neuropsychological theory.* New York: Wiley.

Hier, D. B., Mondlock, J., & Caplan, L. R. (1983). Recovery of behavioral abnormalities after right hemisphere stroke. *Neurology, 33*, 345–350.

Jacobs, B., Schall, M., & Scheibel, A. B. (1993). A quantitative dendritic analysis of Wernicke's area: II. Gender, hemispheric, and environmental factors. *Journal of Comparative Neurology, 237*, 97–111.

Kennard, M. A. (1940). Relation of age to motor impairment in man and in subhuman primates. *Archives of Neurology and Psychiatry, 44,* 377–397.

Kertesz, A., Harlock, W., & Coates, R. (1979). Computer tomographic localization, lesion size, and prognosis in aphasia and nonverbal impairment. *Brain and Language, 8*, 34–50.

Kimura, D. (1983). Sex differences in cerebral organization for speech and practice functions. *Canadian Journal of Psychology, 37*, 19–35.

Kinsbourne, M. (1993). Orientation bias model of unilateral neglect: Evidence from attentional gradients within hemispace. In I. H. Robertson & J. C. Marshall (Eds.), *Unilateral neglect: Clinical and experimental studies* (pp. 63–86). Hillsdale, NJ: Erlbaum.

Kolb, B. (1995). *Brain plasticity and behavior.* Mahwah, NJ: Erlbaum.

Kolb, B., & Gibb, R. (1999). Neuroplasticity and recovery of function after brain injuries. In D. T. Stuss, G. Winocur & I. H. Robertson (Eds.), *Cognitive neurorehabilitation* (pp. 9–25). Cambridge, England: Cambridge University Press.

Lam, C. S., McMahon, B. T., Priddy, D. A., & Gehred-Schultz, A. (1988). Deficit awareness and treatment performance among traumatic head injury adults. *Brain Injury, 2*, 235–242.

LeVere, N. D., & LeVere, T. E. (1982). Recovery of function after brain damage: Support for the compensation theory of the behavioral deficit. *Physiological Psychology, 10,* 165–174.

Luria, A. R. (1973). *The working brain.* New York: Basic Books.

Mateer, C. A., & Dodrill, C. (1993). Neuropsychological and linguistic correlates of atypical language lateralization: Evidence from sodium amytal studies. *Human Neurobiology, 2,* 135–142.

Mateer, C. A., & Sohlberg, M. M. (1988). A paradigm shift in memory rehabilitation. In H. Whitaker (Ed.), *Neuropsychological studies of nonfocal brain injury: Dementia and closed head injury* (pp. 202–225). New York: Springer-Verlag.

Mateer, C. A., Sohlberg, M. M., & Youngman, P. (1990). The management of acquired attention and memory disorders following closed head injury. In R. Wood (Ed.), *Cognitive rehabilitation in perspective* (pp. 68–95). London: Taylor & Francis.

Mattson, A. J., & Levin, H. S. (1990). Frontal lobe dysfunction following closed head injury: A review of the literature. *Journal of Nervous and Mental Disease, 178,* 282–291.

Mayer, E., Brown, V. J., Dunnett, S. B., & Robbins, T. W. (1992). Striatal graft-associated recovery of a lesion-induced performance deficit in the rat requires learning to use the transplant. *European Journal of Neuroscience, 4,* 119–126.

Mazzuchi, A., Cattilani, R., Missale, G., Gugliotta, M., Brianti, R., & Parma, M. (1992). Head injured subjects over 50 years: Correlations between variables of trauma and neuropsychological follow up. *Journal of Neurology, 239,* 256–260.

Melamed, S., Grosswasser, Z., & Stern, M. J. (1992). Acceptance of disability, work involvement, and subjective rehabilitation status of traumatic brain-injured (TBI) patients. *Brain Injury, 6,* 233–243.

Melamed, S., Stern, M., Rahmani, L., Grosswasser, Z., & Najenson, T. (1985). Attention capacity limitation, psychiatric parameters and their impact on work involvement following brain injury. *Scandinavian Journal of Rehabilitation Medicine, 12,* 21–26.

Merzenich, M., Jenkins, W. M., Johnston, P., Schreiner, C., Miller, S. L., & Tallal, P. (1996). Temporal processing deficits of language-learning impaired children ameliorated by training. *Science, 271,* 77–81.

Meyer, E., Ferguson, S. S. G., Zatorre, R. J., Alivisatos, B., Marrett, S., Evans, A. C., & Hakim, A. M. (1991). Attention modulates somatosensory cerebral blood-flow response to vibrotactile stimulation as measured by positron emission tomography. *Annals of Neurology, 29,* 440–443.

Mimura, M., Kato, M., Kato, M., Sano, Y., Kojima, T., Naesar, M., & Kashima, H. (1998). Prospective and retrospective studies of recovery in aphasia: Changes in cerebral blood flow and language functions. *Brain, 121,* 2083–2094.

Musso, M., Weiller, C., Kiebel, S., Muller, S. P., Bulau, P., & Rijntjes, M. (1999). Training-induced brain plasticity in aphasia. *Brain, 122,* 1781–1790.

Najenson, T., Grosswasser, Z., Mendelson, L., & Hackett, P. (1980). Rehabilitation outcome of brain damage patients after severe head injury. *International Rehabilitation Medicine, 2,* 17–22.

Nudo, R. J., Wise, B. M., SiFuentes, R., & Milliken, G. W. (1996). Neural substances for the effects of rehabilitation training on motor recovery after ischemic infarct. *Science, 272*, 1791–1794.

Raskin, S. A. (2000). Issues of gender, socio-economic status and culture. In S. A. Raskin & C. A. Mateer (Eds.), *Management of mild traumatic brain injury* (pp. 269–278). New York: Oxford University Press.

Richards, B. (2000). *The effects of aging and mild traumatic brain injury on neuropsychological test performance.* Unpublished doctoral dissertation, York University, Toronto, Ontario, Canada.

Robertson, I. H., Hogg, K., & McMillan, T. M. (1998). Rehabilitation of unilateral neglect: Reducing inhibitory competition by contralesional limb activation. *Neuropsychological Rehabilitation, 8*, 19–29.

Robertson, I. H., Manly, T., Andrade, J., Baddeley, B. T., & Yiend, J. (1997). Oops!: Performance correlates of everyday attentional failures in traumatic brain injured and normal subjects. The Sustained Attention to Response Task (SART). *Neuropsychologia, 35*, 747–758.

Robertson, I. H., & Murre, J. M. J. (1999). Rehabilitation of brain damage: Brain plasticity and principles of guided recovery. *Psychological Bulletin, 25*, 544–575.

Robertson, I. H., & North, N. (1992). Spatio-motor cueing in unilateral neglect: The role of hemispace, hand, and motor activation. *Neuropsychologia, 30*, 553–563.

Robertson, I. H., & North, N. (1993). Active and passive activation of left limbs: Influence on visual and sensory neglect. *Neuropsychologia, 31*, 293–300.

Roof, R. L., Duvdevani, R., Braswell, L., & Stein, D. G. (1992). Progesterone treatment attenuates brain edema following contusion injury in male and female rats. *Restorative Neurology and Neuroscience, 4*, 425–427.

Roof, R. L., Duvdevani, R., Braswell, L., & Stein, D. G. (1994). Progesterone facilitates cognitive recovery and reduces secondary neuronal loss caused by cortical contusion injury in male rats. *Experimental Neurology, 129*, 64–69.

Roof, R. L., Duvdevani, R., & Stein, D. G. (1993). Gender influences outcome of brain injury: Progesterone plays a protective role. *Brain Research, 607*, 333–336.

Seitz, R. J., Huang, Y., Knorr, U., Tellmann, L., Herzog, H., & Freund, H. J. (1995). Large-scale plasticity of the human cortex. *NeuroReport, 6*, 742–744.

Stein, D. G., Brailowsky, S., & Will, B. (1995). *Brain repair.* Oxford: Oxford University Press.

Stein, D. G., Roof, R. I, & Fulop, Z. L. (1999). Brain damage, sex hormones and recovery. In D. T. Stuss, G. Winocur, & I. H. Robertson (Eds.), *Cognitive neurorehabilitation* (pp. 73–93). Cambridge, England: Cambridge University Press.

Stroup, E. (1999). *Locus of control, awareness of deficit, and employment outcomes following vocational rehabilitation in individuals with traumatic brain injury.* Unpublished doctoral dissertation. University of Victoria, Victoria, British Columbia, Canada.

Sturm, W., Willmes, K., Orgass, B., & Hartje, W. (1997). Do specific attention deficits need specific training? *Neuropsychological Rehabilitation, 7*, 81–176.

Sue, S., & Zane, N. (1987). The role of culture and cultural techniques in psychotherapy. *American Psychologist, 42*, 37–45.

Tallal, P., Miller, S. L., Bedi, G., Byma, G., Wang, X. Q., Nagarajan, S. S., Schreiner, C., Jenkins, W. M., & Merzenich, M. M. (1996). Language comprehension in language-learning impaired children improved with acoustically modified speech. *Science, 271,* 81–84.

Taub, E., Uswatte, G., & Pidikiti, R. (1999). Constraint-induced movement therapy: A new family of techniques with broad application to physical rehabilitation—a clinical review. *Journal of Rehabilitation Research and Development, 36,* 237–251.

Teuber, H. L. (1975). Recovery of function after brain injury in man. In *Outcome of severe damage to nervous system* (Ciba Foundation Symposium No. 34, pp. 159–190). Amsterdam: Elsevier/North-Holland.

Vilkki, J., Ahola, K., Holst, P., Ohman, J., Servo, A., & Heiskanen, O. (1994). Prediction of psychosocial recovery after head injury with cognitive tests and neurobehavioral ratings. *Journal of Clinical and Experimental Neuropsychology, 16,* 325–338.

Von Monakow, C. (1914). *Localization in the cerebrum and the degeneration of functions through cortical sources.* Wiesbaden, Germany: Bergmann.

Weiller, C., Chollet, F., Friston, K. J., Wise, R. J. S., & Frackowiak, R. S. J. (1992). Functional reorganization of the brain in recovery from striato-capsular infarction in man. *Annals of Neurology, 31,* 463–472.

Wertz, R. T. (1996). Aphasia in acute stroke: Incidence, determinants, and recovery. *Annals of Neurology, 40,* 129–130.

Willer, B., Abasch, S., & Dahmer, E. (1990). Epidemiology of disability from traumatic brain injury. In R. L. Wood (Ed.), *Neurobehavioral sequelae of traumatic brain injury* (pp. 18–33). New York: Taylor & Francis.

Wilson, J. T. L., Scott, L. C., Wyper, D., Patterson, J., Hadley, D., & Teasdale, G. M. (1993). *Psychological recovery after trauma and patterns of change on MR and SPECT imaging.* Paper presented at the Second Annual International Neurotrauma Symposium, Glasgow, Scotland.

Xerri, C., Merzenich, M. M., Peterson, B. E., & Jenkins, W. M. (1998). Plasticity of primary somatosensory cortex paralleling sensorimotor skill recovery from stroke in adult monkey. *Journal of Neurophysiology, 79,* 2119–2148.

4

Assessment of Individuals with Cognitive Impairments

One of the first steps in developing a rehabilitation plan is to evaluate the client's cognitive strengths and weaknesses, and to see how these map onto his or her premorbid, current, and projected functioning. The level of functioning demonstrated by an individual with brain injury is dependent on many variables, any and all of which can influence levels of adaptive function. These variables include the following:

1. The specific nature of the brain injury and its effects.
2. The client's preinjury history, including premorbid cognitive and behavioral strengths and weaknesses.
3. The specific situational demands/requirements of the client's current living and/or working environment.
4. The supports available to the person in each environment.
5. Premorbid personality factors.
6. Emotional response to injury and residual limitations.
7. Adaptive and coping skills.
8. Beliefs and expectations of the injured individual and his or her family.

The goals of assessment in the context of rehabilitation include the development of an accurate picture of the individual's levels of cognitive, emotional, and interpersonal functioning, including areas of spared ability or compensatory strength; the individual's ability to carry out everyday functional activities; an estimation of the individual's capacity for participation in rehabilitation; and suggestions about what will probably be the most effective means to facilitate learning and cognitive functioning.

The task of sorting out the myriad factors that affect adaptive functioning and the development of appropriate treatment plans is usually a responsibility shared by many professionals on the rehabilitation team. The neurologist, neurosurgeon, and rehabilitation medicine physician typically provide information about the nature and locus of injury; they also direct activities related to ensuring medical stability (including surgical, medical, and/or pharmacological management). Information about the etiology of injury provides valuable information about the nature of the underlying brain damage or disease, the stage of recovery, the short- and long-term prognosis, and commonly associated cognitive and behavioral syndromes that might be anticipated. We have discussed the major medical diagnostic procedures in Chapter 2. In an inpatient rehabilitation setting, the nursing staff provides information about arousal levels, sleep cycles, and behavioral functioning on the treatment unit. Physical therapists provide information regarding muscle tone, strength, range of motion, and postural control (for sitting, standing, and ambulating). Speech pathologists typically evaluate capacities for communication, and safety concerns with regard to eating and swallowing. Occupational therapists evaluate skills in activities of daily living, visuoperceptual ability. Although all therapists typically address aspects of cognition, the neuropsychologist is typically responsible for the comprehensive evaluation of cognitive functioning, attempting whenever possible to relate cognitive and behavioral findings to the underlying brain systems involved. Rehabilitation psychologists are commonly involved in providing emotional support and counseling to the patient and family, assisting in pain management and relaxation skill building, and in developing behavioral interventions. Many programs will also include recreation or activity therapy, social work services, and program management. In practice, the professionals responsible for carrying out these various functions will vary, depending on the structure and size of the facility and the nature of the setting. The entire rehabilitation team, together with the client and family, is involved in developing and implementing the treatment plan.

The process of evaluating cognitive ability is often hampered by a lack of detailed information about the person's functioning before the injury. Some types of cognitive impairment would be considered *pathognomonic* in an adult; that is, that they are specifically indicative of brain injury (e.g., frequent paraphasic errors, disorientation, severe impairments in memory, or left-sided neglect). However, many aspects of cognitive ability fall on a continuum, such that individuals without any history of neurological disease or injury demonstrate a wide range of abilities related to planning, problem solving, attentional capacity, learning efficiency, emotional regulation, and interpersonal effectiveness. Premorbid functioning must often be inferred from educational records, vocational history, and the reports of patients and their families. A careful clinical interview is needed to gather information about premorbid learning difficulties, school history, a history of problems with social behavior, work history, a history or alcohol/substance abuse, and the person's level of competence and independence prior to the injury. Specific measures can also be used to estimate premorbid intellectual functioning from a combination of demographic factors (e.g., the Barona Index; Barona, Reynolds, & Chastain, 1984), and some psychometric measures rely on skills and abilities (e.g., recognition of single written words) that are likely to be retained even after significant injury or deterioration of function (Blair & Spreen, 1989; Nelson, 1976; Yuspeh & Vanderploeg, 2000). Descriptions of these methods, as well as detailed descriptions, normative data, and background research for many of the tests discussed in this chapter, can be found in several texts devoted to neuropsychological evaluation (Lezak, 1995; Spreen & Strauss, 1998).

Every individual has relative strengths and weaknesses in his or her skills and abilities, and each of us functions in the world more or less independently and successfully. It is sometimes difficult to determine what constitutes a condition that requires intervention. In 1980, the World Health Organization (WHO; www.who.int/icidh) adopted a framework for considering the concepts of *impairment, disability,* and *handicap,* which has proven useful in providing a framework for the assessment of individuals with neurological disorders. *Impairment* was defined as the specific physiological function that is altered (e.g., speech, memory function); *disability* was defined as the impact on specific functional abilities (e.g., communicating needs, remembering to take medications); and *handicap* was defined as the alterations in social and role function resulting from the disabilities (e.g., inability to live along or to work). During the 1990s, the WHO model was revised and expanded so that it included the following four components (Brickenbach, Chatterji, Badley, & Ostün, 1999):

• *Pathophysiology* refers to the interruption or interference of normal physiological processes, body functions, or structures through injury or disease. Various impairments can result from pathophysiology.

• *Impairments* are losses or disorders of cognitive, emotional, or physiological functions; they include, for example, difficulties with motor function, attention, memory, or language.

• *Activity/functional limitations* result from impairments, and refer to the effects of the impairments on a person's everyday life activities. Activity limitations involve a restriction or lack of ability to perform an activity as compared to preinjury performance, and include reductions in efficiency and effectiveness in performance-specific tasks and/or the increased effort to accomplish them. For example, as a result of hemiparesis and organizational difficulty, a person may have difficulty getting dressed, using the phone, and/or doing laundry.

• *Participation* is defined as the nature and extent of a person's involvement in life situations in relation to impairments, activity limitations, health conditions, and contextual factors. It deals with societal phenomena and represents both the person's degree of participation and society's response (which either facilitates or hinders that participation). It considers the social disadvantages that arise from the functional limitations and alter the individual's ability to fulfill normally anticipated social roles relevant to his or her age, background, and other social and cultural factors. The seven domains of participation include personal maintenance; mobility; exchange of information; social relationships; areas of education, work, leisure, and spirituality; economic life; and civic and community life.

The assessment needs to consider each of these levels and to determine at what levels the interventions will be directed. Psychometric assessment of cognitive abilities typically addresses the level of impairment. There has been substantial concern that measurement at this level, although certainly useful and important, is insufficient to enable professionals to fully understand a person's functional capacity or to develop a viable and appropriate rehabilitation plan. There has been considerable interest in developing more "ecologically valid" measurement tools and techniques, which can provide better estimates of functional capacity and limitation. There has also been much more research devoted to the development of meaningful outcome measures that capture broad domains of social involvement and life satisfaction.

APPROACHES TO MEASURING ABILITIES AND IMPAIRMENTS

In this section, we describe and discuss some of the principles, advantages, and disadvantages of various approaches to assessment. First, there is a discussion of psychometric approaches, which have historically been the major tools of neuropsychologists. Second, we describe and discuss functional assessment approaches, including functionally oriented psychometric measures, structured observational methods, and structured and semistructured rating scales.

Psychometric Approaches

The majority of individuals who sustain damage or injury to the brain have difficulties in one or more domains of cognitive or behavioral function. The major domains of cognitive ability that are typically evaluated include arousal and alertness; orientation; attention and concentration; memory and new learning; language and communication; praxic functions; academic skills or reading, writing, spelling, and arithmetic; object recognition and other visuoperceptual and visuospatial abilities; reasoning and prob-lem solving; and executive functions. The executive functions incorporate a variety of capacities, including the capacity for initiation and inhibition, planning and organization, mental and behavioral flexibility, and self-awareness. Major domains of behavioral function that are evaluated in-clude the ability to initiate appropriate behaviors, to inhibit inappropriate behaviors, to engage in effective interpersonal communication, and to demonstrate the capacity for self-regulation of mood and emotion. Each of the chapters in this volume deals with some of the theory and diagnostic is-sues related to the particular cognitive domain under discussion. Accord-ingly, this chapter provides a brief review of useful assessment tools for dif-ferent abilities, rather than a detailed discussion of each of the cognitive domains.

Important Considerations in the Use of Psychometric Tests

The assessment of cognitive abilities usually involves the use of standard-ized assessment tools. The term *standardized* carries a number of implica-tions. First, it means that the assessment tool has been administered to a large group of individuals who have no known neurological injury, and that normative data have been developed for individuals based on that sample. Important variables, such as age, gender, and education, must be considered; the majority of published tests have, at a minimum, age-related norms for some specific age range. Blindly applying norms and cutoff scores derived from middle-class college sophomores to the case of a 52-year-old patient with traumatic brain injury (TBI) who has 10 years of edu-cation might suggest that the individual has a variety of moderate to severe deficits as a result of TBI, when in fact the performance may be within nor-mal limits for someone of that age and educational level. Ideally, there will also be data available (either in the manual or in the scientific literature), for clinical populations. Second, there is a detailed protocol that describes exactly how the test is to be administered and how responses will be re-corded and scored. Third, tests should have published information regard-ing important psychometric properties.

The clinical utility of any psychometric test depends on its appropri-ateness for a specific client, and its scientific integrity is expressed in terms of three basic psychometric properties: reliability, validity, and responsive-ness (Table 4.1). The different kinds of *reliability* include the internal con-sistency of items on the test or scale (*internal reliability*), the reproduc-ibility of the scores when the test or scale is applied by the same evaluator (*intrarater reliability*) or different evaluators (*interrater reliability*), and the likelihood that the patient will receive the same or similar score if tested again, assuming that his or her status has not changed (*test–retest reliabil-*

TABLE 4.1. Important Psychometric Properties of Tests

Property	Definition
Reliability	
Internal reliability	The internal consistency of items on the test or scale.
Intrarater reliability	The reproducibility of scores when the test or scale is applied by the *same* rater.
Interrater reliability	The reproducibility of scores when the test or scale is applied by a *different* rater.
Test–retest reliability	The probability that the individual will receive the same or a similar score if tested again, assuming no change in his or her status.
Validity	
Face validity	Agreement by "experts" that the test or scale measures the ability or concept it is intended to measure.
Content validity	The items on a test are representative of the domain that the test purports to measure.
Criterion-related validity	A relationship between test scores and some criterion or outcome, such as ratings classifications, or other test scores widely used to measure the same ability or construct.
Responsiveness	The ability of the test or scale to detect meaningful, clinically relevant change.

ity). *Validity* considers whether the test or scale measures the ability or concept that one intends to measure. It is usually established by "expert" judgments (*face validity* and *content validity*) or by a high correlation between the scale and some "gold standard" (*criterion validity*). For example, if an examiner wants to know how well someone is able to learn and remember what he or she has been told, a test that involves having the client read the information will not have much face validity. *Responsiveness* assesses the ability of the test or scale to detect meaningful, clinically relevant change (from premorbid function or over the course of recovery). In order to assure at least some level of responsiveness, the scores of a test or scale should have a near-"normal" distribution, with no *floor* or *ceiling* effects when applied to a large population. In a normal distribution, the majority of normal individuals (68%) will score in the middle range of scores—that is, within two standard deviations of the mean, or between the 16th and the 84th percentile. In order for this to occur, the test items must not be so easy that everyone gets them (ceiling effects) or so difficult that no one or very few would do well (floor effects). Although some items may be easy or hard, performance on the test overall by a large group of people should show substantial variability.

Test Selection and Interpretation

Neuropsychological testing typically involves the use of multiple tests that evaluate a large number of different cognitive abilities, as well as a variety of perceptual and motor functions. It also commonly includes some assessment of more global intellectual functioning, academic achievement, and personality and emotional functioning.

Test selection also varies according to the examiner's training and experience, the purpose of the assessment, the time since injury, the overall status of the patient, and the time available. There are two traditional approaches to assessment: the *fixed-battery* approach and the *flexible, process-oriented* approach. The fixed- or standard-battery approach uses a large, predetermined group of tests that assess a variety of abilities and have been shown to be sensitive to brain damage. The most well-known and widely used of these is the Halstead–Reitan Neurological Test Battery (HRB; Reitan & Wolfson, 1993). This approach has the advantages of a very large normative data base and considerable information about the performance of subjects with brain injuries on the various measures. Having the same test measures on clients facilitates comparison across individuals and groups. Disadvantages of the HRB and other fixed batteries are that some of the specific measures may not be appropriate for a particular client or referral question, and/or that the battery does not adequately evaluate the full range of relevant functions. In fact, the HRB is almost always supplemented with other measures, including measures of memory, which it does not adequately address. The HRB also relies heavily on cutoff scores, which may play a role in diagnosis, but often do not provide enough information for rehabilitation planning.

The second primary approach to assessment is a more flexible, process-oriented approach (Kaplan, 1988; Lezak, 1995; Spreen & Strauss, 1998). There are a very large number of psychometrically sound tests that have been shown to be sensitive and useful in evaluating a broad range of cognitive abilities. Neuropsychologists select tests that will evaluate relevant cognitive abilities and concerns. This approach allows much more in-depth analysis of particular functions, such as attention, language, memory, and executive functions. It also allows clinicians to respond to and incorporate new theoretical constructs, new technology, and new and improved measures of cognitive ability. A criticism of the flexible approach is that since all of the tests potentially used in an assessment, although normed individually, have not been normed together as a group or perhaps on relevant clinical populations, it is harder to draw conclusions about patterns of strength amd weakness within an individual test profile.

In a rehabilitation context, we have found that a flexible, process-oriented approach to assessment is most useful. The selection of measures can be based (at least in part) on a patient's presenting problems, and test selection can be further modified based on the patient's performance during the evaluation to provide a more in-depth analysis of cognitive functioning. By adopting a flexible, process-oriented approach, the examiner can select tests that best fit individual client variables (e.g., physical condition, motor and sensory functioning, communication skills, degree of cognitive impairment, and attentional capabilities). With this approach, the examiner is also free to adopt new, theoretically driven, and clinically relevant tools as they become available. This becomes crucially important, for example, in the case of assessment of attention, memory, and executive functions, which are only cursorily examined in the HRB but which are fundamental in the assessment of effects from ABI. In actual practice, most neuropsychologists adopt a relatively fixed, standard battery of tests they routinely administer in order to sample cognitive ability broadly, and then supplement this battery with additional measures as needed or indicated. In the case of TBI, a mixed-model approach utilizing both a fixed battery and flexible measures allows for useful assessments that are relatively brief, yet appropriate for different phases of recovery and for rehabilitation planning. Tests selected should be responsive, in that they are helpful in identifying underlying problems and are sensitive to change over time and treatment. Yet another approach to assessment has been evolving in the context of rehabilitation: the tracking evaluation. This is a brief, noncomprehensive evaluation focusing on tracking key performance domains over time.

Other important considerations with regard to the selection and use of psychometric tests are *testing of limits* and *qualitative interpretation*. In a rehabilitation context, in particular, an examiner is often not as much concerned about whether there *is* a deficit as he or she is about the degree and nature of the deficit. Some patients get the right answer if given extra time, or get the right answer but by a very unusual or idiosyncratic means. Some patients may be able to complete the tasks with some minimal cueing or support, or with a repetition or minor clarification of instructions. After a client achieves a poor score, the examiner may get a better idea of what went wrong by trying the task again and probing, repeating, or providing some other support for correct responding. In some cases, for example, it may be useful to conduct a specific test first with the examining room door closed and then with it open, to see how extraneous noise affects performance. Kaplan (1988), who has written extensively in this area, has developed tests and test procedures designed to closely attend to and explore the ways in which a person responds in order to tease out specific processes. Such information can be extremely valuable in identifying and understanding underlying cognitive difficulties or limitations. Valuable qualitative information can be lost if a psychologist does not attend to it, or relies on a psychometrist who is not trained or skilled in observation of relevant behaviors. It must be recognized, however, that patients with brain injury often are so impacted by physical, cognitive, perceptual, and behavioral changes that slavishly holding to standardized test procedures and norms is not possible or practical. Of course, modifying standardized test procedures may render norms inapplicable.

Finally, assessment must never be too narrowly focused, or significant deficits may be overlooked altogether. In addition, the efficacy of some cognitive abilities is dependent on the integrity of other processes. For example, impairment of a basic ability (such as attention) frequently results in impairment of other, more complex abilities (such as learning or problem solving). These issues are particularly important in the assessment of individuals with TBI, since the nature of the damage tends to be diffuse, even when focal deficits are present.

Appreciating Base Rate Phenomena

When an examiner is faced with a patient who is demonstrating problems on psychometric tests, it is compelling to attribute problems to the disease or trauma in question. It is important, however, to be aware of *base rate phenomena*. For example, among normal individuals with no neurological history and with intellectual functioning in the average range of intelligence, Dodrill (1997) has estimated that approximately 15% of scores on the HRB will fall in the mildly deficient range, and that 3% will fall in the moderately to severely deficient range. These estimates increase as a subject's intellectual level decreases. Given such findings, it is important to be sensitive to the number of test scores obtained, and to be aware of base rates for impairment on the tests that have been used. It is also important to obtain multiple indicators of impairment across separate tests tapping into the same kind of ability before deciding that there is impairment in that domain. Convergence of evidence from multiple sources is an important principle in interpreting tests of cognitive ability (Lezak, 1995).

Sensitivity of Tests

The ability to detect impairments is only as powerful as the tools that have been developed for this purpose. It is important to recognize that the major neuropsychological tests and test batteries were not designed specifically to identify the cognitive and adaptive problems experienced by individuals with TBI. Many tests may not be sensitive enough to detect cognitive problems that are common in a particular population. The difficulty in assessing executive functions through use of traditional psychometric tests, for example, is particularly well documented (Lezak, 1995). Although it is apparent from clinical experience that many individuals with frontal lobe dysfunction have difficulty with organization, planning, and self-regulation, these same individuals often do well on psychometric measures designed to evaluate executive functions. Another concern with regard to test sensitivity involves practice effects. Repeated test administrations are likely to reduce the sensitivity of a particular test. Many patients with TBI have undergone repeated testing on neuropsychological batteries that have not been modified to contain new items or material. The effectiveness of these tests after multiple exposures must be seriously questioned. Finally, there are very few tools to evaluate a number of areas of difficulty that are commonly reported by individuals with brain injury, such as cognitive vulnerability in the presence of distraction.

Noncognitive Factors Influencing Psychometric Assessments

There are many factors that can influence performance on a test, but that have little or nothing to do with the function being investigated. These include a variety of nonspecific factors that are often difficult even to identify, much less quantify. Potential physical influences include hunger, fatigue, headache, and other sources of pain. A complicating factor with respect to pain is that analgesic pain medications often have a sedating effect, which can have a negative impact on processing speed and attentional capacity. The examiner should always note any medications a person is taking during the assessment, to help in determining the basis for findings.

Other physical factors that can greatly affect test performance include visual field difficulties, hemiparesis, poor visual acuity, and hearing problems, to name just a few. In addition, emotional factors such as anxiety, worry, boredom, and/or preoccupation with thoughts or concerns unrelated to the task at hand can affect performance. If antidepressant or antianxiety medications are regularly prescribed, it is usually advised to have the person stay on medication for the testing, as this will provide a better estimate of his or her current, routine level of functioning. Motivational factors—from lack of effort to outright purposeful malingering—also need to be considered, particularly when there are issues of compensation or secondary gain. Measures designed specifically to assess motivational effort can be helpful if concerns arise in this area. In addition, close inspection of patterns of test results may reveal suspicious inconsistencies on various measures, or between test performance and reports of everyday functioning. Under such circumstances, test results need to be interpreted extremely cautiously. Any of the above-mentioned factors can significantly influence test performance. The examiner should ask about these factors, review records for additional information, use measures of symptom validity when appropriate, and closely watch and monitor the person's behavior and appearance over the course of the evaluation (see Slick, Sherman, & Iverson, 1999, for a recent review of this topic). Clients should be made aware whether evaluations consider the question of symptom validity. While this is an important domain of inquiry, it can neverthe-less involve deception and pose a potential ethical dilemma.

Functional Approaches

Psychometric measures differ substantially in terms of how distant or close the specific tasks making up the tests are to typical real-life demands. For example, repeating a string of digits is somewhat comparable to writing down a telephone number after getting it from the operator, whereas ver-batim recall of a short paragraph, recall of word pairings, and reproduc-tion of abstract designs are very unlike typical day-to-day behavior. This is not to say that the tests may not correlate with, and give some indication of, memory capacity. The Trail Making B Test, for example, is very unlike life activities, but it fares well in predicting everyday functional abilities (Heaton & Pendleton, 1981). Quite often, however, psychometric tests have been shown to have poor predictive power in terms of estimating the nature or degree of difficulty a person is experiencing in everyday func-tional activities.

Whereas psychometric measures are by nature designed to isolate cog-nitive abilities so that specific functions can be analyzed in detail, most ac-tivities of daily living involve many integrated cognitive abilities and are done in a functional and familiar context, where the person may have ad-ditional cues for completing tasks and/or can use compensations for areas of weakness. From this perspective, psychometric tasks will tend to *overes-timate* functional impairments. Alternatively, individual tests of cognitive ability typically take only a very short period of concentration; the rules and goals of the task are made very explicit; distractions are reduced; and the examiner provides cues and support to maintain motivation. These fac-tors will tend to improve test performance, but they often *underestimate* the level of impairment the individual may have in a functional context.

Functionally Oriented Psychometric Measures

As a result of these factors, current methods of standardized psychometric assessment may not yield adequate estimates of functional capacity unless they are combined with more naturalistic, quasi-experimental methods that can tie assessment procedures more closely to the process of rehabili-tation. Assessment procedures that attempt to capture this more functional perspective utilize tasks that more closely approximate activities in natural contexts. For example, remembering someone's name, or remembering where a personal possession (such as eyeglasses) has been put, is a very common real-life memory demand. Tests have been developed that incor-porate such "ecologically valid" measures, yet that also specify a standard administration, scoring procedures, and normative data. A number of functionally oriented psychometric measures that have been developed for evaluating attention, memory, and executive functions are discussed later in this chapter.

Structured Observations and Functional Rating Scales

Although the development of tests with more functional face validity has been useful, structured tasks that appear to be more naturalistic are still only approximations of real-life activity. It is necessary and important to rely on other means to measure actual functioning in everyday contexts outside the formal testing situation. One way of doing this is to make observations of the person as he or she is actually performing everyday activities, and to determine how and why the results are effective or ineffective. Because behavior is so variable, observational data can become both unwieldy and unreliable. Structured observational rating measures, however, have been shown to be very useful in evaluating such complex behaviors as dressing, preparing meals, using public transportation, and many other functional activities. The measures should specify specific behaviors that are fundamental to the activity, compensatory strategies adopted by the client, and the nature and frequency of cues or prompts that are needed for successful completion of the task. Structured observations can be used to evaluate how and when adaptive behavior breaks down; to determine how the individual makes use of aids and assists; and to identify how well he or she can dynamically adjust to environmental factors (e.g., distractions, disruptions, and/or the need to make a change in plans). In this context, we have found that collaborations with family members, job coaches, coworkers, and many others can be very valuable (and indeed crucial) to gathering accurate and useful information. More detailed discussions of this approach, and a broad grounding of these techniques in what has been termed *ethnographic assessment*, can be found in work by Simmons-Mackie and Damico (1996).

Although direct observations in a functional setting can be extremely useful, they are often impractical, costly, or infeasible. An alternative approach involves the use of rating scales. Rating scales are used to determine the kind and degree of difficulty an individual is having in a particular domain. Through responses to a structured rating scale, others who have the opportunity to observe the individual in a functional setting can rate a variety of functions. There are rating scales for attention, memory, pragmatic skills, emotional regulation, executive functions, and many other areas of ability. Rating scales can be a particularly effective way to examine differences in ability across different settings. For example, a patient's attentional capacities may appear to be quite good in a quiet, one-on-one setting with a speech pathologist, but may appear quite poor in an open physical therapy exercise area in which there are many distractions. Alternatively, a patient may demonstrate little or no initiation in an unfamiliar setting, but may initiate play with and caretaking for a favorite pet while on home visits. Use of rating scales by therapists, teachers' aides, or job coaches is likely to provide a more accurate and comprehensive picture of the person's capacities in different settings than a set of psychometric tests alone can do. Family members, in particular, can provide valuable information about how the person functions at home. Through their eyes, it is possible to get a much richer picture of the individual's initiation, level of independence for various activities, and capacity for regulation of mood and emotion in a familiar environment. Many scales are also designed with a self-rating form. Having patients rate their own level of functioning, and comparing those ratings to the ratings of family members, caregivers, and/ or professionals, can be useful in determining the patients' level of awareness with regard to their functioning (see Chapter 9 on awareness).

In summary, functional rating scales can facilitate identification of impairments, functional limitations, and participation, and can provide tools to monitor changes over time and response to interventions. However, although these instruments are potentially quite useful, it is important to recognize that their measurement characteristics and psychometric properties are often not well established, and particularly subject to observer bias. Rating and observational scales need to come under the same scrutiny as psychometric measures in terms of their reliability, validity, sensitivity, and specificity. In the absence of adequate information, such measures should not be relied upon in isolation.

ASSESSMENT OF SPECIFIC COGNITIVE ABILITIES

Any area of cognitive ability can be affected after an acquired neurological insult, but certain areas of cognitive ability will be more susceptible, depending on the nature, location, and degree of injury. Disorders of orientation/arousal, attention, memory/new learning, and executive functions are among the most common impairments following diffuse acquired brain injuries, and these are addressed here. The discussion includes psychometric measures, observational approaches, and functional assessment techniques in each area. Approaches to the assessment of general intellectual function and functional outcome are also discussed.

Orientation and Arousal

The Agitated Behavior Scale (Corrigan, 1989; Corrigan & Bogner, 1994) is useful in serial assessments for individuals recovering from severe injuries who demonstrate slow emergence of cognition. It is also helpful in monitoring time-related patterns of agitation and restlessness. Factor-analytic studies have resulted in a *Disinhibition* score, an *Aggression* score, and a *Lability* score. Individuals who demonstrate significant levels of either agitation or impulsivity require increased supervision (including one-to-one structure), and may benefit from involvement in such simple tasks as sorting or repetition tasks. The scale is useful for documenting aggression when it is a product of agitation and confusion. When cognitive abilities have stabilized, overt aggression is more effectively measured through an applied behavior analysis or a measure such as the Overt Aggression Scale (Yudofsky, Silver, Jackson, Endicott, & Williams, 1986).

Posttraumatic amnesia (PTA) is a state characterized by confusion, disorientation, and an inability to remember information for even a short period, despite alertness and an apparent ability to comprehend spoken language. PTA is common following TBI (see Chapter 2), and the longer the duration of PTA (i.e., over 1 week), the greater the likelihood of residual memory deficit. The Galveston Orientation and Amnesia Test (Levin, O'Donnell, & Grossman, 1979) is a questionnaire designed to evaluate, and track over time, a client's orientation to person, place, time, and circumstances.

General Cognitive/Intellectual Abilities

The Wechsler Adult Intelligence Scale—III (WAIS-III; Wechsler, 1997a) is the latest version of the WAIS, undoubtedly the most widely used measure of general intellectual ability. The Full Scale IQ provides a global index of overall intellectual status. It is commonly used in both clinical and research settings. The WAIS-III represents a composite of performance on a large number of subtests; subtests involve such skills as retrieval of general information, vocabulary knowledge, abstract reasoning, both verbal and nonverbal problem-solving/reasoning tasks, rote recall, and tasks involving psychomotor speed. Moderate to severe ABI frequently affects a variety of cerebral functions and results in lowered intellectual scores compared to premorbid levels. In general, the verbal subtests tend to be less sensitive to acquired brain damage in adults than do the nonverbal subtests. The verbal subtests tend to require more overlearned, well-established, and "crystallized" cognitive abilities, and are less susceptible to the effects of ABI. In contrast, the nonverbal subtests tend to rely on more "fluid" abilities that require novel problem solving, and they are often timed. Individuals with slower and/or less efficient processing tend to do more poorly on these measures.

The WAIS-III yields four factor scores: Verbal Comprehension, Perceptual Organization, Working Memory, and Speed of Processing. The test is still too new for many studies that incorporate it to have been published, but early observations indicate that the Working Memory and Speed of Processing factors appear to be most sensitive to the effects of ABI. In the evaluation of individuals with neurological impairments, the focus is typi-

cally directed toward interpreting individual subtests, relationships between subtests, or factor scores, rather than toward the overall IQ score.
Ultimately, a normal-range IQ provides little information about other cognitive abilities. Indeed, many individuals with neurological impairment do
not demonstrate significant declines on a measure of intellectual function,
despite demonstrating areas of significant cognitive difficulty.

Attention

The construct of attention incorporates a wide range of cognitive functions, including immediate span of attention; focused, sustained, and divided attention; as well as speed of information processing. Although specific measures are listed below for each component, most measures of
attention are multifaceted and cannot easily be categorized into distinct
components.

Immediate Span of Attention

Measures of forward and backward digit span are often considered part of
an attention battery. Forward digit span is a relatively passive measure,
usually considered to measure immediate memory and sustained attention
for a brief period. Backward digit span requires storage and manipulation
of numerical information. Because of the demands made on controlled
processing and working memory by backward digit span, it is sometimes
considered a measure of divided attention or working memory. There are
also nonverbal measures of spatial span.

Focused Attention

Measures of focused attention usually require an individual to reject irrelevant information while attending to relevant input, and consist of tasks
that require rapid scanning and identification of targets. They include a variety of cancellation tasks, such as the Concentration–Endurance Test (d2
Test; Brickenkamp, 1981); and the Symbol Search subtest of the WAIS-III
(Wechsler, 1997). Cancellation tasks vary in complexity, but usually consist of rows of characters containing randomly interspersed targets to be
canceled (i.e., crossed out) as quickly as possible. The Trail Making Test
(TMT; Reitan, 1958; Reitan & Wolfson, 1995) is also used as a measure of
focused attention. Part A of the TMT consists of randomly distributed
numbers that must be connected in ascending order; Part B requires sequential alternation between randomly dispersed numbers and letters (e.g.,
1-A-2-B, etc.). Parts A and B of the TMT do not correlate highly, as TMT
Part B requires set shifting (from one sequence to another) and some degree of divided attention. As such, performance differences between TMT
Parts A and B have been interpreted as resulting from a large executive

component demanded in Part B. Performance on Part B has been found to be closely related to other tests of timed executive function, and it is often considered in that manner. All of these tasks are multifactorial, with such requirements as processing speed, visual scanning, quick motor response, and both set maintenance and shifting.

Sustained Attention

Sustained attention, or vigilance, is most commonly measured by auditory or visual continuous-performance tests, which require the individual to monitor a set of external stimuli for the occurrence of a selected target over prolonged periods of time. Computer-based tasks have become widely used in this domain (e.g., the Conners Continuous Performance Test, Conners & Multi-Health Systems Staff, 1995; Test of Variables of Attention, Greenberg, 1998). The computerized measures require sustained attention for periods of up to 20 minutes or more on relatively boring tasks, which require persistent vigilance to stay on task and maintain high levels of accuracy. Other psychometric measures considered to involve sustained attention include a variety of digit symbol substitution tests such as the Digit Symbol Coding subtest of the WAIS-III (Wechsler, 1997). This test consists of rows of blank squares paired with randomly assigned numbers or letters. Above the rows is a key that pairs each number with a symbol. Symbols must be written in the empty squares according to the key as quickly as possible. This does involve some switching of attention and visuomotor speed and coordination as well as sustained attention.

Divided Attention

Tests of divided attention require the individual to engage in more than one cognitive task simultaneously, and typically require a high level of working memory. The Brief Test of Attention (BTA; Schretlin, Bobholz, & Brandt, 1996) requires the individual to listen to a string of numbers and letters, and to count the number of letters in the string. In the second part of the test, the sequences are repeated, but now the individual must count the numbers presented. Thus it is a dual task involving listening and identifying targets, while at the same time keeping a running tally in mind. The Letter-Numbering Sequencing subtest of the WAIS-III (Wechsler, 1997) requires the individual to listen to a set of mixed letters and numbers and recite back first the numbers and then the letters in order.

Speed of Information Processing

Processing speed is most commonly measured by simple and complex reaction time tests. It is inferred from performance on timed tasks (e.g., TMT

Part A) or tasks that require keeping up with paced, continuous stimuli (e.g., BTA, PASAT). The Paced Auditory Serial Addition Task (PASAT; Gronwall, 1977; Gronwall & Sampson, 1974) requires the individual to carry out sequential additions over four trials at increasing speeds. Numbers are presented one at a time by a taped recording. Subjects add pairs of numbers, such that each number is added to the one that immediately precedes it. Numbers must be held in mind while listening to the tapes, and then the addition must be calculated and a response given. Findings are sometimes difficult to interpret in individuals with limited mathematical skill or experience. The advantages of the test are that it has been shown to be quite sensitive to brain injury and that it provides a wide range of variability, with few floor or ceiling effects.

There have also been attempts to develop potentially more ecologically relevant ways of assessing attention. Robertson, Ward, Ridgeway, and Nimmo-Smith (1996) developed the Test of Everyday Attention. This test is designed to measure attention-demanding skills through the use of tasks that closely approximate a variety of common activities, such as searching a map, counting floors in an elevator, searching a telephone directory, and listening for lottery numbers.

Yet another approach to the evaluation of attention is the use of "self" and "other" rating scales of attentional functioning. Ponsford and Kinsella (1991) reported on use of the Attention Rating Scale, a self-report measure of attention in patients with TBI, which lists common attentional problems conforming to a hierarchical view of attention. Information regarding a patient's perception of his or her attentional abilities, in comparison to ratings and direct observations of functioning by staff and caregivers, can provide valuable information about the everyday impact of attention deficits; this can lead to more effective rehabilitation activities (see Attention Questionnaire in Appendix 5.1). Table 4.2 provides a listing of the attention measures discussed in this section.

Memory and New Learning

In clinical neuropsychology, standard evaluations assess at least three aspects of memory: (1) encoding, which is inferred from the acquisition of new information; (2) retention of information over time, which is typically assessed by delayed recall; and (3) recognition, which is typically assessed by yes–no responses to previously presented items interspersed among new items. A very commonly used approach to measure these different aspects of memory and new learning involves learning a list of words. The California Verbal Learning Test (Delis, Kramer, Kaplan, & Ober, 1987), for example, comprises two word lists containing shopping items from four different semantic categories. The first list is presented five times, with an immediate recall following each presentation. The second list is then pre-

TABLE 4.2. Common Procedures for Assessing Attention, Memory/New Learning, Executive Functions, and Behavior/Adjustment/Outcome

Attention

Immediate span of attention
Wechsler Adult Intelligence Scale—III (WAIS-III) subtest: Forward Digit Span (Wechsler, 1997a)

Focused attention
Wechsler Adult Intelligence Scale—III (WAIS-III) subtests: Digit–Symbol Coding, Symbol Search (Wechsler, 1997a)
Concentration–Endurance Test (d2 Test) (Brickenkamp, 1981)
Trail Making Test (Reitan, 1958; Reitan & Wolfson, 1995)

Sustained attention
Conners Continuous Performance Test (Conners & Multi-Health Systems Staff, 1995)
Test of Variables of Attention (Greenberg, 1998)
Wechsler Adult Intelligence Scale—III (WAIS-III) subtests: Digit Symbol Coding, Letter–Number Sequencing (Wechsler, 1997a)

Divided attention
Brief Test of Attention (Schretlin, Bobholz, & Brandt, 1996)
Paced Auditory Serial Addition Task (Gronwall, 1977)
Wechsler Adult Intelligence Scale—III (WAIS-III) subtest: Letter–Number Sequencing (Wechsler, 1997a)

Speed of processing
Various reaction time tests and timed or paced tasks

Mixed batteries
Test of Everyday Attention (Robertson, Ward, Ridgeway, & Nimmo-Smith, 1996)

Attention rating scales
Attention Rating Scale (Ponsford & Kinsella, 1991)

Memory/new learning

General memory scales
Wechsler Memory Scale—III (Wechsler, 1997b)

Verbal learning measures
California Verbal Learning Test (Delis, Kramer, Kaplan, & Ober, 1987)
Selective Reminding Test (Buschke, 1973)

Nonverbal memory measures
Rey Complex Figure—Recall and Recognition (Rey, 1941)
Revised Visual Retention Test (Benton, 1974)
Tactual Performance Test: Memory and Location (Reitan & Wolfson, 1993)

Recognition memory
Recognition Memory Test (Warrington, 1984)
Facial Recognition Test (Benton, Sivan, Hamsher, Varney, & Spreen, 1994)

Additional memory measures
Rivermead Behavioural Memory Test (Wilson, Cockburn, & Baddeley, 1985)
Prospective Memory Screening (Sohlberg, Mateer, & Geyer, 1985)

TABLE 4.2. (*continued*)

Executive functions

Inhibitory and interference control
Stroop Color and Word Test (Golden, 1978; Stroop, 1935)
Consonant Trigram Test (Kaplan, 1988; Stuss, Stethem, Hugenholtz, & Richard, 1989)

Problem solving and planning
Wisconsin Card Sorting Test (Heaton, 1981)
Category Test (Reitan & Wolfson, 1993, 1995)
Rey Complex Figure—Copy (Rey, 1941)
Porteus Maze Test (Porteus, 1959)

Fluency measures
Controlled Oral Word Association Test (Spreen & Benton, 1977)
Ruff Figural Fluency Test (Ruff, Light, & Evans, 1987)
Design Fluency (Jones-Gotman & Milner, 1977)

Observational methods/rating scales
Executive Function Route Finding Task (Boyd & Sauter, 1994)
Six Elements Test (Shallice & Burgess, 1991a)
Multiple Errands Task (Shallice & Burgess, 1991b)
Brock Adaptive Functioning Questionnaire (Dywan & Segalowitz, 1996)
Profile of the Executive Control System (Braswell et al., 1993)

Executive function batteries
Behavioral Assessment of the Dysexecutive Syndrome (Wilson, Alderman, Burgess, Emslie, & Evans, 1996).
Executive Interview (Royall, Mahurin, & Gray, 1992)

Behavior, adjustment, and outcome measures

Functional Independence Measure (Granger & Hamilton, 1987)
Functional Assessment Measure (Hall, Hamilton, Gordon, & Zasler, 1993)
Glasgow Outcome Scale (Jennett & Bond, 1975)
Disability Rating Scale for Severe Head Trauma (Rappaport, Hall, Hopkins, Belieza, & Cope, 1982)
Katz Adjustment Scale (Katz & Lyerly, 1963)
Sickness Impact Profile (Bergner, Bobbitt, Carter, & Gibson, 1981)
Neurobehavioral Rating Scale (Levin et al., 1987)
Portland Adaptability Inventory (Lezak, 1987)
Craig Handicap Assessment and Reporting Technique (Whiteneck, Carlifue, Gerhart, Overholser, & Richardson, 1992)
Mayo–Portland Adaptability Inventory (Malec & Thompson, 1994)
Supervision Rating Scale (Boake & High, 1996)

sented once for immediate recall. Following this interference trial, free- and cued-recall trials of the first list are elicited. Following a 20-minute delay interval filled with nonverbal testing, free and cued recall are again measured, and then a yes–no recognition trial is presented, with words from the first list imbedded with distractors. Various scores can be derived, including measures of immediate recall (List A Trial 1, List B), learning efficiency (total recall, Trials 1 to 5), learning slope, percentage of information retained over time, recall versus recognition scores, spontaneous semantic clustering, ability to benefit from semantic cueing, susceptibility to interference, and response consistency, to name but a few. Another commonly used measure of word list learning is the Selective Reminding Test (Buschke, 1973). There are parallel tests for assessment of nonverbal design learning and memory (e.g., the Revised Visual Retention Test; Benton, 1974). There is also a test on the HRB that examines tactile learning and memory by having subjects place differently shaped blocks in a puzzle board while blindfolded (the Tactual Performance Test; Reitan & Wolfson, 1993). This test also includes an incidental measure of spatial memory.

Neuropsychological studies in individuals with ABI have suggested various patterns of memory impairment. Poor recall after the initial presentation of a word list is commonly seen. This may reflect a problem with attention to the task, with adequate processing of the information in the time allowed, or with memory span, rather than (or in addition to) a problem with retaining information in memory. Poor recall and recognition scores can also be caused by poor initial learning, and/or by limited ability to retain information in memory once it has been processed and encoded. Therefore, it is important to use measures that can help to establish whether poor overall performance is due primarily to impaired encoding, limited attention, limited span, or additional impairments in the retention–recall–recognition process. Individuals with moderate to severe TBI typically demonstrate slow rates of learning and impaired delayed recall, cued recall, and recognition memory (Crosson, Novack, Trenerry, & Craig, 1989). With moderate to severe TBI, moreover, the percentage of information initially retained over time is typically low, indicating that information has not been stored. In contrast, in a large group of individuals with persistent effects from mild TBI (MTBI), Raskin, Mateer, and Tweeten (1998) reported that while initial recall (List A Trial 1) was somewhat low, recall levels by Trial 5 were within normal limits. In addition, there was no drop in recall levels over a delay, and the subjects demonstrated normal facilitation with a recognition format. This suggests that the basis for memory difficulties after MTBI is likely to be attentional in nature, whereas more severely injured individuals are likely to demonstrate impaired memory storage and retrieval, as well as attentional problems. Indeed, one recent study has shown that when initial levels of learning were equated across

TBI and control groups, subsequent forgetting rates were essentially equivalent across the groups (DeLuca, Schultheis, Madigan, Christodoulou, & Averill, 2000). Findings suggest that, at least within a young population of patients with TBI, verbal learning deficits may be in large part secondary to disruption of frontally mediated executive processes, resulting in decreased self-initiated strategic encoding, less effective retrieval strategies, and/or reduced self-monitoring of performance (Richards, 2000).

There are also some tests that use just a recognition format. The client is shown words, faces, or designs; later, these and foils that have not been seen are shown, and the client is asked to indicate which were seen previously. Such tests include the Recognition Memory Test (Warrington, 1984) and the Facial Recognition Test (Benton, Sivan, Hamsher, Varney, & Spreen, 1994). These measures can be particularly useful in the testing of individuals who have a difficult time drawing, copying, or responding verbally.

Other aspects of memory typically addressed in a neuropsychological evaluation are differences between memory for verbal and nonverbal information, as the processing and memory networks for different kinds of information tend to be dependent on different hemispheres and brain regions. Verbal learning, which is primarily dependent on left-hemisphere systems, is typically examined through stimuli consisting of words, sentences, word lists, paired words, and/or short paragraphs. Nonverbal learning and memory paradigms tend to use visual designs, spatial positions, and faces. Material-specific differences in memory can suggest underlying differences in hemispheric functioning, and can possibly identify strengths on which to build rehabilitation strategies. Related to, but not synonymous with, material-specific impairments are modality-specific impairments. These relate to whether information is presented visually or auditorily. It is important to remember that verbal information (e.g., words, stories) can be presented in either modality.

The Wechsler Memory Scale—III (WMS-III; Wechsler, 1997b) is a commonly used measure that samples many of these aspects of memory. It provides normative data for immediate and delayed recall and recognition of short paragraphs, a word list, unfamiliar faces, and abstract designs. It also includes measures of immediate and working memory, including digit span, spatial span, and letter–number sequencing. Another useful feature of the WMS-III is that when it is used in conjunction with the WAIS-III (a very common practice), relationships between the tests can be examined. For example, given a particular level of intelligence and pattern of performance on IQ subtests, certain levels of memory and patterns of memory strength and weakness can be calculated. This is useful in determining the pattern, existence, and degree of neuropsychological impairment.

A number of measures have been developed in an attempt to better estimate memory functioning in everyday living. The Rivermead Behavioural Memory Test (RBMT; Wilson, Cockburn, & Baddeley, 1985) measures such common activities as learning someone's name, asking for an object that has been hidden from view, and recalling a route and sequence of actions. Wilson and colleagues have shown that performance on the RBMT is more related to functional independence in the community than are more traditional psychometric measures of memory and new learning (Wilson, Baddeley, Cockburn, & Hiorns, 1989). The RBMT also includes several tasks that require remembering to do something later in the session without being explicitly told to do so. This kind of ability has been termed *prospective memory*, and the concept has generated a significant amount of research and clinical interest in the last decade.

We ourselves have developed a clinical measure of prospective memory, the Prospective Memory Screening Test (PROMS; Sohlberg, Mateer, & Geyer, 1985), which samples prospective responding to both time and event cues. Prospective memory has also been shown to relate to attention and to a variety of executive functions. It is a particularly relevant concept with regard to everyday memory demands, and is thus an important consideration in rehabilitation (see Chapters 6 and 7 for further discussion and related interventions). A recent modification of this test, which has been used for experimental purposes, is the Prospective Memory Test (Raskin & Buckheit, 1998). This test is based on very similar prospective tasks, but it provides a larger number of tasks, includes both action tasks and verbal tasks, and provides a system for scoring a number of different types of errors.

In addition to the components of memory discussed in this section, many other different kinds of memory have been described in the literature. Some of these include *semantic* and *episodic* memory, *declarative* and *procedural* memory, and executive aspects of memory (e.g., *time tagging, confabulation, priming source memory, recency memory,* and *metamemory*). Although standardized tests do not exist for many of these kinds of memory, they should be considered in the assessment process in the course of interview and observation, and clinicians are encouraged to use or adapt experimental methods described in the literature.

Memory functions are complex, interactive, and dependent on a widely distributed neural network. In order to evaluate the functioning of the memory system, many different abilities must be sampled. The memory "profile" can then be compared to patterns that have been reported in association with specific neurological disorders and diseases. The major memory scales discussed here are listed in Table 4.2; ways in which the information derived from these scales can be used to select and implement treatment and management strategies for memory difficulties are discussed in Chapters 6 and 7.

Executive Functions

Executive functions refer to cognitive abilities involved in the initiation, planning, sequencing, organization, and regulation of behavior (Stuss & Benson, 1986). They constitute a superordinate system that mediates self-initiated behavior and governs the efficiency and appropriateness of task performance. Executive function deficits emerge most clearly in circumstances where strong response sets are developed and appropriate set shifting depends on the monitoring of outcomes. Executive functions are also stressed when successful performance requires maintenance of attention over time, prevention of distraction, and organization of information. It is useful to recognize that executive functions is a catch-all term for some very disparate skills, probably because this domain of ability is a relative newcomer to the taxonomy of human mental abilities (Lezak, 1993). It incorporates basic capabilities, such as working memory and inhibitory control, as well as complex overarching abilities, such as planning, organization, and self-monitoring. Commonly used tests that incorporate these features include the Wisconsin Card Sorting Test (WCST; Heaton, 1981), the Consonant Trigrams Test (CTT; Kaplan, cited in Lezak, 1995), verbal and nonverbal fluency measures, and the Stroop Color and Word Test (Golden, 1978; Stroop, 1935; Trenerry, Crosson, DeBoe, & Leber, 1989). Although these tests tend to push for executive functions, defective executive functions can emerge on a wide variety of tasks in the form of perseverations, disinhibition, distractibility, inefficient strategy selection, loss of set, and poor response monitoring (Richards, 2000). At the same time, it is important to recognize that testing protocols typically provide structure, cues for initiation and maintenance of on-task behavior, minimization of distractions, and explicit goals; these factors reduce the likelihood of seeing impaired executive abilities that the client may be experiencing in everyday functioning, and/or in the absence of such factors. In addition, although a number of psychometric tests have some sensitivity to frontal executive functions, the specificity of the measures is often poor (i.e., individuals with damage to other areas of the brain also do poorly), and their sensitivity is variable (i.e., individuals with obvious executive dysfunction may perform well on the tasks, and vice versa).

A few of the more commonly used executive function measures are discussed here and listed in Table 4.2. On the CTT, randomly ordered strings of three consonants must be recalled following a brief period of engagement in a distracting task (counting backward by 3's). This test is sometimes described as a Brown–Peterson paradigm, in that it relies on short-term, postdistraction recall. The test captures the everyday experience of momentary distraction that results in a loss or disruption of very recent information. Performance on the CTT has been shown to be impaired in frontally lesioned individuals with otherwise solid memory performance (Stuss, Stethem, Hugenholtz, & Richard, 1989). The task appears to require the executive maintenance of directed attention and control of interfering stimuli, and is sensitive to MTBI as well as moderate to severe TBI.

The WCST is an abstract problem-solving task that requires the individual to discover rules governing what constitutes correct performance. The client sorts cards with designs of different number, shape, and quantity. It requires the ability to form abstract concepts, to shift and maintain set, to inhibit established prepotent responses, and to utilize feedback. Substantial evidence of impaired WCST performance exists following moderate to severe ABI (Anderson, Bigler, & Blatter, 1995; Anderson, Damasio, Jones, & Tranel, 1991; Segalowitz, Unsal, & Dywan, 1992). However, even in mild brain injury, or in patients with ABI of varying severity but good recovery, WCST performance is characterized by loss of set and a larger than expected number of perseverative errors (Mateer, 1992; Richards, 2000). The Category Test is another measure of reasoning and problem solving that is often considered in the executive domain (Reitan & Wolfson, 1993, 1995). However, neither the WCST nor the Category Test are sensitive to every "frontal lobe" function and may be performed well even by individuals with significant executive function impairment.

Another measure that is used to assess planning and problem solving, and that requires inhibition, is the Porteus Maze Test (Porteus, 1959). To do well, the client must look ahead to what is coming up and plan moves to get through the maze without running into blind alleys. Planning is also required on the Rey Complex Figure Copy and Recall tests (Lezak, 1995; Rey, 1941). The individual is asked to copy a complex geometric design, and then later to redraw it from memory. The examiner looks for an organized approach to the task and an appreciation of both global and local detail in the figure.

The Stroop Test invokes interference effects by having individuals read the color of ink in which the names of colors are written under timed conditions. Thus, in response to the word *blue* written in red ink, the correct response is *red*. Control conditions, which do not contain interference, typically consist of reading color names written in black ink and naming blocks of color. A comparison of performance under these different conditions allows the examiner to make a determination about the client's ability to inhibit prepotent responding (reading word stimuli) and his or her ability to deal with interference.

Another common measure of executive function involves list generation or verbal fluency. In phonemic fluency tasks, such as the Controlled Oral Word Association Test (Spreen & Benton, 1977) words are generated according to initial letter (e.g., F, A, S), but with some rules about what classes of words can be used. In semantic fluency tasks, words are generated according to a semantic category (e.g., animals) as quickly as possible within a specified period of time. Fluency tasks require retrieval from long-term memory and sustained attention; they also require executive control of retrieval processes to organize retrieval in terms of specific cues, monitor reported responses to avoid repetitions, and inhibit responses that do not fit. There has been some suggestion that phonemic fluency is more sensitive to frontal lobe lesions (Coslett, Bowers, Verfaellie, & Heilman, 1991), whereas semantic fluency is more sensitive to temporal lobe lesions (Newcombe, 1969). Individuals with brain injury tend to produce fewer words and make more errors than controls (Raskin & Rearick, 1996). Nonverbal analogues of these tasks are nonverbal fluency measures, in which the individual is asked to create as many designs as possible within a certain time period and within certain rules or constraints. Examples of these measures include Design Fluency (Jones-Gotman & Milner, 1977) and the Ruff Figural Fluency Test (Ruff, Light, & Evans, 1987).

In addition to individual psychometric measures such as these, there are a number of batteries that group several tasks purported to assess executive functioning. The Executive Interview (Royall, Mahurin, & Gray, 1992) was designed for use as a clinical bedside screener, programmed to monitor for frontal involvement in individuals who have severe functional limitations. It screens for frontal release signs, motor or cognitive perserveration, verbal intrusions, disinhibition, loss of spontaneity, environmental dependency, and utilization behavior. The Behavioural Assessment of the Dysexecutive Syndrome (BADS; Wilson, Alderman, Burgess, Emslie, & Evans, 1996) includes six subtests designed to address everyday problems in organization, planning, and problem solving. The BADS also incorporates a modified version of the Six Elements Test, originally described by Shallice and Burgess (1991a, 1991b). These authors reported that some patients with frontal lobe lesions—who had average or even above-average intellectual ability, and who performed normally on most, if not all, standardized tests of executive function—performed very poorly on open-ended tasks with multiple subgoals. The Six Elements Test requires that six easy (but different) activities be initiated during a specified time period, and carried out in accordance with a few simple rules. Although the individual tasks are very easy, individuals with executive function impairments often demonstrate difficulty starting and stopping tasks, developing a workable plan, performing the tasks according to the rules, and maintaining an awareness of time limits. Although the BADS can be used with a broad range of clients, our experience suggests that it is not usually sensitive to executive function impairments in relatively high-functioning individuals.

Because executive functions have proven so difficult to quantify, a number of less formal, but often very useful, observational approaches have been developed. These identify a task or set of activities to be done, and provide a structured way of scoring and recording detailed information on how the client is going about the task. Examples of this approach include the Six Elements Test discussed above, the Multiple Errands Task (Shallice & Burgess, 1991b), and the Executive Function Route-Finding Task (EFRT; Boyd & Sauter, 1994). In the Multiple Errands Task, the individual is asked to complete a set of different activities within a naturalistic setting such as a shopping mall. Activities involve buying items and finding out information, and doing so within a particular set of rules or constraints and within a particular time frame. The examiner shadows the person, making systematic observations of how efficiently the person goes about the task and how he or she seeks out and uses information.

The EFRT involves asking the person to find a particular place (e.g., a particular office in a medical center). Observational scoring criteria provide an evaluation of performance characteristics on a 4-point scale. Areas evaluated include (1) Task Understanding, (2) Incorporation of Information Seeking, (3) Retaining Directions, (4) Error Detection (self-monitoring), (5) Error Correction, and (6) On-Task Behavior. (The EFRT is provided in Appendix 8.2 of this text.) Both the Multiple Errands Task and the EFRT have been reported to have good predictive ability in terms of functional independence and ability to benefit from rehabilitation.

Yet another approach to estimating executive function abilities involves the use of structured rating scales. One portion of the BADS (Wilson et al., 1996), for example, consists of a 20-item Dysexecutive Questionnaire (DEX; Wilson et al., 1996), which is completed by the client and a family member or caregiver. Items on the DEX tap various aspects of executive function, such as initiation, planning, and functional problem solving. Another example of such a scale is the Profile of the Executive Control System (PRO-EX; Braswell et al., 1993). The PRO-EX structures staff and family ratings of behavior on seven scales (Goal Selection, Planning/Sequencing, Initiation, Executive, Timesense, Awareness of Deficits, and Self-Monitoring). Yet another such scale, the Brock Adaptive Functioning Questionnaire (BAFQ; Dywan & Segalowitz, 1996), provides for "self" and "other" reports on 12 scales designed to tap into different domains of executive functioning. Preliminary research with this instrument has identified two factors—one reflecting capacity for planning and initiation (believed to be primarily dependent on dorsolateral prefrontal systems), and one reflecting social monitoring and control of arousal (thought to be more orbitofrontally mediated). Dywan and Segalowitz (1996) reported that scores on the BAFQ were related to frontally generated electrophysiological measures. A summary sheet for the PRO-EX, and examples of items from the BAFQ scales, are provided in the Appendices to Chapter 8. Finally, several measures have been designed to look at level of awareness, motivation for change, and commitment to involvement in rehabilitation. These include the Change Assessment Questionnaire (Lam, McMahon, Priddy, & Gehred-Schultz, 1988) and the Self-Awareness of Deficits Interview (Fleming, Strong, & Ashton, 1996). (A more detailed discussion of awareness is provided in Chapter 9.)

General Measures of Disability and Outcome

Consistent with the WHO's emphasis on participation, recent years have shown a dramatic shift in rehabilitation in terms of developing reliable functional outcome measures and more global indicators of adaptation to disability. There is a great deal of interest in developing more valid and effective ways of looking at the natural history of disability and the long-term impact of rehabilitation efforts. A few of the more commonly used measures are discussed here and listed in Table 4.2.

The Functional Independence Measure (FIM; Granger & Hamilton, 1987), one of the most widely used outcome measures in North America and Europe, is an 18-item ordinal scale that rates the level of assistance required to perform various activities of daily living. It uses a seven-level scoring system, with scores ranging between 126 (normal status) and 18 (totally dependent). Although the FIM purports to sample both mobility and cognitive capacities, the cognitive items typically account for only a small amount of the total variance on the test, and it does not rate visual, speech, swallowing, or affective disabilities. In general, the FIM correlates moderately well with other disability and handicap scales, such as the Glasgow Outcome Scale (GOS; Jennett & Bond, 1975) and the Barthel Index (Mahoney & Barthel, 1965). All of these correlate well with burden of care, but all are very blunt measures of outcome. They also have some notable floor and ceiling effects: They are unlikely to detect changes of the magnitude that are typically seen following successful rehabilitation or other therapeutic interventions in the postacute phase, and they have less relevance for individuals with less severe injury. In many settings, the FIM is used together with the Functional Assessment Measure (FAM; Hall, Hamilton, Gordon, & Zasler, 1993), a 12-item extension of the FIM that addresses cognitive and psychosocial issues. Combining the FIM with the FAM results in a somewhat more sensitive and broadly based measure, but it is still very gross in its ratings. The Disability Rating Scale for Severe Head Trauma (Rappaport, Hall, Hopkins, Belieza, & Cope, 1982) is much more sensitive than the GOS, and has fewer ceiling effects than the FIM and FAM, although its sensitivity to change in the postacute stage is again extremely limited. Most of these measures are best suited to the acute end of inpatient cognitive and behavioral rehabilitation. Although these scales have limited usefulness with individual patients, they do allow for at least a rough comparison of outcome across different rehabilitation settings.

Other measures of disability provide more sensitive assessment of abilities in the postacute and long-term stages. Some of the more widely used measures that have been extensively used in reporting outcomes are as follows:

• The Katz Adjustment Scale (Katz & Lyerly, 1963) has been used to look at personality changes following brain injury and their psychosocial effects. The scale consists of 127 items and has both patient and relative report forms. It has been shown to detect change following rehabilitation (Prigatano et al., 1986), and it compares well with other measures of social outcome.

• The Neurobehavioral Rating Scale (Levin et al., 1987) measures a wide range of cognitive, behavioral, and psychiatric symptoms, and has been used in the diagnosis of organic personality syndrome or personality change following ABI. It has also been shown to be sensitive to change over time, and to detect different patterns of psychopathology related to frontal lobe injury.

• The Portland Adaptability Inventory (Lezak, 1987) was introduced to determine psychosocial outcome following brain injury. It was adapted by Malec and Thompson (1994) and renamed the Mayo–Portland Adaptability Inventory. Areas of function addressed include temperament and emotionality (e.g., anxiety, agitation, depression), activities and social behavior (e.g., social contacts, leisure activities, alcohol use), and physical capabilities (e.g., use of hands, dysarthria).

• The Sickness Impact Profile (Bergner, Bobbitt, Carter, & Gibson, 1981; Temkin et al., 1988) is a measure that addresses impact of illness or injury on many life domains from the perspective of the injured person. It has been used in a number of large ABI outcome studies (e.g., Dikmen, Ross, Machamer, & Temkin, 1995), and many of the scales are quite relevant to meaningful outcome; however, it is very long, and there is a heavy weighting on physical limitations.

• The Supervision Rating Scale (Boake & High, 1996) identifies 13 levels of supervision, reflecting all forms of activity that require the caregiver to be in the physical vicinity of the client to ensure safety. It is completed by informants who are acutely aware of what level of supervision is received and required.

• The Craig Handicap Assessment and Reporting Technique (Whiteneck, Charlifue, Gerhart, Overholser, & Richardson, 1992) addresses issues of handicap with respect to a broad range of independence and social integration, including the ability of the individual to fulfill roles in the family, at work, and in social and leisure pursuits.

SUMMARY

Assessing outcomes remains a challenging task, because so many variables enter into long-term adaptation and adjustment for all individuals—not just those who are injured. Nevertheless, it is an important task, and the use of standardized instruments will allow a better understanding of the natural recovery from brain injury, as well as the effects of rehabilitation efforts. The following principles should guide the assessment of individuals with cognitive impairment:

- An examiner must be knowledgeable about cognitive systems and the instruments selected for use in assessment.
- Test instruments must be appropriate to an individual's age, education level, linguistic and cultural background, and current cognitive and functional status.
- Tests should be chosen for both their sensitivity and specificity with respect to the cognitive domain of interest and to the etiology of the client's problems.
- Because the effects of brain injury are dependent on multiple factors, assessment must be comprehensive; it should include evaluation of both preinjury and postinjury physical, cognitive, emotional, personality, social, and contextual variables.
- A combination of psychometric tests; structured observations in functional settings; and standardized ratings by the client, family, caregivers, and therapists is likely to yield the most accurate and complete information with regard to current functional capacity.
- Examiners should be aware of the psychometric strengths and weaknesses of the instruments they employ for assessment.
- Assessment findings, with respect to the effects of the injury or disease, should make sense from a pathophysiological, neurological, and neuropsychological perspective, and should be consistent with major findings in the literature.
- It is just as important to identify areas of strength and functional ability as it is to identify weaknesses and functional limitations
- Assessment must span the WHO-identified domains of impairment, activity limitation, and participation to achieve a comprehensive and contextual perspective.
- Collaborative assessment involving the individual, the family, and the entire evaluation and treatment team will yield the most integrated and realistic assessment for the purpose of rehabilitation planning.

One of the most challenging aspects of assessment is deciding how much testing to do and when to do it. It is important to obtain a comprehensive evaluation, but there are good arguments against comprehensiveness, at least early on, because the patient may change rapidly and you can "burn" measures that can't be repeated well (e.g., memory tests). Early on it is probably most useful to track a few key cognitive domains over time, perhaps making more use of observational ratings and scales. The timing for a more comprehensive evaluation should coincide with some plateau of gains and/or need for information to aid in making an important transition (e.g., to home, school, work). Careful decision making with regard to the timing of assessments can also mitigate, to some degree, decreasing lengths of hospital stays and shrinking reimbursements.

Finally, it is important to remember that formal or psychometric assessments are only indications of what an individual can do at a particular time and in a particular context. These can serve as approximations to what is possible or likely in other settings or contexts. Although they are useful and potentially revealing, they never tell the full story. It is critical not to reify any procedure or test, but rather to gather information from many sources in a truly investigative and diagnostic endeavor. In rehabilitation, the process of assessment is ongoing. The incorporation of systematic observations and ratings during the course of treatment extends and refines the more formal assessment process. The assessment is facilitated by an open and collaborative approach, which involves therapists, the family, other caregivers, and the client in a process of understanding the nature of the client's impairments and their relationship to functional limitations and community participation.

REFERENCES

Anderson, C. V., Bigler, E. D., & Blatter, D. D. (1995). Frontal lobe lesions, diffuse damage, and neuropsychological functioning in traumatic brain-injured patients. *Journal of Clinical and Experimental Neuropsychology, 17*, 900–908.

Anderson, C. V., Damasio, H., Jones, R. D., & Tranel, D. (1991). Wisconsin Card Sorting Test performance as a measure of frontal lobe damage. *Journal of Clinical and Experimental Neuropsychology, 13*, 909–922.

Barona, A., Reynolds, C. R., & Chastain, R. (1984). A demographically based index of pre-morbid intelligence for the WAIS-R. *Journal of Consulting and Clinical Psychology, 52*, 865–887.

Benton, A. L. (1974). *Revised Visual Retention Test* (4th ed.). New York: Psychological Corporation.

Benton, A. L., Sivan, A. B., Hamsher, K., Varney, N., & Spreen, O. (1994). Facial Recognition Test. In *Contributions to neuropsychological assessment: A clinical manual* (2nd ed., pp. 35–52). New York: Oxford University Press.

Bergner, M., Bobbitt, R. A., Carter, W. B., & Gibson, B. G. (1981). The Sickness Impact Profile: Developmental and final revision of a health status measure. *Medical Care, 19*, 787–805.

Blair, J. R., & Spreen, O. (1989). Predicting premorbid IQ: A revision of the National Adult Reading Test. *The Clinical Neuropsychologist, 3*, 129–136.

Boake, C., & High, W. M. (1996). Functional outcome from traumatic brain injury. *American Journal of Physical Medicine and Rehabilitation, 75*, 1–9.

Boyd, T. M., & Sautter, S. W. (1994). Route-finding: A measure of everyday executive functioning in the head-injured adult. *Applied Cognitive Psychology, 72*, 171–181.

Braswell, D., Hartry, A., Hoornbeek, S., Johansen, A., Johnson, L., Schultz, J., & Sohlberg, M. M. (1993). *Profile of the Executive Control System.* Puyallup, WA: Association for Neuropsychological Research and Development.

Brickenbach, J. E., Chatterji, S., Badley, E. M., & Ostün, T. B. (1999). Models of disablement, universalism and the ICIDH. *Social Science and Medicine, 48,* 1173–1187.

Brickenkamp, R. (1981). *Test d2: Concentration–Endurance Test* (5th ed.). Göttingen, Germany: Verlag für Psychologie.

Buschke, H. (1973). Selective reminding for analysis of memory and learning. *Journal of Verbal Learning and Verbal Behavior, 12,* 543–550.

Conners, C. K., & Multi-Health Systems Staff. (1995). *Conners Continuous Performance Test.* Toronto: Multi-Health Systems.

Corrigan, J. D. (1989). Development of a scale for assessment of agitation following traumatic brain injury. *Journal of Clinical and Experimental Neuropsychology, 11,* 261–277.

Corrigan, J. D., & Bogner, J. A. (1994). Factor structure of the Agitated Behavior Scale. *Journal of Clinical and Experimental Neuropsychology, 16,* 205–210.

Coslett, H. B., Bowers, D., Verfaellie, M., & Heilman, K. M. (1991). Frontal verbal amnesia: Phonological amnesia. *Archives of Neurology, 48,* 949–955.

Crosson, B., Novack, T. A., Trenerry, M. R., & Craig, P. L. (1989). Differentiation of verbal memory deficits in blunt head injury using recognition trials of the California Verbal Learning Test: An exploratory study. *The Clinical Neuropsychologist, 3,* 29–44.

Delis, D. C., Kramer, J. H., Kaplan, E., & Ober, B. A. (1987). *California Verbal Learning Test: Adult Version.* San Antonio, TX: Psychological Corporation.

DeLuca, J., Schultheis, M. T., Madigan, N. K., Christodoulou, C., & Averill, A. (2000). Acquisition versus retrieval deficits in traumatic brain injury: Implications for memory rehabilitation. *Archives of Physical Medicine and Rehabilitation, 81,* 1327–1333.

Dikmen, S., Ross, B. L., Machamer, L. E., & Temkin, N. R. (1995). One year psychosocial outcome in head injury. *Journal of the International Neuropsychological Society, 1,* 67–77.

Dodrill, C. (1997). Myths of neuropsychology. *The Clinical Neuropsychologist, 11,* 1–17.

Dywan, J., & Segalowitz, S. (1996). Self- and family ratings of adaptive behavior after traumatic brain injury: Psychometric scores and frontally generated ERPs. *Journal of Head Trauma Rehabilitation, 11,* 79–95.

Fleming, J. M., Strong, J., & Ashton, R. (1996). Self-awareness of deficits in adults with traumatic brain injury: How best to measure? *Brain Injury, 10,* 1–15.

Golden, J. C. (1978). *Stroop Color and Word Test.* Chicago: Stoelting.

Granger, C. V., & Hamilton, B. B. (1987). *Uniform data set for medical rehabilitation.* Buffalo: Research Foundation, State University of New York.

Greenberg, L. M. (1998). *Test of Variables of Attention.* Edmonton, Alberta: Universal Attention Disorders.

Gronwall, D. (1977). Paced Auditory Serial Addition Task: A measure of recovery from concussion. *Perceptual and Motor Skills, 44,* 367–373.

Gronwall, D., & Sampson, H. (1974). *The psychological effect of concussion.* Auckland, New Zealand: Oxford University Press.

Hall, K., Hamilton, B., Gordon, W., & Zasler, N. (1993). Characteristics and comparisons of functional assessment indices: Disability Rating Scale, Functional Independence Measure and Functional Assessment Measure. *Journal of Head Trauma Rehabilitation, 8,* 60–74.

Heaton, R. K. (1981). *Wisconsin Card Sorting Test.* Odessa, FL: Psychological Assessment Resources.

Heaton, R. K., & Pendleton, M. G. (1981). Use of neuropsychological tests to predict adult patients' everyday functioning. *Journal of Consulting and Clinical Psychology, 46,* 807–821.

Jennett, B., & Bond, M. (1975). Assessment of outcome after severe brain damage: A practical scale. *Lancet, i,* 480–484.

Jones-Gotman, M., & Milner, B. (1977). Design fluency: The invention of nonsensical drawings after focal cortical lesions. *Neuropsychologia, 15,* 653–674.

Kaplan, E. (1988). A process approach to neuropsychological assessment. In T. Boll & B. K. Bryant (Eds.), *Clinical neuropsychology and brain function: Research, measurement, and practice* (pp. 125–167). Washington, DC: American Psychological Association.

Katz, M. M., & Lyerly, S. B. (1963). Methods for measuring adjustment and social behaviour in the community: Rationale, description, discriminative validity and scale development. *Psychological Reports, 13,* 503–535.

Lam, C. S., McMahon, B. T., Priddy, D. A., & Gehred-Schultz, A. (1988), Deficit awareness and treatment performance among traumatic head injury adults. *Brain Injury, 2,* 235–242.

Levin, H. S., Mattis, S., Ruff, R. M., Eisenberg, H. M., Marshall, L. F., & Tabaddor, K. (1987). Neurobehavioral outcome following minor head injury: A three center study. *Journal of Neurosurgery, 66,* 234–243.

Levin, H. S., O'Donnell, V. M., & Grossman, R. G. (1979). The Galveston Orientation and Amnesia Test. *Journal of Nervous and Mental Disease, 167,* 675–684.

Lezak, M. D. (1987). Relationship between personality disorders, social disturbances, and physical disability following traumatic brain injury. *Journal of Head Trauma Rehabilitation, 2,* 57–69.

Lezak, M. D. (1993). Newer contributions to the neuropsychological assessment of executive functions. *Journal of Head Trauma Rehabilitation, 8,* 24–31.

Lezak, M. D. (1995). *Neuropsychological assessment* (3rd ed.). New York: Oxford University Press.

Mahoney, F. I., & Barthel, D. W. (1965). Functional evaluation: The Barthel Index. *Maryland Medical Journal, 14,* 61–65.

Malec, J. F., & Thompson, J. M. (1994). Relationship of the Mayo–Portland Adaptability Inventory to functional outcome and cognitive performance measures. *Journal of Head Trauma Rehabilitation, 9,* 1–15.

Mateer, C. A. (1992). Systems of care for post-concussive syndrome. *Physical Medicine and Rehabilitation, 6,* 143–160.

Nelson, H. (1976). *The National Adult Reading Test (NART).* Windsor, England: National Foundation for Educational Research.

Newcombe, F. (1969). *Missile wounds of the brain.* London: Oxford University Press.

Ponsford, J., & Kinsella, G. (1991). The use of a rating scale of attentional behavior. *Neuropsychological Rehabilitation, 1,* 241–257.

Porteus, S. D. (1959). *The maze and clinical psychology.* Palo Alto, CA: Pacific Books.

Prigatano, G. P., Fordyce, D. J., Zeiner, H. K., Roueche, J. R., Pepping, M., & Wood, B. C. (1986). *Neuropsychological rehabilitation after brain injury: Theoretical and clinical issues.* Baltimore: Johns Hopkins University Press.

Rappaport, M., Hall, K. M., Hopkins, K., Belieza, T., & Cope, D. N. (1982). Disability Rating Scale for Severe Head Trauma: Coma to community. *Archives of Physical Medicine and Rehabilitation, 63,* 118–123.

Raskin, S. A., & Buckheit, C. A. (1998). *Prospective memory in traumatic brain injury.* Paper presented at the annual meeting of the Cognitive Neuroscience Society, San Francisco.

Raskin, S. A., Mateer, C. A., & Tweeten, R. (1998). Neuropsychological assessment of individuals with mild traumatic brain injury. *The Clinical Neuropsychologist, 12,* 21–30.

Raskin, S. A., & Rearick, E. (1996). Verbal fluency in individuals with mild traumatic head injury. *Neuropsychology, 10,* 416–422.

Reitan, R. M. (1958). The validity of the Trail Making Test as an indicator of organic brain damage. *Perceptual and Motor Skills, 9,* 127–130.

Reitan, R. M., & Wolfson, D. (1993). *The Halstead–Reitan Neuropsychological Test Battery: Theory and clinical interpretation.* Tuscon, AZ: Neuropsychology Press.

Reitan, R. M., & Wolfson, D. (1995). Category Test and Trail Making Test as measures of frontal lobe functions. *The Clinical Neuropsychologist, 9,* 50–55.

Rey, A. (1941). L'examen psychologique dans les cas d'encephalopathie traumatique. *Archives de Psychologie, 28,* 286–340.

Richards, B. (2000). *The effects of aging and mild traumatic brain injury on neuropsychological test performance.* Unpublished doctoral dissertation, York University, Toronto, Ontario, Canada.

Robertson, I. H., Ward, T., Ridgeway, V., & Nimmo-Smith, I. (1996). The structure of normal human attention: The Test of Everyday Attention. *Journal of the International Neuropsychological Society, 2,* 525–534.

Royall, D. R., Mahurin, R. K., & Gray, K. F. (1992). Bedside assessment of executive dyscontrol: The Executive Interview (EXIT). *Journal of the American Geriatric Society, 40,* 1221–1226.

Ruff, R. M., Light, R. H., & Evans, R. W. (1987). The Ruff Figural Fluency Test: A normative study with adults. *Developmental Neuropsychology, 3,* 37–52.

Schretlin, D., Bobholz, J. H., & Brandt, J. (1996). Development and psychometric properties of the Brief Test of Attention. *The Clinical Neuropsychologist, 10,* 80–89.

Segalowitz, S. J., Unsal, A., & Dywan, J. (1992). CNV evidence for the distinctiveness of frontal and posterior neural processes in a traumatic brain-injured population. *Journal of Clinical and Experimental Neuropsychology, 14,* 545–565.

Shallice, T., & Burgess, P. W. (1991a). Higher-order cognitive impairments and frontal-lobe lesions in man. In H. S. Levin, H. M. Eisenberg, & A. L. Benton (Eds.), *Frontal lobe function and injury* (pp. 125–138). Oxford: Oxford University Press.

Shallice, T., & Burgess, P. W. (1991b). Deficits in strategy application following frontal lobe damage in man. *Brain, 114,* 727–741.

Simmons-Mackie, N., & Damico, J. S. (1996). Accounting for handicaps in aphasia:

Communicative assessment from an authentic social perspective. *Disability and Rehabilitation, 18,* 540–549.

Slick, D. J., Sherman, E. M. S., & Iverson, G. L. (1999). Diagnostic criteria for malingered neurocognitive dysfunction: Proposed standards or clinical practice and research. *The Clinical Neuropsychologist, 13,* 545–561.

Sohlberg, M. M., Mateer, C. A., & Geyer, S. (1985). *Prospective Memory Screening (PROMS) and Prospective Memory Process Training (PROMPT).* Puyallup, WA: Association for Neuropsychological Research and Development.

Spreen, O., & Benton, A. L. (1977). *Neurosensory Center Comprehensive Examination for Aphasia (NCCEA).* Victoria: University of Victoria Neuropsychology Laboratory.

Spreen, O., & Strauss, E. (1998). *A compendium of neuropsychological tests: Administration, norms, and commentary* (2nd ed.). New York: Oxford University Press.

Stroop, J. R. (1935). Studies of interference in serial verbal reaction. *Journal of Experimental Psychology, 18,* 643–662.

Stuss, D. T., & Benson, F. B. (1986). *The frontal lobes.* New York: Raven Press.

Stuss, D. T., Stethem, L. L., Hugenholtz, H., & Richard, M. T. (1989). Traumatic brain injury: A comparison of three clinical tests and analysis of recovery. *The Clinical Neuropsychologist, 3,* 145–156.

Temkin, N., McClean, A., Dikmen, S., Gale, J., Bergner, M., & Almes, M. J. (1988). Development and evaluation of modifications to the Sickness Impact Profile for head injury. *Journal of Experimental Epidemiology, 41,* 47–57.

Trenerry, M. R., Crosson, B., DeBoe, J., & Leber, W. R. (1989). *Stroop Neuropsychological Screening Test.* Odessa, FL: Psychological Assessment Resources.

Warrington, E. K. (1984). *Recognition Memory Test.* Windsor, England: National Foundation for Educational Research.

Wechsler, D. (1997a). *Wechsler Adult Intelligence Scale—III.* San Antonio, TX: Psychological Corporation.

Wechsler, D. (1997b). *Wechsler Memory Scale—III.* San Antonio, TX: Psychological Corporation.

Whiteneck, G. C., Charlifue, S. W., Gerhart, K. A., Overholser, D., & Richardson, G. N. (1992). Quantifying handicap: A new measure of long-term rehabilitation outcomes. *Archives of Physical Medicine and Rehabilitation, 73,* 519–526.

Wilson, B. A., Alderman, N., Burgess, P. W., Emslie, H. C., & Evans, J. J. (1996). *The Behavioural Assessment of the Dysexecutive Syndrome.* Burry, St. Edmunds, England: Thames Valley Test Company.

Wilson, B. A., Baddeley, A. D., Cockburn, J., & Hiorns, R. (1989). The development and validation of a test battery for detecting and monitoring everyday memory problems. *Journal of Clinical and Experimental Neuropsychology, 11,* 855–870.

Wilson, B. A., Cockburn, J., & Baddeley, A. D. (1985). *The Rivermead Behavioral Memory Test.* Burry, St. Edmunds, England: Thames Valley Test Company.

Yudofsky, S. C., Silver, S. M., Jackson, W., Endicott, J., & Williams, D. (1986). The Overt Aggression Scale for the objective rating of verbal and physical aggression. *American Journal of Psychiatry, 143,* 35–39.

Yuspeh, R. L., & Vanderploeg, R. D. (2000). Spot-the-Word: A measure for estimating premorbid intellectual functioning. *Archives of Clinical Neuropsychology, 15,* 319–326.

II

MANAGEMENT APPROACHES FOR COGNITIVE IMPAIRMENTS

Management of
Attention Disorders

Together with problems in memory, problems in attention and concentration are the most commonly reported symptoms following brain damage (McKinlay, 1981). Even mild attentional symptoms tend to persist and contribute to long-term dysfunction, and they are correlated with poor outcome in persons with traumatic brain injury (TBI) and strokes (Brooks & McKinlay, 1987). This chapter focuses on methods for managing impairments in this critical cognitive process. It begins with a review of theoretical constructs important for understanding attention. This is followed by a discussion of the assessment of attention. The remainder of the chapter is devoted to describing four distinct approaches for remediating or managing attentional problems.

THEORY REVIEW

Models of Attention

Attention is usually described as a wide assortment of skills, processes, and cognitive states. Among the more consistent findings in individuals with brain injury are decreased reaction time and reduced speed of information processing (Gronwall, 1987, 1991; Ponsford & Kinsella, 1992; Stuss et al., 1989; Van Zomeren, Brouwer, & Deelman, 1984). Patients with acquired brain injury (ABI) report problems with concentration, distractibility, forgetfulness and the ability to do more than one thing at a time (Hinkeldey & Corrigan, 1990; Mateer, Sohlberg, & Crinean, 1987).

Chapter 1 reviewed the different types of models that are used to describe cognitive functions such as attention. There is considerable overlap among factor-analytic, cognitive processing, and clinical models of attention. Most attention models, regardless of their theoretical orientation, include functions related to sustaining attention over time (vigilance), capacity for information, shifting attention, and screening out nontarget information. For example, in their factor-analytic model, Mirsky, Anthony, Duncan, Ahearn, and Kellam (1991) identify four attention factors: (1) focus–execute, (2) sustain, (3) encode, and (4) shift. In a clinical model of attention, Mapou (1995) includes the following components: deployment of attention, capacity, resistance to interference, and mental manipulation. Cognitive processing models incorporate the concepts of vigilance, selection, dual-task performance, and automaticity (Baddeley, 1986). A review of various attention models with consideration of attentional symptoms commonly occurring following brain injury suggests that maintenance of attention, selectivity, capacity, and shifting of attention are key theoretical concepts with a high degree of clinical relevance.

Working memory is another concept critical to conceptualizing attention. The notion of *working memory* proposed by Baddeley and Hitch (1974) recognizes the contributions of multiple systems for the successful storage and retrieval of information. Simplistically speaking, working memory is the set of processes that permits us to hold on to information until it is utilized or encoded, or to keep stored information readily accessible. For example, working memory allows us to hold on to information long enough to write it down and to temporarily divert our attention to a new task, and then successfully return to the original activity. Working memory is associated with an active set of control processes, including rehearsal, coding, decision, and retrieval strategies. These processes encourage information to be encoded or held in a temporary store. Working memory requires not only the storage and retrieval of information, but also the manipulation of that information for task purposes. Therefore, it depends upon storage, rehearsal, and executive processes.

Baddeley and Hitch (1974) describe a construct related to working memory termed the *central executive*. It forms an interface between a long-term permanent memory store and working memory, the temporary, active storage of information. The key attention components identified above—maintenance of attention, selection of target information, capacity of information-processing ability, and alternating attention between tasks—rely on working memory and central executive processes. Figure 5.1 illustrates how working memory depends on information retrieval and storage.

Neuroanatomical substrates for various attention functions have been identified. Posner and Petersen (1990) suggest that three separate but interrelated brain circuits control attentional functions in humans—*orienting of attention in space, target selection and conflict resolution*, and *alerting/sustained attention*—in addition to working memory processes.

The first circuit, spatial orienting, depends on the *posterior attentional system*, which includes the posterior parietal lobe, the superior colliculus,

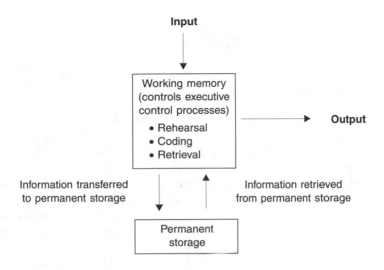

FIGURE 5.1. Working memory: How it facilitates information retrieval and storage.

and the lateral pulvinar nucleus. This is a primitive attention system responsible for low-level orientation to simple stimuli; it is not addressed in clients with sufficient attention to participate in a cognitive intervention program.

The second circuit, target selection and conflict resolution, is performed in anterior areas of the brain that include the anterior cingulate gyrus and supplementary motor areas. The thalamus is a brain structure that has also been closely associated with the selection of target information. Thalamic nuclei play a role in analyzing information received from ascending brainstem tracts and selecting what will continue for higher-level processing, as well as selecting what information descending from the cortex will be integrated and sent for further analysis (Mateer & Ojemann, 1983). The capacity to shift or alternate attention is a related function, which is primarily associated with activation of the anterior cingulate (Bakay Pragay, Mirsky, Ray, Turner, & Mirsky, 1978).

The alerting and sustained attention network, the third circuit, is employed when attention needs to be sustained in the absence of salient novel external stimuli. The right hemisphere—in particular, right prefrontal regions—and the norepinephrine system are involved in maintaining vigilance.

Finally, working memory processes, which help temporarily hold on to information, have been shown to activate a brain network that includes areas of the dorsolateral prefrontal cortex—with different localization for verbal and spatial material—and posterior areas (Awh, Smith, & Jonides,

1995; Cabeza & Nyberg, 1997). When the neuroanatomical correlates of different attentional functions are reviewed, the complexity and diversity of the circuitry are striking.

A Useful Clinical Model

In this section, we describe a clinical, componential model of attention that incorporates many of the aforementioned theoretical concepts and the types of attentional symptoms present in the population with brain injuries. It is a rational model based on analysis of task performance, errors, and subjective complaints by persons with brain injury (Sohlberg & Mateer, 1987, 1989). Over the years other researchers (e.g., Mapou, 1995; Mirsky et al., 1991) have employed similar taxonomies of attention, providing corroborative support for the clinical utility of dividing attention into the various components described below.

The clinical model consists of the following five components of attention, summarized in Table 5.1 and discussed below.

1. *Focused attention.* This is the ability to respond discretely to specific visual, auditory, or tactile stimuli. Although almost all patients with brain injuries recover this level of attention, it is often disrupted in the early stages of emergence from coma. A patient may initially be responsive only to internal stimuli (e.g., pain, temperature).

2. *Sustained attention.* This refers to the ability to maintain a consistent behavioral response during continuous and repetitive activity. It is divided into two subcomponents. One subcomponent incorporates the notion of *vigilance*. Disruption of vigilance can be observed in a patient who can only focus on a task or maintain responses for a brief period (i.e., seconds to minutes), or who fluctuates dramatically in performance over even brief periods (i.e., variable attention or attentional lapses). It also incorporates the notion of *mental control* or *working memory* with tasks that involve manipulating information and holding it in mind.

TABLE 5.1. Clinical Model of Attention

Focused attention	Basic responding to stimuli (e.g., head turning to auditory stimuli)
Sustained attention	• Vigilance: maintenance of attention over time during continuous activity • Working memory: actively holding and manipulating information
Selective attention	Freedom from distractibility
Alternating attention	Capacity for mental flexibility
Divided attention	Ability to respond to two tasks simultaneously

3. *Selective attention.* This level of attention refers to the ability to maintain a behavioral or cognitive set in the face of distracting or competing stimuli. It thus incorporates the notion of *freedom from distractibility.* Individuals with deficits at this level are easily drawn off task by extraneous, irrelevant stimuli. These can include external sights, sounds, or activities, as well as internal distractions (worry or rumination). Examples of problems at this level include an inability to perform therapy tasks in a stimulating environment (e.g., an open treatment area) or to prepare a meal with children playing in the background.

4. *Alternating attention.* This level of attention refers to the capacity for mental flexibility that allows individuals to shift their focus of attention and move between tasks with different cognitive requirements, thus controlling which information will be selectively processed. It thus involves working memory processes. Problems at this level are evident in the patient who has difficulty changing treatment tasks once a "set" has been established, and who needs extra cueing to pick up and initiate new task requirements. Real-life demands for this level of attentional control are frequent. Consider the student who must shift between listening to a lecture and taking notes, or the secretary who must continuously alternate between answering the phone, typing, and responding to inquiries.

5. *Divided attention.* This level of attention involves the ability to respond simultaneously to multiple tasks or multiple task demands. Two or more behavioral responses may be required, or two or more kinds of stimuli may need to be monitored. This level of attentional capacity is required whenever multiple simultaneous demands must be managed. Performance under such conditions (e.g., driving a car while listening to the radio, or holding a conversation during meal preparation) may actually reflect either rapid and continuous alternating attention or dependence on more unconscious automatic processing for at least one of the tasks. Modeling divided attention as a separate component of attention highlights its importance in the rehabilitation context.

These five components of attention provide a framework for organizing attention assessment and treatment activities.

ASSESSMENT OF ATTENTION

Attention abilities will usually be evaluated as part of a larger cognitive assessment. A useful cognitive assessment (see Chapter 4) provides a detailed description of an individual's specific cognitive profile and indicates how that profile will probably interact with behavioral and environmental variables to affect functional capacity in a variety of real world situations. Initially, a patient may receive a diagnostic workup (e.g., a neuropsychological evaluation) prior to remediation. However, there is no absolute division between assessment and treatment. Treatment itself is diagnostic, and evaluation needs to continue throughout the intervention process. Furthermore, given current service delivery constraints, a complete diagnostic workup is often not an option because it will not be reimbursed. Hence it is important for all rehabilitation specialists who address problems in attention to have an appreciation of assessment practices.

Useful tools for the assessment process include standardized psychometric tests, rating scales and questionnaires, and interview plus behavioral observation. Each of these are reviewed with respect to evaluating attention.

Standardized Testing

Several standardized tests are known for their ability to assess theoretically grounded aspects of attention function. Chapter 4 lists standardized tests that are particularly sensitive to the types of attention difficulties present in the population with brain injuries, and that tap several of the components of attention described above (see Table 4.2). It is noted there that interpretation of performance on these tests is founded on both the normative statistical base for each measure and an approach to testing that incorporates extensive observational information about how an individual approaches the test—particularly with respect to successes and failures. The use of multiple measures of attention should thus provide information on the nature of an attentional disorder and the degree to which the person is impaired by this disorder.

Kinsella (1998) writes about the difficulty of using multifactorial neuropsychological tests, and calls for standardized measures to evaluate discrete components of attention. She also discusses the need for further study of the relationship between neuropsychological tests of attention and different theoretical components of attention in order to improve our assessment practices. From a research perspective, having standardized instruments that measure discrete types of attention (e.g., sustained attention and selective attention) should increase our understanding of how attention operates in the brain. Clinically, such instruments can assist us in pinpointing underlying attention deficits that warrant intervention.

The Test of Everyday Attention (Robertson, Ward, Ridgeway, & Nimmo-Smith, 1996), discussed in Chapter 4, responds to some of the needs outlined by Kinsella (1998). This test was developed in order to improve clinical and research assessment of attention. It contains eight tasks designed to measure abilities in four different attention functions (sustained attention, selective attention, attentional switching, and auditory–verbal working memory). It uses some materials that simulate real-world activities, although it is not a functional assessment. Initial data suggest adequate reliability and validity.

Formal assessment using standardized neuropsychological tests provides valuable information on a person's attentional functioning, which can be compared to the levels of performance that would be expected if there were not neurological problems. In addition to pinpointing the level of impairment, tests can also provide information relative to the nature of the problem (e.g., identifying difficulty with sustained vs. alternating attention). Furthermore, standardized attention tests are efficient. One shortcoming of standardized tests, however, is their difficulty in predicting how well an individual will function in real-world activities. The ecological validity of cognitive assessment is often questioned, as the relationship between standardized tests and daily tasks is not well defined (Sbordonne & Long, 1996). Thus the use of standardized tests in conjunction with observation and interview will be critical in order to identify disabilities and prioritize treatment options.

Rating Scales/Questionnaires

A number of rating scales and questionnaires can help organize clinicians' observations and questions about attention functioning. Responses can then help identify directions for therapy. Examples of three questionnaires relevant to attentional functioning are described below. (Chapter 4 describes the second and third of these as measures of executive functions, but they are also useful in the assessment of attention.)

The Attention Questionnaire (Sohlberg, Johnson, Paule, Raskin, & Mateer, 1994) is based in part on Ponsford and Kinsella's (1991) attention questionnaire and asks clients to rate the frequency of occurrence for different attention problems. The attention problems are related to difficulty in sustaining, switching, and dividing one's attention, as well as screening out distractions; all of these attention functions are theoretically and clinically motivated. The questionnaire supplies a numerical indicator summarizing the overall frequency of perceived attention problems. (See Appendix 5.1.)

The Dysexecutive Questionnaire (DEX) is a subtest on the Behavioural Assessment of the Dysexecutive Syndrome (Burgess, Alderman, Wilson, Evans, & Emslie, 1996). It contains 20 questions related to decreased attention and executive control that commonly occur following brain injury. The respondent rates each problem on a frequency of occurrence scale. The DEX has rating forms for self and others.

The Brock Adaptive Functioning Questionnaire (BAFQ; Dywan & Segalowitz, 1996) contains 68 questions that were developed through clinical practice with the help of community volunteers who had sustained brain injuries, as well as their families. It asks subjects to rate degree of difficulty with specific functions in five different behavioral domains: planning, initiation, attention/memory, arousal/inhibition, and social monitoring. The BAFQ has forms for self and a significant other.

Questionnaires give an indication of different individuals' perceptions of functioning. This is particularly useful in prioritizing treatment goals as a questionnaire may reveal what is most bothersome to a client and/or significant other. However, it is important to remember that questionnaires do not produce authentic data—only impressions. For example, if there is no question on a rating scale that corresponds to an individual's problem area, it may go unidentified (Sohlberg, McLaughlin, Pavese, Heidrich, & Posner, 2000). Also, given the frequency of reduced awareness in the population with brain injuries, as well as issues specific to families, data provided by questionnaires can be misleading (Hillier, 1997).

Structured Interviews/Observations

Structured interviews may provide information not revealed in questionnaire data. Sohlberg and colleagues (2000) completed a study looking at changes in attentional functioning following attention intervention. The data from the structured interviews proved to be the most revealing source of change in abilities. For example, there were subjects who showed no change in attention function based on questionnaire data, but when they were asked structured questions such as "What kinds of changes have you experienced since coming to the clinic?", they provided specific, relevant examples of improved functioning that relied on increased attentional abilities. Transcripts from the structured interviews showed that only after attention treatment did subjects report changes in real-world activities that related to attention (e.g., "I can drive and listen to music," "I remember phone numbers better"). It appeared that reported changes were not evident on questionnaire data because the particular everyday functions that were meaningful to the clients were not always made explicit on the rating sheets. For example, a client did not relate "increased sustained attention" to "ability to read for longer time periods." Asking clients to describe specific tasks that were difficult and easy provided critical information. It is thus quite helpful to interview clients and significant others to obtain their perspectives on abilities and disabilities. Responses from structured interviews may be less susceptible to expectancy effects. Interview data may also suggest the most important contexts for further observation.

Observation of behavior is perhaps the most functionally relevant assessment tool; however, it is time-consuming and subjective. If possible, a combination of observation, interview, and standardized tests may be the most helpful in elucidating attentional deficits. Structured observations where the clinician observes relevant behaviors may be the most useful. For example, if a client has identified sustained attention as an issue, the clinician may document time on task for a variety of activities.

Assessment: A Summary

Given clinicians' limited time with patients, it is not always feasible to complete a full neuropsychological battery, to administer a structured interview and questionnaires, and to complete structured observations. Clinicians may need to prioritize assessment activities based upon their hypotheses of what is impaired and the treatment goals set by the clients and their families. Clinicians can administer attentional tests to sample the types of attention problems that observation and interview data suggest are most problematic. It is helpful to have redundant measures that sample a specific type of attention in order to test clinical hypotheses. When a hypothesis is generated (e.g., "The client has the most difficulty with selective attention or distractibility"), the clinician can continue to test the hypothesis during diagnostic interventions, where changes in real-world activities are the primary measure of the interventions' efficacy.

Alternative assessment paradigms that offer an ecological means to measure real-world functioning are needed. Some of the up-and-coming models are described in Chapter 4. For example, assessment models that use interpretive research methods to evaluate the impact of impairments on an individual's daily life may be very helpful, if they can be made less time-intensive (Simmons-Mackie & Damico, 1996).

APPROACHES TO MANAGING
PROBLEMS IN ATTENTION

Chapter 1 reviews several important underlying assumptions guiding our approach to the management of cognitive impairments. One of these assumptions is that rehabilitation specialists should not isolate cognition. In order to address problems in a client's attentional functioning, a clinician will need to consider social, behavioral, and emotional issues along with the cognitive effects. A related assumption is the importance of adopting an eclectic management approach and drawing upon a broad range of traditions—including behavioral, sociological, psychological, and neuropsychological disciplines. The options for managing attention impairments described in this section are based upon a broad range of disciplines.

Four approaches to addressing difficulties in attention are listed below. Most often a clinician will implement some combination of these approaches, either simultaneously or at different times in the recovery process.

- *Attention process training* involves the use of cognitive exercises that are designed to remediate and improve attentional systems. It is primarily based on neuropsychological theory.
  - *Use of strategies and environmental supports* includes both self-

management strategies and modifications to the environment to help a client compensate for attention problems. Self-management strategies may also work to remediate attention problems. This management approach draws upon behavioral and neuropsychological traditions.

• *Use of external aids* refers to the various aids that are available to help individuals track and organize information. This approach to managing attention problems draws upon behavioral and neuropsychological principles.

• *Psychosocial support* addresses the emotional and social factors that can result from and/or exacerbate an attentional deficit. Therapeutic practices in this domain come from sociological and psychological traditions.

Attention Process Training

Most attention process training programs are based on the notion that attentional abilities can be improved by providing opportunities for stimulating a particular aspect of attention. The aspects of attention that are addressed vary widely among programs and depend upon the model of attention that drives a particular program. Treatment usually involves having patients engage in a series of repetitive drills or exercises that are designed to provide opportunities for practice on tasks with increasing attentional demands. Repeated activation and stimulation of attentional systems are hypothesized to facilitate changes in cognitive capacity (Neimann, Ruff, & Baser, 1990; Sohlberg & Mateer, 1987; Sohlberg et al., 2000; Sturm, Willmes, Orgass, & Hartje, 1997).

There are several commercially available attention training packages and computer programs, motivated by the assumption that discrete components of attention can be selectively rehabilitated through targeted stimulation. One example is the Attention Process Training (APT) program (Park, Proulx, & Towers, 1999; Sohlberg & Mateer, 1987; Sohlberg et al., 1994, 2000), which is a widely used cognitive rehabilitation program designed to remediate attention deficits in individuals with brain injury. The APT materials consist of a group of hierarchically organized tasks that exercise different components of attention commonly impaired after brain injury, including sustained, selective, alternating, and divided attention. The program tasks place increasing demands on complex attentional control and working memory systems.

Treatment Activities

The treatment activities in most attention training programs are usually not functional and tend to resemble laboratory tasks. This is because most functional activities (e.g., meal planning, vocational tasks) are multifaceted and require activation of many different cognitive processes. Discrete attention tasks permit the stimulation of isolated components of attention. Examples of attention process training exercises include listening for descending number sequences on auditory attention tapes, alphabetizing words in an orally presented sentence, detecting targets with the presence of distractor noise, and performing complex semantic categorization tasks that require switching sets. A number of tasks combine auditory and visual activities.

The clinician will want to have a rationale for selecting specific tasks and for organizing an attention process training program. Helpful questions for promoting an organized selection of tasks are as follows:

1. What component of attention does this task activate?
2. What other tasks could it be grouped with to allow me to stimulate the same type of processing?
3. What are my methods for scoring objective and subjective performance parameters, such as accuracy, speed, and type of errors?
4. How could I alter the administration procedures to make the task easier or harder, or what other tasks would form a hierarchy with this activity?

Examples of specific treatment activities corresponding to particular components of attention are listed below. Clinicians can review available treatment packages and computer programs to ascertain what type of attention a particular task addresses. The exercises listed below are from the APT program and serve as examples. Appendices 5.2 to 5.4 provide examples of clinical protocols used to record patient performance on some of these tasks.

Sustained attention

- Exercises that require listening for target words or sequences on attention tapes, and pressing a buzzer when the target is identified
- Paragraph-listening comprehension exercises
- Exercises that require sequencing an auditorily presented number series in ascending or descending order
- Mental math activities

Alternating attention

- Exercises that require listening for one type of target word or sequence on attention tapes, and then switching to listening for a different type of word or sequence
- Paper-and-pencil tasks that require alternating between generating numbers or letters that come before or after the presented target in a number line or alphabet

- Activities where the respondent begins with a designated number and then switches between adding and subtracting selected numbers

Selective attention

- Any of the sustained attention tasks with background distractor noise or movement
- Tasks involving placement of visual distractor overlays (e.g., an plastic overhead sheet with distractor lines) on top of a paper-and-pencil activity

Divided attention

- Reading paragraphs for comprehension and simultaneously scanning for a target word (e.g., while reading, client has to count the number of *ands*)
- Completing a sustained attention task while simultaneously performing a reaction time computer task
- Completing a time-monitoring task (requiring tracking elapsed time) while simultaneously engaging in a sustained attention activity

Therapy Principles

Therapy principles relevant to providing attention process training focus on how to select exercises and when to stop or modify a program. The six treatment principles described below are recommended for effective administration of the APT program or other process-oriented therapies designed to boost impaired attentional systems (Sohlberg et al., 1994; Sohlberg & Mateer, 1989).

- *Principle 1. Use a treatment model that is grounded in attention theory.* Working from a theoretical model ensures a rational basis for the treatment hierarchies being utilized. It also promotes the systematic delivery of a therapy regimen. The clinical model described earlier in this chapter (focused, sustained, selective, alternating, and divided attention) is an example of a theoretically motivated treatment model.
- *Principle 2. Use therapy activities that are hierarchically organized.* Arranging exercises in a hierarchical fashion can allow repeated stimulation and activation of the target underlying process. As a client progresses, the same components can be stimulated at increasingly higher levels.
- *Principle 3. Provide sufficient repetition.* Tasks need to be completed with enough intensity to stimulate improved attentional processing. If a therapy schedule does not permit sufficient repetition, enlisting caregivers to provide extra practice outside of established clinical hours or establishing a home therapy program may be important.

- *Principle 4. Treatment decisions should be based upon client performance data.* Data-based treatment allows clinicians to make informed decisions about when to start, stop, or modify a therapy program. For example, examination of accuracy or speed may reveal that a client needs easier or more challenging activities. Examination of error profiles may show that all errors are at the beginning of a task (difficulty with achieving a "ready set") or at the end of a task (difficulty with sustained attention or fatigue). In addition, showing a client his or her performance on a graph can be an objective, powerful illustrator of progress. Appropriate decisions about treatment can only be made through careful evaluation of client performance.

- *Principle 5. Actively facilitate generalization from the start of treatment.* Clinicians must plan for and measure generalization from attention therapy tasks to real-world activities. Clients need to be given opportunities to apply retrained attentional skills to everyday activities. Since the therapy tasks are chosen because they target very select components of attention, it is important to actively facilitate generalization to real-world functional activities that involve many cognitive processes. For example, if a client is working on sustained attention tasks, he or she might develop a list of real-world activities (e.g., the number of minutes the client can attend while reading the newspaper) that should improve as sustained attention increases. The client can engage in these activities and monitor changes. The clinician and client can review performance on these generalization activities as part of the therapy process. It is usually helpful to involve a significant other from the beginning of therapy to facilitate the generalization process. See Appendix 5.5 for an example of a generalization activity for an individual who is working primarily on improving selective attention to decrease vulnerability to distraction.

- *Principle 6. Be flexible in adapting the therapy format.* Each client and each clinical setting are unique. Attention process training may be adapted to a number of formats, including individual sessions and group therapy. In addition, given current service delivery constraints, home programs may be the only way for a client to receive enough repetitive stimulation with tasks. Clinicians can train family members to administer tasks.

Treatment Efficacy

Attempts to measure the effects of attention process training may evaluate changes at three different levels: (1) a training task itself, (2) psychometric tests related to the task, and (3) everyday functioning. Improvements following attention process training at the first level, the training task, have been consistently demonstrated across studies. Even in subjects with severe brain injury, improvements have been noted on activities involving maintenance of attention during tasks, accuracy and speed of visual search, and a wide range of other tasks requiring increasingly complex stimulus-response demands (Ben-Yishay, Piasetsky, & Rattock, 1987; Wood & Fussey, 1987). It is unclear from the literature how task-specific the training effects have been and whether training has generalized to any other domain.

Results from studies that have evaluated attention process training on unpracticed psychometric measures of attention are more mixed. A number of studies do report significant posttreatment improvements on standard measures of attention following exercise-oriented training (Diller et al., 1974; Gray, Robertson, Pentland, & Anderson, 1992; Ruff et al., 1989; Sivak et al., 1984a; Sohlberg & Mateer, 1987; Sturm, Hartje, Orgass, & Willmes, 1993; Sturm et al., 1997). Findings by Sturm and colleagues (1997) support the effectiveness of attention process training for improving discrete components of attention. They reported improved performance on neuropsychological tests specific to the type of attention that was trained. They further suggested that only patients with higher-level vigilance abilities may respond to training involving more complex components of attention.

A more recent study (Park et al., 1999) compared performance on two neuropsychological tests (the Paced Auditory Serial Addition Task [PASAT] and the Consonant Trigrams Test [CTT]) in subjects with brain injury who received the APT program versus a normal control group. Both groups received the outcome measures twice, but the controls received no training. Results showed that the performance of the experimental group improved on both the neuropsychological measurements. The control group improved on one of the measures (PASAT) but not the other (CTT). The authors suggest that the cognitive processes involved in the CTT are different from those stimulated by the training tasks in the APT, and conclude that the APT resulted in learning of new skills rather than improved processing.

There have also been a few reports of negative findings. Malec, Rao, Jones, and Stubbs (1984) failed to demonstrate psychometric changes, but they utilized only a very short training period and a limited number of training tasks. Ponsford and Kinsella (1988) demonstrated improvements on attention-dependent tasks in a group with severe head injuries, but not at a level exceeding spontaneous recovery levels.

Measurement of improvement at the level of everyday functioning is the most important indicator of the success or failure of attention training. Several studies have attempted to look at real-world indicators of changes in attention. Wood and Fussey (1987) reported improved "attention to task" during therapy activities. Sivak, Hill, and Olson (1984b) reported improved driving performance following perceptual skills and attention training. In a series of studies, we and our colleagues (Mateer & Sohlberg, 1988; Mateer, Sohlberg, & Youngman, 1990; Mateer, 1992) reported improvement following attention training, not only on measures of attention, memory, and learning, but on levels of independent living and return to work.

In an evaluation of APT treatment effects, Sohlberg and colleagues (2000) compared the influence of APT to that of another intervention (brain injury education) on tasks of daily life and on performance on attentional networks involving vigilance, orienting, and executive function in 14 subjects with acquired brain injury. The overall results suggested that the brain injury education was most effective in improving self-reports of psychosocial function and facilitated some cognitive benefits when it followed APT. Figure 5.2 shows the average number of reported changes in three categories during a structured interview that was conducted after subjects had completed 10 weeks of brain injury education and 10 weeks of APT training. As shown, APT influenced the extent of improvement on self-report of cognitive function.

APT also appeared to modify performance on some measures of executive attention and working memory. An initial good level of alertness appeared necessary for improvements in executive functions and high-level attention. Subjects who received APT followed by brain injury education or the reverse order of treatment were divided into groups according to whether they demonstrated high- or low-level vigilance abilities. Figure 5.3 shows changes in improvement scores on tests assessing attention and executive function networks, such as the PASAT (see Chapter 4). Results in-

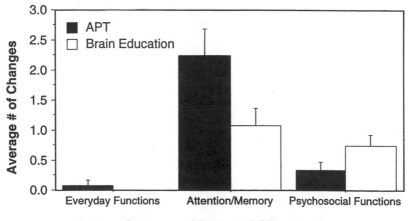

Category of Reported Change

FIGURE 5.2. Average number of subject-reported functional, cognitive, and psychosocial changes following APT (APT in the figure) and brain injury education. APT appears to influence self-report of cognitive changes. From Sohlberg, McLaughlin, Pavese, Heidrich, and Posner (2000). Copyright 2000 by Swets & Zeitlinger. Reprinted by permission.

dicated that PASAT scores increased over time and that improvement after APT was greater than improvement after brain injury education, suggesting that APT had a specific effect on the cognitive functions measured by the PASAT. Performance on the PASAT also depended upon the vigilance levels of the subjects; those with higher vigilance levels had higher PASAT scores and showed a greater improvement over time. However, both groups, regardless of vigilance level, benefited more from APT than from brain injury education. The study encourages clinicians to consider individual attention profiles when designing cognitive interventions. Overall, the results of this study suggest that APT may be effective for improving certain types of executive and working memory functions in patients with specific attention profiles (e.g., high vs. low vigilance levels).

In summary, the majority of published studies have reported positive findings with attention process training. We still have much to learn about what types of patients can benefit from this type of therapy. Increased understanding of how and when attentional functions can improve is an important research focus. The literature on brain recovery mechanisms is beginning to offer possible explanations for how attention process training might operate to improve functioning. There are increasing numbers of reports demonstrating the plasticity of the adult central nervous system (e.g., Nudo, 1996) and experience-dependent recovery processes due to changes in synaptic connectivity (Tallal et al., 1996). Advances in neuroimaging may help elucidate these mechanisms.

To illustrate the important clinical aspects of attention process train-

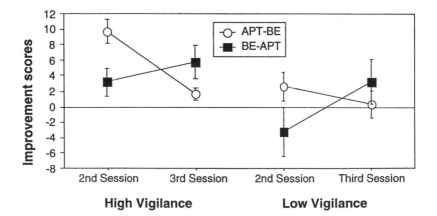

FIGURE 5.3. Improvement scores on the PASAT following APT (APT in the figure) and brain injury education (BE in the figure) in subjects with high and low vigilance levels. APT appears to have a specific effect on functions measured by the PASAT, especially for subjects with high vigilance levels. From Sohlberg, McLaughlin, Pavese, Heidrich, and Posner (2000). Copyright 2000 by Swets & Zeitlinger. Reprinted by permission.

ing more fully, we end our discussion of this option for managing attention impairments with an actual case example.

Case Example of Attention Process Training

Gary was a 35-year-old male who was injured in a car accident at the age of 33. Computed tomography (CT) and magnetic resonance imaging (MRI) scans suggested diffuse damage indicative of a high-velocity shearing injury. He was unconscious for 11 days, and the length of his posttraumatic amnesia (PTA) was estimated at about 2 weeks. He received inpatient rehabilitation for physical therapy, cognition, and behavior management. He also attended a community reentry program for 1 month. At the time of his accident, Gary worked in retail sales. Following rehabilitation, he attempted to return to his sales job on a part-time basis. He experienced difficulties tracking orders and interacting appropriately with colleagues, primarily due to decreased attention, organization, and impulsivity. His employer attempted to simplify his job, and his sister assisted with home management tasks. It was felt that attention process training might be helpful in improving Gary's performance at work.

Gary received 10 weeks of attention process training. He came in for treatment three times a week for 1 hour each visit. (This regimen could have been altered to do 1 hour of treatment with 2 hours of home practice, had his sister been available to assist.) He experienced the most difficulty with high-level sustained attention (mental control or holding on to information) and with selective attention (distractibility). This was determined through neuropsychological evaluation and an interview.

His initial attention process training program consisted of three sustained attention exercises and three selective attention exercises. The sustained attention exercises included listening to attention tapes that required him to press a buzzer when he heard a target and a variety of mental math activities. For example, one tape required him to press the buzzer every time he heard one letter followed by another letter that came before it in the alphabet. He also had an exercise that required him to give back the words in an orally presented sentence in alphabetical order. Examples of selective attention exercises were paragraph-listening exercises with background noise. As Gary improved his accuracy and speed on tasks, their difficulty level was increased, and several new sustained and selective attention tasks were added to his program.

Gary and his clinician developed a generalization home program. Together, they generated a log for recording the amount of time he could sit and concentrate on mock vocational tasks (filling out order sheets), and he worked to increase the time. He also kept a log where he rated his level of distractibility during home chores when he was listening to music. Performance on these activities was reviewed during therapy.

Results of both neuropsychological testing and self-report suggested significant improvements in attention following the attention process training. He showed increases at or greater than 0.65 standard deviations on five neuropsychological attention and executive function tests (the PASAT, the Dichotic Listening Test, the Stroop Test, the Controlled Oral Word Association Task, and the Gordon Diagnostic System). Maintenance of improvement was demonstrated, as these scores remained stable when Gary was tested 10 weeks following cessation of attention process training. (During that period he received counseling.)

Self-report suggested improved performance on everyday tasks. Scores improved on both questionnaires (the Attention Questionnaire and the DEX, described earlier) that were completed prior to and following the attention process training. Unlike the improved neuropsychological test performance, improvements on the questionnaire reporting were not maintained during the ensuing 10-week phase when Gary was receiving counseling support and no attention process training. Although it was not a desirable clinical outcome that he did not perceive his attention abilities to be as high, it supports a functional relationship between the attention process training and improved daily functioning. Only when he was receiving the attention process treatment did he report increases in functioning on the questionnaire. It may have been that he needed a longer course of training.

Responses to a structured interview were also striking. After the attention process training, Gary offered five specific examples of "recent changes in his functioning," all of which suggested improved attention abilities. He noted, "Work is a lot easier because I can read the orders better and pay attention more . . . my memory has improved . . . speed of processing seems to be quicker . . . "

It should be noted, however, that although his employer reported improved performance following the attention process training, Gary continued to need job accommodations, such as more time for completing tasks and written checklists. He also sought counseling to deal with self-esteem issues. Hence the attention process training appeared to be useful at improving select cognitive skills that did generalize to everyday functioning. It did not, however, dramatically change the level of support Gary required to perform his job.

Use of Strategies and Environmental Supports

Another option for managing attention deficits is the use of compensatory strategies and/or environmental supports. Sometimes strategies are used in conjunction with attention process training. Alternatively, they may be used later in the recovery phase, when a person is reintegrating into home or work environments that are suited to the adoption of task-specific strategies. If decreased attention is problematic for particular tasks or settings, identifying an appropriate strategy or form of environmental support may be the most efficient method for mitigating problems. We divide our discussion into self-management strategies (which the client learns to initiate) and environmental supports (where the environment is modified in some way to lessen the effects of an attention problem).

Self-Management Strategies

Self-management strategies mostly encompass self-instructional routines that help an individual focus attention on a task. One of the most common symptoms following brain injury is an inability to process information automatically. Tasks that used to be automatic (e.g., driving, reading) may now require deliberate, effortful concentration. Individuals tend to have difficulty concentrating and experience a reduced capacity to process information. Some clients are helped by strategies that encourage them to be more deliberate in focusing their attention. Examples of these types of strategies are described below.

Orienting Procedures. Orienting procedures may be helpful for clients who have difficulty sustaining attention or screening out distractions. The goal of these procedures is to encourage clients to monitor their activities consciously, thereby avoiding attentional lapses. A general orienting procedure that we frequently use is to teach clients to ask themselves orienting questions at specified times. For example, a client may be trained to ask the following three orienting questions each time his or her watch beeps on the hour: (1) "What am I currently doing?" (2) "What was I doing before this?" (3) "What am I supposed to do next?" If successful, this orienting routine will prevent a client from experiencing gaps in focusing his or her attention.

Orienting procedures may be designed for specific tasks or environments. For example, a driving routine can be helpful for clients who have a tendency to drive and temporarily forget where they are driving. A car memo pad is installed, and a client is trained to write down three items on the pad before turning the key: (1) destination, (2) estimated time of arrival, and (3) time at which it would be appropriate to pull over and ask for help if feeling unsure of whereabouts.

Another example of a task-specific orienting procedure is a reading routine. The special education literature is full of research-backed strategies that can be applied to the brain injury population. Winograd and Hare (1988) review seven studies showing how direct instruction of reading comprehension strategies can improve performance. For example, Adams, Carnine, and Gersten (1982) taught fifth-grade students an effective study skills strategy composed of six steps: previewing subheadings, reciting subheadings, asking questions, reading for detail, rereading subheadings, and rehearsing. We have adapted this routine for clients with acquired brain injuries who have difficulty with sustained attention for reading.

Pacing. Clients with attention problems often experience difficulty with fatigue and/or with maintaining concentration over an extended period of time. It can be helpful to teach them pacing strategies. The goal of pacing is twofold. First, it is important to help clients develop realistic expectations for productivity. Some clients feel continually frustrated as they attempt to achieve the same activity level as before their brain injury. Second, pacing allows clients to keep going for a longer period of time. Training clients to pace themselves appropriately needs to be individualized. Sometimes it is helpful to build in breaks at set time intervals in a particular environment. Another option is to build in breaks based on task completion (e.g., taking a break after reading 10 pages). Higher-functioning clients may benefit from self-monitoring fatigue or attention levels and then learning to take a break when they begin to rate themselves with higher levels of fatigue or reduced attention.

Time of day can be a helpful aspect of pacing. Many individuals find that they function well in the morning but are "used up" in the afternoon. It may be useful to teach people to complete more demanding household or vocational tasks in the morning, and to schedule only light activities for the latter part of the day.

Setting up an appropriate pacing strategy obviously relies on careful assessment of when and where attention problems interfere. Involving the client and relevant family members, employers, or other key persons in the design and piloting of a pacing strategy will be imperative.

Key Ideas Log. Another attention problem that interferes with day-to-day functioning is difficulty in switching between tasks (i.e., alternating attention). A common complaint is that people lose their train of thought or cannot resume an activity if they are interrupted or must temporarily divert their attention. To manage this difficulty, individuals can learn to quickly jot (or tape-record on a voice messenger) key questions or ideas that come to mind but can be addressed later. This allows them to continue with a particular task, rather than going to confer with a colleague or family member on another issue as it comes to mind and having to return to the task at hand.

Increasing the Success of Strategies. One might imagine any number of strategies that can be used in myriad circumstances to help people manage decrements in sustaining, switching, or focusing their attention. Several reminders serve to increase the chance that the strategies will be useful:

• More time spent assessing a client's attention problem will increase the likelihood of selecting useful strategies. It is important to understand *how, when,* and *where* the attention problem is troublesome. This will require careful observation and interview.
• There should be a plan for measurement. How will the clinician or the client know whether a strategy is working? What are the indicators of problems? What are the expectations for improvement?
• Clients should be involved as much as possible in strategy selection

and development. The more ownership clients have over the strategies adopted, the more likely they are to invest the time to learn to use them.

• Remember that establishing a strategy usually means training someone who may have difficulties with memory, learning, or organization to implement a new habit. Habit formation is difficult even without concomitant cognitive problems. Hence clinicians should build in systematic training with adequate support, a reasonable expectation for sufficient time to establish a habit, and an expectation that the client will need periodic refreshers as use of the habit wanes. (See Chapter 6 on training the use of metacognitive strategies for memory problems, and Chapter 7 on training the use of external aids.)

Environmental Supports

The addition of environmental supports can be very effective in managing attention difficulties. Careful assessment of the environment should be part of any cognitive management plan. Consideration of how to set up the environment to minimize the effects of an attention deficit can result in significant improvement in functioning. Environmental supports can be grouped into two categories: task management strategies and environmental modifications.

Task Management Strategies. During the interview process, the clinician will learn what tasks are affected by the attention disorder. Together, the clinician and client can then generate strategies to deal with these issues. A common example of an attention problem is difficulty attending in distracting environments. The clinician and client can make a list of "difficult" and "helpful" environments. This may result in a list of restaurants that are "noisy or busy" and those that are "quiet," and stores that produce disorientation (typically in malls) and those that are more helpful (often smaller stores). The client can be reminded that, when possible, he or she should choose the more helpful environment in each case. Examples of other strategies to eliminate distractions when completing a task that requires concentration include turning off the television or stereo, shutting a door or curtains, using earplugs, and turning off the ringer for the phone or answering machine.

Environmental Modifications. Most environmental modifications involve organizing clients' physical space to reduce the load on their attention, memory, and organizational abilities. Setting up filing systems, message centers, and bill payment systems, and organizing and labeling cupboards, are all examples of environmental modifications that might assist an individual with an attention disorder. Helping people to reduce clutter and eliminate visual distractions can be quite useful.

Posting directions to others in an individual's environment may also lessen task demands. For example, we have had a number of clients who were greatly helped by posting various forms of "do not disturb" signs that gave them uninterrupted time to work on an activity. These have been used in both home and vocational environments.

Increasing the Success of Environmental Supports. Establishing environmental supports requires the same planning as establishing self-management strategies. Carefully assessing the context, having a plan for measuring success or lack of success, investing the client and others in the supports, and building in time for the client to get accustomed to using the supports are critical to the effectiveness of this type of intervention. See Appendix 5.6 for a sample patient handout. Together, the client and clinician can review the handout and select the strategies that will be most useful for that client.

Given the individual nature of strategies and environmental supports, the research literature is restricted to case reports sharing the procedures and outcomes of particular strategies (Mateer, 1997). We now provide an example of a client whose attention deficits were addressed by environmental supports and the adoption of self-management strategies.

Case Example of Using Strategies and Environmental Support

Matt was a 24-year-old graduate student who had suffered a serious brain injury in a ski accident when he was 18. He was in coma for a week and suffered PTA for an estimated additional week. CT scans suggested right frontal lesions and suspected diffuse axonal shearing. After taking a year off from college, Matt returned and was able to complete his undergraduate degree. His grade point average was significantly lower, however, and he reported that schoolwork was much more difficult. He put in many extra hours and was unable to pursue extracurricular activities. Most of his difficulties were related to decreased new learning abilities and reduced attention. He also exhibited a slightly blunted affect. Prior to his accident, he had been a very high-performing student. He had not received any previous cognitive rehabilitation.

When Matt entered a 1-year teacher graduate education program, he sought cognitive rehabilitation because he was no longer able to "barely get by in classes." Upon interview, he said his greatest difficulty was in following lectures. He would periodically "zone out" and miss about 10 minutes of a lecture before he realized he was lost. He brought in some sample lecture notes, which he and the clinician analyzed. It was observed that the gaps in information often occurred at the beginning of a lecture; it appeared as if Matt had trouble getting back on track once he experienced being lost. He and the clinician decided to try a strategy whereby he would come to class at least 10 minutes early and establish a "ready set." He would assemble his materials (notepaper, pencil, and handouts) and look over the notes from the previous lecture and the associated reading for that day. At the end of the lecture, he filled out a rating form designed to record any "zone-outs"; he made notations about when they occurred and for about how long. Matt implemented the strategy with little difficulty. After 2 weeks, however, it became apparent that it was not helpful in reducing the attention lapses, so Matt and the clinician discussed trying a new strategy.

The next strategy was to have Matt audiotape his lectures. He purchased a microcassette recorder and began taping lectures and listening to them at home to fill in any gaps. Matt also continued to log the attention lapses. Unfortunately, this strategy was not successful either, because the amount of time it took to listen to every lecture outside of class was too burdensome. Next, the clinician helped Matt qualify for "disabled student" status and obtain a peer to take notes for him. Again, however, this was not successful, as Matt could not integrate the student's notes with the readings.

The clinician went to observe Matt in a lecture and then reviewed his lecture notes. She observed that he asked quite a few questions in class. They both discovered that the segments surrounding the time when he asked questions contained the most complete notes. They developed a new strategy whereby Matt would jot down relevant questions that he might ask the professor in the margin while he was listening to the lecture. This produced a dramatic improvement, and the attention lapses became less frequent and shorter in duration. Certainly he continued to struggle with school performance, but he was able to attend to lectures and achieve passing grades.

Matt's case illustrates the importance of careful assessment, involving the client in strategy selection, and having a method to measure the success of a strategy.

Use of External Devices

A number of external devices can assist individuals in tracking information and initiating planned activities. Chapter 7 reviews principles and procedures for selecting and training the use of external devices to help people compensate for decreased memory and executive functions. This information is also relevant for individuals whose attention problems may be lessened by using an external aid to help them track and respond to information. Devices that can be particularly useful for individuals with attention impairments include the following:

- Written calendar systems with day planners
- Written checklists
- Electronic organizers
- Voice-activated message recorders
- Task-specific devices such as pill box reminders, key finders, and watch alarms

The reader is referred to Chapter 7 for a description of device options, as well as methods for selecting and teaching people to use these devices.

Psychosocial Support

The importance of psychosocial support for managing cognitive difficulties cannot be underestimated. The connection between emotional states and cognitive functioning is well established (Kay, 1992). Individuals who have experienced a life-altering change in functioning may display reactive effects (including grief, anger, and denial) that affect their information-processing capacity. The source of an attentional deficit may be organic brain damage (i.e., changes in the neural circuitry that subserves attention abilities), psychoemotional (e.g., inability to process information adequately due to overwhelming grief), or a combination of these.

Effective management of cognitive impairments requires a clinician to be skilled at providing psychosocial support as well as neurocognitive intervention. Approaches to psychosocial support include supported listening, brain injury education, relaxation training, psychotherapy, and grief therapy (see Chapter 12).

Decreased attention ability may be the result of an interaction between neurological impairment and psychosocial factors; individuals can become paralyzed by even very subtle symptoms. Kay (1992) discusses possible dysfunctional scenarios arising from a person's "shaken sense of self" after a brain injury. He describes problems due to "the fear of going crazy" and "conditioned anxiety" responses about one's performance. He acknowledges the importance of neuropsychological rehabilitation such as attention process training, as well as psychosocial therapies including stress management, family systems therapy, and psychotherapy. It is important to acknowledge the interaction between neurological dysfunction and psychoemotional difficulties when designing a remediation program. Therapists need to link psychosocial treatment to changes in neuropsychological functioning.

In recent years, the benefits of self-efficacy and personal empowerment have begun to be realized within the realm of cognitive rehabilitation. Therapists have gradually moved away from traditional medical models (where we are the experts and prescribe the treatment) toward a therapy process where we "partner" with our clients and, together, determine what activities and goals may be most helpful (Andrews & Andrews, 2000). Such partnering helps individuals take control of their situation and reduces feelings of victimization and discouragement (Sohlberg, 2000). Behavioral logs and facilitated self-observation are among the methods used to empower individuals to make changes. Sohlberg (2000) describes how patients with mild brain injuries benefit from assistance in tracking their successes and their concerns, and from discussing their observations with a therapist. Helping clients focus and track the contexts where their attention processes break down, as well as situations where attention is functioning well, often leads to a perception that attention is improving. It may be that people inadvertently do things to improve their functioning due to increased self-monitoring. Alternatively, people may feel more in control when they are assisted to pay attention to their own functioning during their day-to-day lives (Sohlberg, Glang, & Todis, 1998).

The effectiveness of psychosocial support is illustrated in a recent study comparing the effects of psychosocial support and attention process training on persons with acquired brain injury (Sohlberg et al., 2000). Whereas the attention process training was associated with greater improvement on neuropsychological test performance, as well as with more robust patient perceptions of improved attention functioning on a day-to-day basis, the power of the psychosocial support was unanticipated. Some improvement in cognitive functioning was noted following the psychosocial treatment, which consisted of brain injury education and supported listening. The authors suggest that some individuals may have been significantly depressed; the information about their brain injury combined with the supportive listening may have lessened depression or anxiety symptoms, which may have been one cause of their reduced attention abilities. Another explanation may be that supplying individuals with information about the nature of their disabilities helps them engage in behaviors that compensate for difficulties. The medical community may benefit from changing the traditional perception of a placebo effect as a research method to determine whether an intervention *really* worked, to encouraging therapies that produce and build upon a so-called "placebo effect." Interventions that empower individuals to understand and modify their circumstances may be surprisingly efficacious.

An actual case report illustrates the potential for psychosocial support to be an effective intervention for attention problems.

Case Example of Using Psychosocial Support

Maria was a 45-year-old woman with an acquired brain injury due to a motor vehicle accident. She was unconscious for 2 days, and the length of her PTA was estimated at 1 week. She received 2 weeks of inpatient rehabilitation and 7 follow-up outpatient visits for speech, occupational therapy, and physical therapy. At 20 months after her injury, she sought additional help for her "thinking problems." At that time, she was unemployed and living in her own house. She was unable to drive. Her daughter assisted with groceries and money management. Maria indicated that she mostly just watched television or sat. The only activity that she could describe doing was occasional baking, which both she and her daughter reported was usually not successful. Prior to her accident, she had been a receptionist at the same medical office for 15 years.

Cognitive testing revealed significant impairments on attention tests. The cognitive rehabilitation plan was to begin with brain injury education and supportive listening to improve Maria's depression and increase her self-esteem. This would be followed by selecting self-management strategies with Maria and teaching her to implement them. Maria received nine 1-hour sessions where she learned about her brain injury and its cognitive consequences. She also had an opportunity to share feelings about her loss of independence and how much she missed work. These thoughts were incorporated into a journal. She was further supported in discovering what had not been affected by her brain injury. She initiated developing some advocacy materials for people with brain injuries, based on what she had learned.

Before the self-management portion of the cognitive rehabilitation plan was begun, the cognitive tests were readministered. Significant improvements were noted on the attention tests. Maria's scores on the PASAT, the Gordon Diagnostic System, and the Dichotic Listening Test all increased by more than 1 standard deviation. She and her daughter also endorsed improved cognitive functioning on rating scales.

The improvements in Maria's neuropsychological performance were unanticipated, since they were administered following psychosocial support. However, Maria had received little support following her injury and had become quite isolated. She also exhibited little understanding of the changes in her abilities due to her accident. At the beginning of treatment she indicated how much she missed her work and friends, but she did not like to bother her daughter by asking her to take her places. She also expressed lingering anger at the drunk driver who had caused her accident. Maria presented as depressed. It is likely that the education and support helped lessen the effects of her depression, and that this resulted in improved cognitive functioning.

Also, simply getting out and coming to therapy may have been a significant factor in improving her psychosocial status. Hence the therapist worked with Maria's daughter to develop some community involvements and reduce barriers to transportation.

Individualized Programming

In this part of the chapter, four different approaches to managing attention impairments have been discussed: attention process training, training use of strategies and environmental support, training use of external aids, and the provision of psychosocial support. The selection of therapeutic approaches depends upon individual patient factors such as stage of recovery, responsiveness to diagnostic therapy, and amount of authorized services. Most often, several therapies are used in combination. For example, a therapy regimen for attention deficits might include attention process training for specific components of attention (e.g., sustained attention), in conjunction with training in pacing techniques and psychosocial support (where the client keeps behavioral logs and discusses insights gained from tracking attention successes and attention lapses). An hour-long treatment session might contain 30 minutes devoted to attention exercises (which are also supplemented in a home program), 15 minutes devoted to practicing pacing techniques, and 15 minutes spent reviewing behavioral logs. Programming will ultimately be driven by individual client profiles.

SUMMARY

The importance of attentional functioning in all aspects of daily functioning is well established. Attention can be divided into discrete components that can be differentially affected by brain damage (i.e., focused, sustained, selective, alternating, and divided attention). Although the attentional system appears quite vulnerable to disruption, it also appears to be amenable to treatment. Indeed, studies examining the effectiveness of attention process training are some of the most compelling in the cognitive rehabilitation literature. In addition, training individuals in the use of strategies and providing environmental and psychosocial supports are useful methods for addressing attentional impairments. Whether therapy involves a direct process-oriented approach, strategy training, or some combination of techniques, the ultimate measure of therapeutic success is improved functioning in real-world activities that are dependent upon attention.

REFERENCES

Adams, A., Carnine, D., & Gersten, R. (1982). Instructional strategies for studying content area texts in the intermediate grades. *Reading Research Quarterly, 18,* 27–55.

Andrews, J. R., & Andrews, M. A. (2000). *Family-based treatment in communicative disorders: A systematic approach.* DeKalb, IL: Janelle Publications.

Awh, E., Smith, E. E., & Jonides, J. (1995). Human rehearsal processes and the frontal lobes: PET evidence. *Annals of the New York Academy of Sciences, 769,* 97–117).

Baddeley, A. D. (1986). *Working memory.* Oxford, England: Clarendon Press.

Baddeley, A. D., & Hitch, G. (1974). Working memory. In G. A. Bower (Ed), *The psychology of learning and motivation* (Vol. 8, pp. 47–89). New York: Academic Press.

Bakay Pragay, E., Mirsky, A. F., Ray, C. L., Turner, D. F., & Mirsky, C. V. (1978). Neuronal activity in the brainstem reticular formation during performance of a "go–no go" visual attention task in the monkey. *Experimental Neurology, 60,* 83–95.

Ben-Yishay, Y., Piasetsky, E. B., & Rattock, J. (1987). A systematic method for ameliorating disorders of basic attention. In M. J. Meyer, A. L. Menton, & L. Diller (Eds.), *Neuropsychological rehabilitation* (pp. 165–181). Edinburgh: Churchill Livingstone.

Brooks, D. N., & McKinlay, W. (1987). Return to work within the first seven years of severe head injury. *Brain Injury, 1,* 5–15.

Burgess, P. W., Alderman, N., Wilson, B. A., Evans, J. J., & Emslie, H. C. (1996). The Dysexecutive Questionnaire (DEX). In B. A. Wilson, N. Alderman, P. W. Burgess, H. C. Emslie, & J. J. Evans (Eds.), *Behavioural assessment of the Dysexecutive Syndrome.* Burry, St. Edmunds, England: Thames Valley Test Company.

Cabeza, R., & Nyberg, L. (1997). Imaging cognition: An empirical review of PET studies with normal subjects. *Journal of Cognitive Neuroscience, 9*(1), 1–26.

Diller, L., Ben-Yishay, Y., Gerstman, L. J., Goodkin, R., Gordon, W., & Weinberg, J. (1974). *Studies of cognition and rehabilitation in hemiplegia* (Rehabilitation Monograph No. 50). New York: New York University Medical Center.

Dywan, J., & Segalowitz, S. J. (1996). Self and family ratings of adaptive behavior after traumatic brain injury: Psychometric scores and frontally generated ERPs. *Journal of Head Trauma Rehabilitation, 11*(2), 79–95.

Gray, J. M., Robertson, I., Pentland, B., & Anderson, S. (1992). Microcomputer-based attentional retraining after brain damage: A randomized group controlled trial. *Neuropsychological Rehabilitation, 2,* 97–115.

Gronwall, D. (1987). Advances in the assessment of attention and information processing after head injury. In H. S. Levin, J. Grafman, & H. M. Eisenberg (Eds.), *Neurobehavioral recovery from head injury* (pp. 355–395). New York: Oxford University Press.

Gronwall, D. (1991). Minor head injury. *Neuropsychology, 5,* 235–265.

Hillier, S. L. (1997). Awareness and perceptions of outcomes after traumatic brain injury. *Brain Injury, 11,* 525–536.

Hinkeldey, N. S., & Corrigan, J. D. (1990). The structure of head-injured patients' behavioral complaints: A preliminary study. *Brain Injury, 4,* 115–134.

Kay, T. (1992). Neuropsychological diagnosis: Disentangling the multiple determinants of functional disability after mild traumatic brain injury. *Physical Medicine and Rehabilitation State of the Art Reviews,* 109–127.

Kinsella, G. (1998). Assessment of attention following traumatic brain injury: A review. *Neuropsychological Rehabilitation, 8*(3), 351–375.

Malec, J., Rao, N., Jones, R., & Stubbs, K. (1984). Video game practice effects on sustained attention in patients with craniocerebral trauma. *Cognitive Rehabilitation, 2,* 18–23.

Mapou, R. (1995). A cognitive framework for neuropsychological assessment. In R. Mapou & J. Spector (Eds.), *Clinical neuropsychological assessment: A cognitive approach* (pp. 295–337). New York: Plenum Press.

Mateer, C. A. (1992). Systems of care for post-concussive syndrome. In L. J. Horn & N. D. Zasler (Eds.), *Rehabilitation of post-concussive disorders* (pp. 143–160). Philadelphia: Henley & Belfus.

Mateer, C. A. (1997). Rehabilitation of individuals with frontal lobe impairment. In J. Leon-Carrion (Ed.), *Neuropsychological rehabilitation: Fundamentals, innovations and directions* (pp. 285–300). Delray Beach, FL: GR Press/St. Lucie Press.

Mateer, C. A., & Sohlberg, M. M. (1988). A paradigm shift in memory rehabilitation.

In H. Whitaker (Ed.), *Neuropsychological studies of nonfocal brain injury: Dementia and closed head injury* (pp. 202–225). New York: Springer-Verlag.

Mateer, C. A., Sohlberg, M. M., & Crinean, J. (1987). Perceptions of memory functions in individuals with closed head injury. *Journal of Head Trauma Rehabilitation, 2,* 79–84.

Mateer, C. M., Sohlberg, M. M., & Youngman, P. (1990). The management of acquired attention and memory disorders following closed head injury. In R. Wood (Ed.), *Cognitive rehabilitation in perspective* (pp. 68–95). London: Taylor & Francis.

Mateer, C. M., & Mapou, R. L. (1996). Understanding, evaluating and managing attention disorders after traumatic brain injury. *Journal of Head Trauma Rehabilitation, 11*(2), 1–16.

Mateer, C. A., & Ojemann, G. A. (1983). Thalamic mechanisms in language and memory. In J. Segalowitz (Ed.), *Language functions and brain organization* (pp. 171–191). New York: Academic Press.

McKinlay, W. M. (1981). The short-term outcome of severe blunt head injury as reported by relatives of the injured persons. *Journal of Neurology, Neurosurgery and Psychiatry, 44,* 527–533.

Mirsky, A., Anthony, B. J., Duncan, C. C., Ahearn, M. B., & Kellam, S. G. (1991). Analysis of the elements of attention: A neuropsychological approach. *Neuropsychological Review, 2,* 109–145.

Neimann, H., Ruff, R. M., & Baser, C. A. (1990). Computer-assisted attention training in head injured individuals: A controlled efficacy study of an outpatient program. *Journal of Clinical and Consulting Psychology, 58,* 811–817.

Nudo, R. (1996). *Functional plasticity in primate motor cortex: Implications for stroke rehabilitation.* Paper presented at the Towards a New Science of Cognitive Rehabilitation convention, St. Louis, MO.

Park, N., Proulx, G. B., & Towers, W. M. (1999). Evaluation of the Attention Process Training programme. *Neuropsychological Rehabilitation, 9*(2), 135–154.

Ponsford, J. L., & Kinsella, G. (1988). Evaluation of a remedial programme for attentional deficits following closed head injury. *Journal of Clinical and Experimental Neuropsychology, 10,* 693–708.

Ponsford, J. L., & Kinsella, G. (1991). The use of a rating scale of attentional behavior. *Neuropsychological Rehabilitation, 1,* 241–257.

Ponsford, J. L., & Kinsella, G. (1992). Attention deficits following closed head injury. *Journal of Clinical and Experimental Neuropsychology, 14,* 822–838.

Posner, M., & Petersen, S. E. (1990). The attention system of the human brain. *Annual Review of Neuroscience, 13,* 25–42.

Robertson, I., Ward, T., Ridgeway, V., & Nimmo-Smith, I. (1996). The structure of normal human attention: The Test of Everyday Attention. *Journal of the International Neuropsychological Society, 2,* 525–534.

Ruff, R. M., Baser, C. A., Johnson, J. W., Marshall, L. F., Klauber, S. K., Klauber, M. R., & Minteer, M. (1989). Neuropsychological rehabilitation: An experimental study with head injured patients. *Journal of Head Trauma Rehabilitation, 4*(3), 20–36.

Sbordone, R., & Long, C. J. (1996). *Ecological validity of neuropsychological testing.* Delray Beach, FL: GR Press/St. Lucie Press.

Simmons-Mackie, N., & Damico, J. S. (1996). Accounting for handicaps in aphasia: Communicative assessment from an authentic social perspective. *Disability and Rehabilitation, 18,* 540–549.

Sivak, M., Hill, C. S., Henson, D. L., Butler, B. P., Siber, S. M., & Olson, P. (1984a). Improved driving performance following perceptual retraining in persons with brain damage. *Archives of Physical Medicine and Rehabilitation, 65,* 163–167.

Sivak, M., Hill, C. S., & Olson, P. (1984b). Computerized video tasks as training techniques for driving related perceptual deficits in persons with brain damage: A pilot evaluation. *International Journal of Rehabilitation Research, 7,* 389–398.

Sohlberg, M. M. (2000). Psychotherapy approaches. In S. Raskin & C. Mateer (Eds.), *Neuropsychological management of mild traumatic brain injury* (pp. 137–156). New York: Oxford University Press.

Sohlberg, M. M., Glang, A., & Todis, B. (1998). Improvement during baseline: Three case studies encouraging collaborative research when evaluating caregiver training. *Brain Injury, 12*(4), 333–346.

Sohlberg, M. M., Johnson, L., Paule, L., Raskin, S. A., & Mateer, C. A. (1994). *Attention Process Training II: A program to address attentional deficits for persons with mild cognitive dysfunction.* Puyallup, WA: Association for Neuropsychological Research and Development.

Sohlberg, M. M., & Mateer, C. A. (1987). Effectiveness of an attention training program. *Journal of Clinical and Experimental Neuropsychology, 19,* 117–130.

Sohlberg, M. M., & Mateer, C. A. (1989). *Introduction to cognitive rehabilitation: Theory and practice.* New York: Guilford Press.

Sohlberg, M. M., McLaughlin, K., Pavese, A., Heidrich, A., & Posner, M. (2000). Evaluation of attention process training and brain injury education in persons with acquired brain injury. *Journal of Clinical and Experimental Neuropsychology, 22*(1), 656–676.

Sturm, W., Hartje, W., Orgass, B., & Willmes, K. (1993). Computer-assisted rehabilitation of attention impairments. In F. Stachowiak (Ed.), *Developments in the assessment of rehabilitation and brain-damaged patients.* Tübingen, Germany: Narr.

Sturm, W., Willmes, K., Orgass, B., & Hartje, W. (1997). Do specific attention deficits need specific training? *Neuropsychological Rehabilitation, 7,* 81–103.

Stuss, D. T., Stethem, L. L., Hugeholtz, N., Picton, T., Pivik, J., & Richard, M. T. (1989). Reaction time after head injury: Fatigue, divided and focused attention and consistency of performance. *Journal of Neurology, Neurosurgery Psychiatry, 52,* 742–748.

Tallal, P., Miller, S. L., Bedi, G., Byma, G., Wang, X. Q., Nagarajan, S. S., Schreiner, C., Jenkins, W. M., & Merzenich, M. M. (1996). Language comprehension in language-learning impaired children improved with acoustically modified speech. *Science, 271,* 81–84.

Van Zomeren, A. H., Brouwer, N. H., & Deelman, B. G. (1984). Attention deficits: The riddle of selectivity, speed and alertness. In N. Brooks (Ed.), *Closed head injury: Psychological, social, and family consequences* (pp. 74–107). Oxford: Oxford University Press.

Winograd, P., & Hare, V. C. (1988). Direct instruction of reading comprehension strategies: The nature of teacher explanation. In C. Weinstein, E. Goetz & P. Alexander (Eds.), *Learning and study strategies: Issues in assessment, instruction and evaluation* (pp. 121–138). New York: Academic Press.

Wood, R. L., & Fussey, I. (1987). Computer assisted cognitive retraining: A controlled study. *International Disability Studies, 9,* 149–153.

APPENDIX 5.1

APT-II ATTENTION QUESTIONNAIRE

Client Name_____

Rater's Name and Relationship to Client (if applicable)_____

Therapist_____   Date_____

I. RATING SCALE*: Please answer the following questions about your (or _____'s) attention as it applies to daily functioning by ticking the box which offers the best description.

DESCRIPTION	Not a problem or no change from before	Only gets in the way on occasion (less than once a week)	Sometimes gets in the way (about 1-3 times per week)	Frequently gets in the way (is a problem most days)	Is a problem all the time (affects most activities)
1. Seem to lack mental energy to do activities					
2. Am slow to respond when asked a question or when participating in conversations					
3. Can't keep mind on activity or thought because mind keeps wandering					
4. Can't keep mind on activity or thought because mind feels "spacy" or "blank"					
5. Can only concentrate for very short periods of time					
6. Miss details or make mistakes because level of concentration decreased					
7. Easily get off track if other people milling about nearby					
8. Easily distracted by surrounding noise					
9. Trouble paying attention to conversation, if more than one other person					
10. Easily lose place if task or thinking interrupted					
11. Easily overwhelmed if task has several components					
12. Difficult to pay attention to more than one thing at a time					
13.					
14.					

Scoring: a) total number of items ticked in second column multiplied by (1)_____

b) total number of items ticked in third column multiplied by (2) _____

c) total number of items ticked in fourth column multiplied by (3)_____

d) total number of items ticked in fifth column multiplied by (4) _____

Total Score: add a) through d) _____

II. INDIVIDUALIZED ATTENTIONAL PROBLEM LIST: In the space provided below describe the five most frequent and frustrating breakdowns in your attention ability. The first line has been filled out with an example description.

Describe Attention Breakdown (include setting and approx. freq.)	What do you do when it occurs?
Example: I cannot concentrate when I am preparing dinner because the noise from the children playing around my feet and even in the next room distracts me. I forget ingredients or parts of the meal and usually feel totally frustrated during this time. This happens for every dinner.	I often yell or blow up at the children or cry while I am cooking. Sometimes I just give up and make something simple like sandwiches.
1.	
2.	
3.	
4.	
5.	

APPENDIX 5.2

APT-II SUSTAINED ATTENTION SCORESHEET

Name _M.S._

Treatment Activity/Level _Number Sequence Descending_
_4 #s, 0-30_

Percent Correct	Cumulative # of minutes						
100	20						
90	18						
80	16						
70	14						
60	12						
50	10						
40	8						
30	6						
20	4						
10	2						
0	--						

Date/ Trial #'s

7/23	7/24	7/25	7/26	7/27	7/30
1-10	11-20	21-30	31-40	1-10	11-20

Comments

kept interrupting task to discuss family problems

took 1st 5 minutes of session to listen to family update before task

Brought in "attention success log"- very pleased with improvements

KEY

● -- Percent correct out of ten trials
X -- Cumulative # of minutes to complete ten trials

Note. From Sohlberg, Johnson, Paule, Raskin, and Mateer (1994). Copyright 1994 by the Association for Neuropsychological Research and Development. Materials now available from Lash & Associates, 708 Young Forest Drive, Wake Forest, NC 27587. Reprinted by permission.

APPENDIX 5.3

APT-II ALTERNATING ATTENTION SCORESHEET

Name _L. V._

Treatment Activity/Level _serial numbers (series III & IV)_

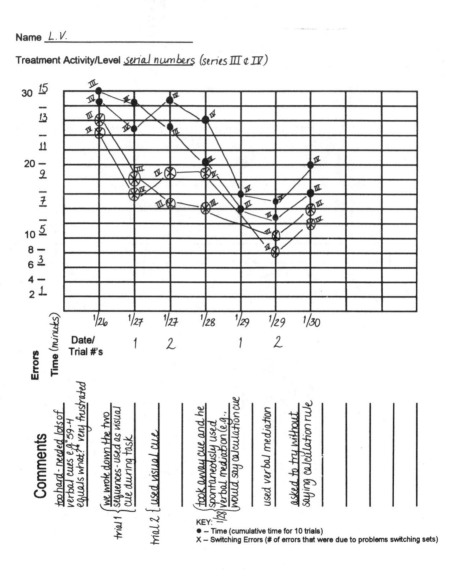

KEY:
● — Time (cumulative time for 10 trials)
X — Switching Errors (# of errors that were due to problems switching sets)

APPENDIX 5.4

APT-II SELECTIVE ATTENTION SCORESHEET

Name _R.D._

Treatment Activity/Level _math worksheets (addition and subtraction using a calculator)_

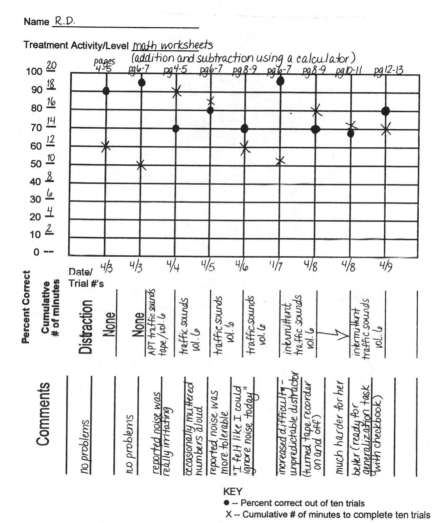

KEY
● -- Percent correct out of ten trials
X -- Cumulative # of minutes to complete ten trials

159

APPENDIX 5.5

APT-II SELECTIVE ATTENTION GENERALIZATION SHEET

Examples of Generalization Activities:

--multistep task with personalized background noise tape (e.g., cooking while playing tape of children noise; office task with typing/phone noise tape; checkbook task with restaurant tape)

--multistep task with actual background distractor (e.g., cooking task with children playing in the kitchen; paying bills with television on; computer entry with unrelated conversation nearby)

Generalization Goal: _Larry will do weekly bill paying/correspondence sitting at desk while listening to tape of children playing at lowest volume and give "irritation rating" of 2 or less for 2 consecutive weeks_

DATE	ACTIVITY (note performance in quiet)	DISTRACTOR (e.g., tape/volume, other)	PERFORMANCE	COMMENTS
10/2	(quiet area - has no problem with task) paying bills, filing mail, answering correspondence	kid tape, lowest volume	Irritation rating - "3"	I got up twice & turned off tape then turned it back on
10/9	→		Irritation rating - "3"	turned off tape 1 time
10/16		→	Irritation rating - "2"	felt better - had practiced using tape twice during the week while cooking

Larry's rating scale :   1 - Do not feel irritated.
2 - Feel mildly irritated - can continue without stopping.
3 - Feel moderately irritated - fists clench, jaw tightens. Have to occasionally stop task.
4 - Feel extremely irritated - swearing. Cannot continue task.

APPENDIX 5.6

PATIENT HANDOUT: ATTENTION STRATEGIES

This handout lists a number of useful strategies you can try to manage persistent attention problems.

1. Reduce distractions.
   - Turn off radios, TVs, etc. when concentrating (e.g., trying to read) or when having a conversation.
   - Use earplugs.
   - Close curtains so you are not tempted to stare out the window.
   - "De-clutter" your environment.

2. Avoid crowds.
   - Plan your day so you can shop and/or drive during "off" hours.
   - If you must be in a crowded situation, don't require yourself to do something that demands a lot of concentration.

3. Manage fatigue.
   - As soon as you begin to feel overwhelmed, take a short break—the sooner the break, the faster you will be able to get back to what you were doing and be effective.
   - Be persistent and keep coming back to what you were doing.
   - Don't push yourself so hard that you get frustrated.
   - Get enough sleep—naps are good as long as you can still sleep during the night.

4. Avoid interruptions.
   - Turn off the ringer on your phone or use an answering machine when you are trying to get something done.
   - Use a "do not disturb" sign if you live in a busy household.

5. Get sufficient exercise.
   - Research is beginning to show that a more efficient body means a more efficient brain.
   - Regular exercise is good for your thinking skills.

6. Ask for help.

Memory Theory
Applied to Intervention

MEMORY THEORY

Memory, like attention, is not a unitary process, but an alliance of interrelated subsystems. We have come a long way in understanding these relationships. In this section, we consider a number of memory models with particular relevance to cognitive rehabilitation.

Stages of Memory and Associated Neuroanatomical Correlates

The evolution in our understanding of memory has resulted in defining stages of memory. Understanding these stages provides a helpful taxonomy for organizing memory assessment and treatment activities. Although there is variation among researchers, most agree that the stages of memory include *attention, encoding, storage,* and *retrieval* (Baddeley, Wilson, & Watts, 1995; Huppert & Piercy, 1982; McDowall, 1984; Posner & Petersen, 1990). These stages are closely linked and interact. Neuroanatomical correlates for different stages of remembering have been identified and are described below.

Attention

The attention stage incorporates a multiplicity of functions described in Chapter 5. At the most fundamental level, it includes alertness and arousal. At higher levels, maintaining concentration over time (sustained attention), resisting interference (selective attention), and being able to allocate attentional resources (alternating and divided attention) are important. The concept of working memory, which allows for temporarily holding on to information, is an integral part of the attention process. Attention is a logical component of any memory model; it is this capacity that initially allows the system to gain access to and ultimately to utilize incoming information.

Decreased alertness, arousal, and sustained attention have been associated with damage to brainstem structures or to diffuse, bilateral subcortical damage. Difficulties with higher levels of attention, such as selective, alternating, and divided attention, are more likely to reflect either disruption of higher-level thalamic structures that have attentional gating functions or disruption of frontal lobe structures that control attention. Patients who have diffuse damage secondary to closed head injury typically display attentional impairments. Theoretical and neuropsychological constructs relevant to attention and working memory are reviewed more fully in Chapter 5.

Encoding

Encoding is also an initial stage of memory. It is the level of analysis performed on material to be remembered. Remembering verbal material depends upon encoding its phonological characteristics, whereas remembering visual information depends upon encoding the graphic representation. Craik and Lockhart (1972) highlighted the importance of encoding to recall ability. They advanced the *levels-of-processing hypothesis*, suggesting that information that is "deeply" processed will have a higher likelihood of being recalled than information that is "shallowly" processed. For example, subjects who processed word lists semantically (a deep level of analysis) by being asked meaning-based questions ("Is it a kind of jungle animal?") had better recall than did subjects who processed the word list phonologically ("Does the word rhyme with *dog*?"). The poorest performance was in subjects who were asked to process words superficially by paying attention to their visual appearance. Encoding has been shown to be enhanced by a number of strategies that result in deeper processing. For example, chunking or categorizing information is a more effective rehearsal strategy than simply repeating the information to be remembered.

Recent work in functional neuroanatomy suggests that information about the meaning of objects and words are stored as clusters of brain networks. For example, different types or classes of objects (e.g., animals and tools) are associated with brain networks located in specific cortical regions (Martin, Wiggs, Lalonde, & Mack, 1994). Tasks requiring naming different categories of objects will activate different cortical networks.

Memory problems secondary to encoding deficits result from damage to a number of brain structures and networks. These include diencephalic structures (e.g., dorsomedial thalamus and frontal lobe systems) and lateralized damage to the hemisphere controlling language systems or visual processing. Such damage disrupts the understanding, organization, and categorization of material to be remembered. Patients with damage to these systems will have difficulty remembering because they have not adequately encoded the material. Thus, under circumstances where they successfully encode information, they demonstrate a normal rate of forgetting. Classic diagnoses for patients who typically display encoding deficits are Korsokoff's syndrome and bilateral thalamic infarcts.

Storage

Storage of memory refers to the transfer of a transient memory to a form or location in the brain for permanent retention or access. The mechanisms accounting for how new learning interacts with old learning are not well understood. We do know that storage can be disrupted when there is interference in the learning process. *Retroactive interference* refers to interference in learning new information due to the presentation of subsequent learning material. *Proactive interference* refers to disruption in memory due to the presentation of learning material prior to the new learning. Several theoretical constructs provide for integration of new memories within the individual's existing cognitive–linguistic schema.

Persons with damage to hippocampal and bilateral medial temporal lobe structures often display difficulty with storage. They may analyze information appropriately (i.e., demonstrate successful encoding), but are unable to maintain it in storage. Their long-term memory is impaired, and their retention of information deteriorates after exposure; in other words, they have an abnormally rapid rate of forgetting. Diagnoses that may result in a medial temporal lobe syndrome include brain damage due to anoxia, herpes encephalitis, and early Alzheimer's disease. Persons who have had electroconvulsive therapy may also have transitory problems with storage.

Retrieval

Retrieval of memory refers to searching for or activating existing memory traces. It requires monitoring the accuracy and appropriateness of memories pulled from storage. Tulving (1966) conducted a classic experiment examining retrieval mechanisms. He showed that simply attempting to recall a previously presented word list facilitated learning; in other words, recall improved with successive administration of lists. Retrieval is often examined by comparing recognition ability to recall ability. Recognition of previously presented information is typically superior to straight recall of that information. A variety of cueing strategies may be used to facilitate recall.

Retrieval is usually linked to frontal lobe contributions to memory ability. Frontal lobe structures are involved in strategy formation, memory for temporal order, self-monitoring, and initiating retrieval. Persons with traumatic brain injury and associated frontal lobe damage often exhibit changes in the ability to efficiently retrieve stored information. Persons with frontal damage are specifically susceptible to memory errors of distortion and confabulation. They may have poor source memory and confuse the source of their learning; they recall facts but not the context of when information was acquired (Shimamura & Squire, 1991).

Various systems and structures in the brain influence different aspects of memory, as indicated above. The type of memory loss that results from brain trauma will depend upon the nature of the pathology and the degree and locus of injury. Often more than one "stage" of remembering is affected. Focal neuropathology that selectively produces a storage or retrieval deficit is less common.

Review of a client's medical record may reveal damage to particular brain structures, which may help a clinician formulate hypotheses about the nature of predicted memory impairment. Figure 6.1 illustrates the major neuroanatomical structures involved in memory and new learning. The hippocampus and hippocampal gyri as well as the parahippocampal gyrus and entorhinal cotrices, all bilateral structures deep in the temporal lobes, are critical for learning. They act as a semi-passive loop that holds information until it is stored (usually by association with existing semantic knowledge) in areas important for semantic memory. Some researchers suggest that the incorporation of new knowledge leads to changes in brain structure. Over the course of many repetitions of the same or substantially similar episodes of information processing, they suggest there will be synaptic changes among connections in neocortical systems (neural substrates involved in higher cognitive processing, including parietal, temporal, and occipital lobe circuits). When there is an accumulation of such changes, a memory or cognitive skill may be acquired (McClelland & McNaughton, 1995). There is substantial evidence that distinct neural systems allow for different types of memory (e.g., long-term versus short-term memory).

There is still much to be learned about the neurocircuitry of memory. For example, the roles of the amygdala and mamillary body are thought to be critical to memories with emotional significance, but this process is not fully understood. As noted in Chapter 5, researchers are increasingly recognizing the very important role of the frontal lobes in allocating attention and organizing memories. Both *time tagging* (the ability to retrieve the temporal order of information from memory) and *source monitoring* (the ability to remember the source of learned information) have been shown to be involved in frontal systems (see Baddeley et al., 1995; Shimamura & Squire, 1991).

Types of Memory

Time-Dependent Forms of Memory

We have described the different levels or stages involved in remembering and their corresponding neuroanatomical correlates. Another clinically im-

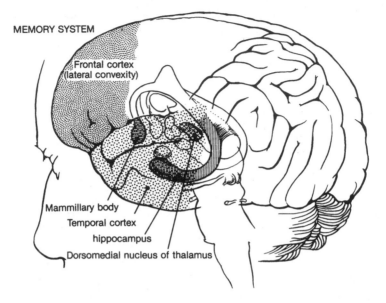

FIGURE 6.1. The major neuroanatomical structures involved in memory and new learning, including the lateral temporal cortex, the hippocampus, the dorsomedial nucleus of thalamus, and the frontal lobe. Copyright 1988 by Biomedical Illustrations, Inc. Reprinted by permission.

portant taxonomy distinguishes between two types of time-dependent memory—*long-term* versus *short-term* memory (see Table 6.1). This distinction is primarily based upon (1) the *duration* of a memory store and (2) the *capacity* of the store. Duration refers to the length of time information is held in store, and capacity refers to the amount of information that can be held in store. Long-term memory (sometimes called *secondary* memory) holds information in a permanent store and has an unlimited capacity. Information can be held in long-term memory from minutes to years after the initial exposure without any active processing. Short-term memory (sometimes called *primary* memory) is what a person can hold in the mind prior to being interrupted. It has a short duration and a very limited capacity. The average individual can hold approximately 3–5 items in short-term memory.

Short-term memory is similar to working memory (see Chapter 5); however, working memory incorporates the dynamic aspects of holding onto and manipulating information. Working memory encompasses multiple systems and constitutes the engine of cognition. It allows us to execute a large array of cognitive routines and to temporarily store information so that cognitive routines can operate (Jonides, 2000). The storage stage of remembering employs long-term memory systems, whereas the attention

TABLE 6.1. Types of Memory
_____

Time-dependent forms of memory

Short-term memory (working memory)	The storage of limited information (3–5 items) for a restricted period of times (up to a few minutes)
Long-term memory	Unlimited memory with no decay

Content-dependent forms of memory (all involve long-term memory)

Declarative memory	Explicit knowledge base
Episodic memory	Storage of events that are tagged in time and place
Semantic memory	Storage of facts
Nondeclarative memory	Implicit memory; does not require episodic memory
Procedural memory	Acquisition of perceptuomotor skills and the learning of rules and sequences
Priming	Increased chance of retrieval when previously exposed to information without explicit learning

Everyday memory

	Functional memory constructs
Prospective memory	Remembering to carry out intentions
Metamemory	Awareness about one's own memory functioning

Amnesia terms

Anterograde amnesia	Inability to acquire new information following brain damage
Retrograde amnesia	The inability to retrieve information stored prior to brain damage
Posttraumatic amnesia	Period of confusion with inability to remember events moment to moment, usually following decreased consciousness

_____

Note. Data from Markowitsch (1998).

stage of remembering is more dependent upon short-term memory. Encoding and retrieval depend upon aspects of both short- and long-term memory.

Content-Dependent Forms of Long-Term Memory

Long-term memory can be further distinguished by the type of information that is processed. We recognize two broad categories of memory that are differentially processed: *declarative* and *nondeclarative* memory (see Table 6.1). The evidence for these two distinct types of memory originated from studies demonstrating that amnesic patients showed some preserved learning ability. Patients with very severe memory impairments could learn procedures or skills, given repeated practice; however, they did not recall participating in the training sessions (see, e.g., Cohen, 1984; Squire, 1992). This line of investigation led cognitive psychologists to classify learning systems into declarative and nondeclarative memory systems (or *explicit* and *implicit* memory), each of which has its own subtypes of memory.

Declarative Learning. The declarative learning system constitutes a person's knowledge base. It implies conscious awareness and the ability to report something explicitly. It is made up of two subsystems: episodic and semantic memory.

Semantic memory refers to a broad domain of cognition composed of knowledge acquired about the world, including word meanings, classes of information, facts, and ideas. It is information that one has learned and knows, but for which one may have no recollection of when or where it was learned (Tulving, 1972). Recalling the dates of World War II and knowing that mangos are a type of fruit are examples of semantic memory.

Episodic memory is the recall of personal experiences that are tagged in time and place. It is the memory for events that one experiences. Recalling a dinner with friends or a shopping expedition relies on episodic memory, whereas semantic memory consists of memories shared by members of a community, episodic memories are unique to an individual and tied to a specific context. Most memory theorists view episodic memories as one vehicle by which semantic memory is created. The notion is that a series of episodes leads to the extraction of meaning and the formulation of knowledge or semantic memory. Hence semantic memory may store information that began as personally experienced, separate events (Baddeley et al., 1995).

The distinction between episodic and semantic memory is particularly important in cognitive rehabilitation. Following brain injury, individuals often present with preserved semantic memory (allowing them to access their old knowledge), but with a poor ability to expand their semantic memory and create new knowledge, due to impaired episodic memory. This is different from the presentation of individuals who have Alzheimer's dementia. While they too have difficulty with episodic memory, they further experience a gradual deterioration in semantic memory. Their knowledge base slowly erodes. For example, a person with dementia may mistake a brightly colored object such as a button for food. Individuals with acquired brain injury, however, do not lose this type of memory. As discussed, memory research (see, e.g., Evans et al., 2000; McClelland & McNaughton, 1995) suggests that typically new learning occurs via episodic memory, which is mediated by the hippocampus and medial temporal lobes. Following severe brain injury, learning may occur through strengthening of neocortical connections and utilize nondeclarative systems, as described below.

Nondeclarative Learning. Research has identified a type of learning that does not rely upon episodic memory. It allows one to learn without having conscious awareness of learning. Nondeclarative or implicit learning encompasses the "learning how" portion of skills, in contrast to declarative learning, which encompasses "learning that" (Squire, 1992). The most important examples of nondeclarative learning for cognitive rehabilitation are priming and procedural learning.

Priming refers to the phenomenon that cues (partial bits of information) can prompt an accurate recall without an individual's even being aware of, or recalling, that the information was previously presented. Stem completion activities are the classic examples of priming (Tulving & Schacter, 1990). If you give someone a list of words that includes the word *chair* and then, after a delay, present the stimulus *ch_ _*, the individual is more likely to say "chair" than to say "chain" or some other word that would fit in the frame, even though the person may not recollect having ever seen that word. The underlying theory is that something in the nervous system has been altered by previous exposure to information (i.e., it has been primed), and the information can be pulled out with appropriate cues or prompts. This ability is often intact in persons with amnesia; the hope is that cognitive rehabilitation efforts can capitalize on this preserved capacity in amnesic patients to achieve functional goals. Spaced retrieval, a technique that utilizes priming effects, is discussed later in this chapter.

Procedural learning refers to the acquisition of skills or action patterns. Individuals with severe memory impairments can learn to do some skills without having to recall the training. Examples include motor tasks (e.g., operating a computer) and perceptual tasks (e.g., reading modified scripts). The clinical implication of this dissociation between declarative and nondeclarative memory is that therapists may be able to tap into nondeclarative memories and assist amnesic patients to learn a functional set of procedures. Certainly, many functional tasks contain both declarative and nondeclarative elements. Future research must strive to distinguish these elements.

Potential Benefits of Errorless Learning. Numerous case studies demonstrate that even densely amnesic individuals can acquire new information. It seems that the nature of this acquisition is different than for typical individuals. Learning is slower and requires more repetition; often severely impaired individuals fail to recall the learning task and may deny that they have the knowledge despite demonstrating mastery. Learning in this population is attributed to relatively preserved nondeclarative learning (Baddeley, 1992).

Errorless learning, a method of instruction that reduces errors in the acquisition phase (Wilson, Baddeley, Evans, & Shiel, 1994), has increased our understanding of memory functioning and encouraged clinicians to be more systematic in their instruction of persons with severe memory impairments. The literature suggests that for some individuals and for certain types of tasks, eliminating the opportunity for making errors when they are initially learning a task will improve learning.

Wilson and colleagues (1994) compared errorless and errorful learning conditions in five people with memory impairments, each of whom learned a different task: names of objects; names of people; steps to program an electronic memory aid; orientation information; and general knowledge items. In all cases, the errorless learning condition was more effective in accuracy of learning and/or efficiency.

Hunkin, Squires, Aldrich, and Parkin (1998a) attempted to evaluate errorless learning for teaching a word-processing program. They demonstrated success for teaching a subject with a severe memory impairment to use a word processor on a microcomputer. The training involved several different stages, including basic errorless training, errorless recognition, errorless search and recognition, and instructed exercise. In spite of a severe anterograde memory deficit, the subject learned the procedures and could perform them as quickly without instruction as he could with instructions, showing that errorless learning can be applied to learning computer skills.

More recently, Evans and colleagues (2000) affirmed the conclusion that errorless learning is beneficial for some clients and with some tasks. In a variety of experiments involving both cued and free recall, they found a benefit of errorless learning in a name-learning task in the cued-recall condition. They did not, however, replicate the Wilson and colleagues (1994) finding showing benefits of errorless learning when teaching the steps to use an electronic organizer. The authors concluded that the benefit of errorless learning depends upon whether the recall condition requires cued recall (implicit memory) or free recall (explicit memory). However, results from a study by Hunkin, Squires, Parkin, and Tidy (1998b) suggest that errorless learning results in improved memory in both cued- and free-recall conditions. These researchers assert that errorless methods facilitate learning because they tap residual explicit memory.

The results of the few experimental studies of errorless learning are difficult to interpret because of differences in task demands (e.g., number of items to remember; procedural vs. semantic tasks) and variation in recall conditions (cued vs. free recall; nature of cues). There is also an emphasis on experimental rather than functional tasks (e.g., memory for word lists vs. practical activities) Furthermore, the training time and testing delays tend to be short; training and testing typically occur on the same day. Because of the tremendous clinical implications, errorless learning is an important area in need of further research. One relatively clear finding in the current literature is that errorless learning is beneficial across a broad range of tasks and affords the most benefit to individuals with more severe memory impairments.

Another reason to focus research efforts in this area is that errorless learning is somewhat antithetical to current rehabilitation practices. Many clinicians train and instruct their patients via a traditional "test and correct" method: They observe clients doing a target task, provide a minimal amount of cueing, and correct clients' behavior when a mistake is committed. Having clients "guess" at answers and then supply them with correct information is frequently how information is taught. As reviewed above, however, recent experimental research clearly supports an alternative training technique using errorless conditions, where therapists prevent clients from making errors by providing systematic guidance in the initial acquisition phase. For example, if a client is learning responses to an orientation questionnaire, the client will be told the correct answer until the clinician judges that the client can respond correctly without assistance. Another example is to model a particular step or procedure for a client and have the client imitate it until he or she can do it without being shown. The idea is to avoid errors during the initial learning phase in order that people do not "practice" error responses. Practice is the presumed route that most people learn.

Other Disorders of Memory

Thus far, we have described two ways to classify potential disruptions in memory. First, we have noted that memory impairment may be captured by considering changes in functioning at a particular stage of information processing (i.e., attention, encoding, storage, and retrieval). Second, memory impairment may be described by looking to see what types of learning systems are preserved and disrupted (e.g., procedural vs. declarative learning). Several other distinctions are important to understanding memory impairments. These are discussed below and summarized in Table 6.1.

Anterograde versus Retrograde Memory Loss

Anterograde memory loss affects the ability to remember events occurring *after* the onset of a memory problem. Most of the references to memory impairment discussed thus far concern difficulty with aspects of anterograde memory, such as impaired information processing. *Retrograde* memory loss refers to the loss of memory for events *prior* to an insult or injury. In many cases, retrograde memory loss, frequently termed *retrograde amnesia* (RA), is temporary; memories of life events gradually fill in until some period until just prior to the event that injured the brain. This is commonly known as *shrinking* RA. A short RA for events immediately preceding a brain trauma is common. People usually do not remember the events just prior to or during an accident, because this information remained in short-term memory and was not yet consolidated into long-term memory.

Permanent, long-term RA is uncommon and occurs only with some degree of anterograde memory loss. In general, RA affects both episodic and semantic memory to various degrees. There is usually a temporal gradient; that is, recent memories are more affected than those from earlier years (Kapur, 1993). Researchers have proposed different types of RA and attempted to pinpoint the associated neuropathology. Most agree that there exists a classic RA, distinguished by the presence of anterograde memory deficits that affect both storage and retrieval processes (Kapur, 1993; Schmidtke & Vollmer, 1997). RA is very disturbing not only for clients, but also for their families. We recall one case of an individual who, after a severe closed head injury, could not recall the process of his divorce; he was devastated by receiving the information that he was no longer married to his wife. Recovery and treatment recommendations are greatly affected by a client's response to losing personal history and the associated loss of sense of prior self.

For some clients with frontal lobe damage, RA may represent a problem with time tagging and source memory rather than an actual loss of remote memory. *Reduplicative paramnesia* is another example of an isolated neurological disturbance (rather than loss) of memory, which usually follows frontal lobe damage. It is a condition in which an individual believes that a familiar place or person has been duplicated. Neuropsychological analyses of cases of reduplicative paramnesia suggest it represents a combination of perceptual and memory deficits as well as an impaired ability to synthesize information (Patterson & Mack, 1985). Conditions such as retrograde amnesia and reduplicative paramnesia remind clinicians that memory is not a unitary function and is part of a highly integrated cognitive system.

Posttraumatic Amnesia

Posttraumatic amnesia (PTA) is a particular type of anterograde amnesia during which an individual cannot remember events from moment to moment. It is the period of confusion or disorientation that occurs following a comatose stage and is characterized by an inability to store or recall information on a day-to-day or even minute-to-minute basis. The duration of PTA is felt to be a better prognostic indicator than the length of coma (Levin, Benton, & Grossman, 1982). Measuring the duration of PTA, however, is not simple. Studies differ in their definition of when PTA begins and whether it is measured prospectively or retrospectively (Ahmed, Bierley, Sheikh, & Date, 2000). Most medical centers with rehabilitation services now attempt to record the duration of PTA using some standardized method. The Galveston Orientation and Amnesia Test, the Picture Test of Amnesia, and the Westmead Scales (see Chapter 4) are all used early following a significant brain injury to help determine when memory is returning.

Material-Specific Memory Loss

Memory loss can be specific to verbal or nonverbal material. Many memory tests assess memory loss by comparing performance on verbal and nonverbal memory tasks. This distinction implies that memory for verbally based information (letters, words, names, paragraphs) is encoded and stored separately from information that is not easily verbally labeled (abstract designs, figures, melodies, faces, spatial position). Individuals with focal deficits are more likely to manifest material-specific memory deficits than are individuals with diffuse involvement. For example, left temporal lobe damage is more likely to result in a memory impairment for words, whereas right temporal lobe damage is more likely to result in a memory impairment for visual information (Milner, 1970).

Due to the design of many memory tests, the diagnosis of a material-specific memory deficit may be overemphasized. It is often the case that differential performance on measures of verbal and nonverbal memory reflects differences in the patient's underlying capacity for the analysis of verbal versus nonverbal information, previously described as an encoding deficit. Care should be taken, however, in making presumptions about how patients are encoding, processing, or analyzing information that is presented to them. For example, a client may verbally encode a visual depiction (e.g., label an abstract drawing a "spider web"). If, however, a client demonstrates pronounced difficulty with learning and recall specific to verbal or nonverbal information, this information will greatly influence the direction of therapy.

Changes in Everyday Memory Ability

The functional implications of an individual's memory impairment ultimately guide the direction of a clinical regimen. As we have emphasized throughout this book, the goal of all neurorehabilitation programs is to improve the day-to-day functioning of individuals challenged by cognitive impairments. This has encouraged the broadening of memory models to incorporate aspects of "everyday memory." *Prospective memory* is perhaps the most practical aspect of everyday memory (Winograd, 1988). It is the ability to remember to carry out intentions. Examples of prospective memory include remembering to take a medication or return a phone call. Performance on prospective memory tasks is more highly correlated with everyday functioning than is performance on traditional recall tasks (Raskin & Sohlberg, 1996; Wilson, 1986).

In the last decade, a modest but promising body of research has begun to explore the nature of remembering intentions and has attempted to create models to organize and increase our understanding of prospective memory (for a review, see Brandimonte, Einstein, & McDaniel, 1996).

There is consensus among researchers that prospective memory is a distinct yet broad type of memory that involves a complex set of cognitive operations, including both retrospective (recall) and prospective (future) memory functions. Many of the cognitive functions associated with prospective memory functioning are described in this text within the context of attention, memory, and executive function theory.

Dobbs and Reeves (1996) clarify the cognitive functions associated with prospective memory and remind us that prospective memory is not a *type* of memory task, but is a set of *processes*. They describe the following interactive components responsible for helping us act on our intentions: (1) metaknowledge (knowledge about the specific intended task); (2) planning (formulating steps to facilitate performance); (3) monitoring (intermittently recalling that the task needs to be performed and evaluating relevant circumstances); (4) content recall (remembering the actual intended action); and (5) output monitoring (remembering whether the action has been carried out). Prospective memory training, which stimulates these functions, has been adapted as a memory rehabilitation technique; it is reviewed in detail in this chapter (Raskin & Sohlberg, 1996).

Metamemory, or people's understanding of their own memory functioning, is also a critical aspect of everyday memory. Most people possess awareness of their own strengths and weaknesses relevant to memory and learning, and this awareness influences their behavior. For example, we know there are certain actions we need to follow in order to avoid memory mishaps (e.g., jot a reminder note, write down navigational directions, use a grocery list, keep an appointment book). We further have some sense of what we know. If someone were to ask, "What was the title of that book you were talking about last month?" and we had forgotten it, we know that we would recognize it. Such judgments about the accuracy of what we know and the likelihood that we will recognize correct information have been termed *feelings of knowing* (Howieson & Lezak, 1995). Some individuals with memory problems have impaired metamemory and do not recognize the extent and/or nature of their memory impairment. They may not have sense of what actions would be useful to mitigate their memory problems and may have changes in their feelings of knowing.

IMPLICATIONS OF MEMORY THEORY FOR MANAGING DEFICITS

Management Options

Research activity has increased our understanding of what aspects of memory may be selectively impaired and preserved. This has led to the development of a variety of memory management techniques. These techniques may be roughly divided into (1) methods that aim to restore or improve memory ability across a variety of tasks and contexts, and (2) methods that are domain-specific or aim to teach a particular skill or body of information. Examples of different methods in these two categories are listed below and are discussed in the remainder of this chapter.

Restorative/generalized memory intervention approaches

- Memory practice drills
- Mnemonic strategy training
- Prospective memory training
- Metamemory training

Domain-specific memory intervention approaches

- Mnemonic strategy training for specific information
- Expanded rehearsal time (spaced retrieval methods)
- Use of preserved priming (method of vanishing cues)
- Creating a personal history (for managing RA)

A third broad category of memory management, training the use of external memory aids, does not fit clearly into either of these two domains. Some external aids may be domain-specific, because they help an individual circumvent a memory impairment and accomplish specific tasks; there is no expectation for generalization of improved memory functioning to other contexts. For example, training an individual to utilize a pill box with an alarm feature is an example of domain-specific training. Other external aids are intended to help with a wide variety of memory difficulties across a number of contexts. For example, a multifunction electronic memory and planning system might allow an individual to compensate for deficits in episodic and prospective memory by facilitating recording information related to ongoing past events and cueing the individual to initiate intended future events. Successful implementation of external memory aids depends upon careful selection and systematic instruction, incorporating what we know about learning and memory. This information is presented in Chapter 7.

Selection of Memory Management Technique(s)

A challenge for clinicians is to select the most effective memory management technique(s) from the available options. Memory tasks usually involve a composite of cognitive operations, and it is difficult to dissociate the required memory processes from other cognitive functions. The majority of patients with brain injury who exhibit memory problems have other cognitive impairments as well. Examination of the individual client's profile and the rehabilitation context will suggest an appropriate place to start. A cognitive rehabilitation plan may simultaneously utilize more than one memory intervention approach as well as other cognitive rehabilitation techniques. The selection process will be facilitated by the results of the cognitive assessment (instruments for assessing memory are described in Chapter 4). Cognitive assessment will reveal which memory processes are preserved and which are impaired, and will help identify the most pressing memory problems. A careful assessment can also assist in the prediction of long-term memory needs.

Let us consider several examples of how memory assessment information can be applied to the selection of an appropriate intervention. If a client manifests difficulty with memory due to attention or encoding, and can remember information in instances when it is successfully encoded, it may be most useful to attempt attention process training (see Chapter 5) or to address the encoding problems (e.g., language-processing therapy or setting up compensation systems to circumvent the encoding problem). If, however, a client is amnesic and cannot consolidate, form, and store new memories, a focus on possible spared procedural learning may be the best therapy direction (e.g., method of vanishing cues or spaced retrieval techniques). If a client has most difficulty with retrieval of memories, the clinician may recommend a focus on organization and metacognitive strategy treatment (see Chapter 8).

In many cases, the best way to select a memory management approach is to implement a trial of diagnostic treatment and determine whether a client responds favorably to a particular approach. A number of variables influence response to memory treatment, some of which are specific to the client (e.g., client's affective state) and some of which are specific to how the treatment is implemented (e.g., schedule and type of prompting, practice). Discussion of relevant variables is infused in the description of specific memory treatments. Wilson and Moffat (1992) offer several guidelines for facilitating information processing when working with clients who have memory disturbances. These guidelines are useful for clinical interactions with people who have memory problems, regardless of the intervention approach.

- *Simplify* information; be clear and concise with instructions.
- *Reduce* the amount of information to be remembered.
- *Check* for understanding.
- Try to help the person *link* information to existing information. Make associations.
- Set up practice regimens with *distributed practice*; it is better to work at learning something a few minutes several times a day than for an hour once a day.
- Help individuals *organize* information that needs to be remembered.

- *Train* individuals to use communication techniques that encourage processing meaning, such as paraphrasing, rehearsal, and question asking.

Restorative Methods

This section discusses four types of restorative memory interventions: memory practice drills, mnemonic strategy training, metamemory training, and prospective memory training.

Memory Practice Drills

The use of memory drills to improve damaged memory suggests that memory can be strengthened as if it were a mental muscle. Over a decade ago, experimental work failed to demonstrate general improvements in memory functioning associated with administration of memory exercises (Schacter & Glisky, 1986). Although there has been no empirical support for this approach, the abundance of memory practice regimens on computer programs and in workbooks suggests that memory drills are still used in clinical practice. If there is improvement in client performance following "memory exercises," we suggest that it is most likely to be due to increases in attention ability. As discussed in Chapter 5, there is experimental work suggesting that isolated components of attention can be selectively improved with drill-oriented attention exercises (Sohlberg, McLaughlin, Pavese, Heidrich, & Posner, in press; Sturm, Willmes, Orgass, & Hartje, 1997).

Clients may complain of memory problems that are actually secondary to attention deficits. We have treated clients whose "memory" impairments have abated following attention process training (Sohlberg & Mateer, 1989). At this time, we do not understand why attention processes respond more favorably to drills than does memory functioning. Attention appears to be widely represented within the brain, and it is the most frequent cognitive disturbance following a variety of neurological diseases and trauma. The organization of attention processes in the brain, coupled with the fact that we have isolated some relevant discrete components of attention (e.g., selective attention), may account for why attention exercises have been more successful than memory exercises. Advances in our ability to measure neurological functioning during performance of cognitive tasks may help us better understand recovery mechanisms and explain treatment outcomes.

Mnemonic Strategy Training

The early memory intervention literature focused on teaching clients to use mnemonic strategies. Examples of mnemonic strategies include visual imagery, verbal organization strategies (e.g., forming acronyms; making paired associations with target words), and semantic elaboration (linking target words or ideas in a story). The most popular and thoroughly researched mnemonic strategy is the use of visual imagery (Wilson, 1986). Teaching clients to construct visual images, or providing them with associated images for information that is to be remembered, appears to be beneficial to some (see, e.g., Cermak, 1975; Wilson, 1982) but not all (see, e.g., Baddeley & Warrington, 1973; Crovitz, Harvey, & Horn, 1979) clients with memory impairments. Mnemonics appear to work best in artificial laboratory situations and often have little benefit in real-life contexts (Miller, 1992). It seems that persons with significant memory impairments have difficulty learning the strategies and implementing them spontaneously. They do not appear to maintain or generalize them beyond the training context (Cermak, 1975; Crovitz et al., 1979; Miller, 1992).

Glisky and Schacter (1986) suggest two possible reasons why persons with brain injury are unlikely to implement spontaneously mnemonic strategies. First, they suggest that there are only a limited number of opportunities in naturalistic contexts to employ techniques. For example, most individuals do not need to try to learn a list of words. Functional activities that lend themselves to the use of mnemonics do not occur with enough frequency. The second barrier is that the learning of mnemonics places considerable cognitive demands on persons with brain injury. They are often difficult to learn, and require memory, abstraction, and effortful processing abilities that are commonly impaired in these patients.

Although the general effectiveness of mnemonic strategies is limited, there may be specific cases where teaching an individual to utilize a mnemonic strategy will help him or her succeed on a specific task. For example, Wilson (1986) successfully used visual imagery to teach people's names to four subjects with severe memory disturbances. The strategy was useful in teaching a specific list of names. Similarly, Oberg and Turkstra (1998) evaluated an elaborative encoding technique to teach two adolescents specific vocabulary required for school. The technique required subjects to formulate their own semantic relationships for target words (e.g., to give personally relevant examples) and to complete synonym and definition recognition tasks. Both subjects learned the treated words and maintained knowledge for 1 month. They could not, however, employ the encoding technique without the assistance of the clinician. Both of these interventions may be considered domain-specific, because they were only useful for learning a specific body of information.

The other situation when a clinician may utilize mnemonics is when treating individuals with mild cognitive impairment. This population is often better able to learn and generalize strategies (Glisky & Schacter, 1986) than are individuals with severe memory impairments. The principles discussed in Chapter 8 for training metacognitive routines are relevant for teaching mnemonic strategies to this group.

Prospective Memory Training

Prospective memory training is an intervention paradigm in which clients with brain injury are administered repetitive prospective memory tasks. An example of a program involving such training is our Prospective Memory Process Training (PROMPT; Sohlberg, Mateer, & Geyer, 1985). In this type of training, the clinician asks the client to remember to carry out a target task in a specified number of minutes. The number of minutes is increased after the client demonstrates repeated success at a particular time interval. Over the course of the training, the clinician systematically lengthens the amount of time a client can remember and act on an assigned task.

Task variables that may be altered in a prospective memory training paradigm include (1) type of prospective memory task (e.g., one-step motor command vs. multistep functional task); (2) time delay (i.e., number of minutes between task administration and task execution); (3) distractor task during time delay (e.g., sitting quietly monitoring the time vs. completing math worksheet, or engaging in conversation); and (4) associated prompts to initiate task (e.g., alarm vs. requirement to monitor the time independently). The client's current level of functioning will determine what variables the clinician selects to start the therapy program. For example, if a client is unable to hold on to an instruction for 30 seconds, the clinician may elect to utilize some type of prompting in the initial training phase. In one study of our PROMPT program (Sohlberg, White, Evans, & Mateer, 1992b), researchers prompted clients to "keep holding on to time and task" until the clients could hold on to the instruction.

The clinician alters one task variable at a time, observes the effects, and waits for stable improvement before altering another variable. For instance, if the clinician increases the complexity of the task to be remembered, he or she will hold the intervening waiting time constant. The overall goal of the program is to increase the intervening delay systematically as the client's prospective memory lengthens. A clinical protocol demonstrating how performance on each of these variables may be documented is provided in Appendix 6.1.

The most common method for managing deficits in prospective memory is to teach people to utilize external aids such as appointment books. (Training the use of external aids is discussed in Chapter 7.) Prospective memory training, on the other hand, is a specific restorative technique designed to improve prospective memory functioning or perhaps to improve processing in associated functions.

Several descriptive and experimental studies have evaluated prospective memory training. Furst (1986) designed a 6-week training program using a functional prospective memory task that involved punching a card in a time clock at set times. Results showed an improvement in accuracy of response for the 12 adults with brain injury who participated in the study. We and our colleagues (Raskin & Buckheit, 1998; Raskin & Sohlberg,

1996; Sohlberg, White, Evans, & Mateer, 1992a, 1992b) evaluated our PROMPT program by examining the outcome of repetitively administering prospective memory tasks (mostly one-step motor commands) requiring patients with brain injuries to initiate an action at future designated times. The initial time delays were selected based on the patients' existing span. The time delay was lengthened as the patients improved. In some cases, intervening distractions were used. Each of these papers described improvements in prospective memory on the training tasks, with varying levels of generalization to real-world tasks and related neuropsychological tests.

The experiment by Raskin and Sohlberg (1996) compared performance on prospective memory tasks following prospective memory training with performance on the same tasks following recall drills in two subjects. Their results showed that both subjects' prospective memory improved in conjunction with prospective memory training; they demonstrated an increase in the length of time they could remember to carry out an assigned task after having received prospective memory training. Also associated with the treatment was improved performance on functional tasks, consisting of assignments to telephone the clinic and of routine home tasks as recorded in diaries kept by significant others. Over the course of the experiment, there was some improvement on neuropsychological measures of attention and working memory. There were no changes on measures of executive functions and time estimation, however, and only slight changes in recall ability. These findings were replicated and extended in a later study, in which 10 subjects with brain injury received prospective memory training and recall drills (Raskin & Buckheit, 1998). All subjects showed an increase in the time they were able to recall the prospective memory tasks, whereas none of the subjects demonstrated improvement on the recall drills. There was significantly improved prospective memory functioning in everyday contexts, as measured by a diary study and a questionnaire of prospective memory.

The authors of studies examining the efficacy of prospective memory training acknowledge the difficulty in determining whether prospective memory training simply teaches a behavior or skill (e.g., monitoring time) or whether there is improvement in the underlying processes that mediate acting on future intentions. It may be that repeated practice with memory for actions has a more robust effect than memory for verbal directions. More research is needed to clarify such issues. We include prospective memory training as an example of a restorative approach, because initial experiments suggest that the effects appear to generalize across contexts and tasks.

Clients for whom this technique may be useful include those with severe memory disturbances who can encode information but do not hold on to it, and who have preserved procedural learning. We have used it with clients who are unsuccessful using an external memory system because they cannot hold on to information long enough to write it down in their system. Lengthening the amount of time an individual can hold on to information from 30 seconds to 5 minutes may allow successful use of an external aid.

Metamemory Training

Some clients with memory disturbances benefit from an improved understanding of the nature and effects of their memory problems. The information about awareness training, discussed in detail in Chapter 9, applies to increasing awareness about memory disturbances. Awareness may be increased via an "educational" approach to learning about one's memory impairments. Other clients may need help "experiencing" the effects of preserved and damaged memory.

One metacognitive training method with particular relevance to improving metamemory functioning consists of prediction exercises. These involve helping clients compare predictions with actual performance. They can easily be adapted for memory tasks. For example, Rebmann and Hannon (1995) reinforced clients for the accuracy of their predictions on tasks. Differences between predicted performance on memory tests and actual test scores decreased over time. Similarly, Schlund (1999) provided feedback and review for a client who predicted performance on recall of personal information. Results suggested that the provision of feedback on accuracy of predicted recall reduced the variability between self-reports and recall performance.

Another aspect of metacognitive training is to teach people self-instructional or self-monitoring routines (i.e., executive strategies) that will help them improve their memory functioning. Strategies can be used to help them review material to be remembered in a way that will increase the likelihood of recall. This approach is discussed in Chapter 8.

Methods to Teach Domain-Specific Knowledge

The experimental literature has shown that people with severe memory disturbances can learn new information and show transfer of this learning (e.g., Evans et al., 2000; Glisky & Schacter, 1989). This has been most successful for the acquisition of domain-specific knowledge or knowledge relevant to a particular function. Glisky and Schacter (1989) describe three defining characteristics of domain-specific training:

- The goal is to alleviate specific problems associated with memory impairment rather than restore memory processes or improve general memory functioning.

- Information learned using instructional techniques has practical value to the client.
- The purpose of the acquisition of domain-specific knowledge is to teach clients information or procedures that they can access or implement independently.

Examples of tasks that may be considered domain-specific are as follows:

Procedures for transferring to and from a wheelchair
Procedures for operating a walker
Procedures for operating a computer
Range-of-motion exercises
Medication schedule
Names of people or objects
Vocabulary specific to a school subject
Route or room location; location of a school locker or classroom
Academic procedures (e.g., spelling rules, math algorithms)
Letter formation for dysgraphia
Orientation information
Swallowing procedures
Oral motor exercises to increase strength and coordination

We have noted earlier that mnemonic strategy training is best used to teach domain-specific knowledge. Three other domain-specific memory approaches to addressing memory deficits are described below: expanded rehearsal techniques, use of priming, and formation of personal history.

Expanded Rehearsal

Spaced retrieval (SR) is an intervention strategy that uses expanded rehearsal. The individual practices successfully recalling information over progressively longer intervals of time. It is based on experimental work in which name–face associations were taught by presenting photographs in a spaced interval sequence; this research demonstrated that the longer the distracting interval from the first to the second successful recall attempt, the greater the likelihood of recall at a third recall attempt (Bjork, 1988).

Brush and Camp (1998a, 1998b) have delineated clinical procedures for using SR to teach clients with memory impairments specific information. During SR training, a client is first told the target information and then asked immediately to recall the information. In subsequent trials, the client is asked to recall the information after time intervals that are doubled as the training progresses. The time intervals between recall attempts are interspersed with conversation or therapy activities. If the client makes an error response, the clinician provides the correct information, asks for immediate recall, and goes back to the last time interval at which the client was correct. Intervals are increased more slowly if the client demonstrates errors. An important component of the training is that it should be error-free. These authors suggest the following checklist for clinicians to follow when using SR techniques to teach a patient information or procedures:

- Learning should be effortless (if the process is onerous for a patient, it is not an appropriate method).
- The information or procedures taught should be concrete.
- Errors should be limited.
- One piece of information should be taught at a time.
- Data sheets should be used to track intervals, but the length of intervals does not have to be exact.
- If clients cannot recall target information longer than 6 minutes after six sessions, chances for retention are limited.

A sample therapy sequence and a therapy protocol illustrating use of the SR techniques are described in Boxes 6.1 and 6.2, respectively.

The following are examples of behaviors that have been targeted using SR techniques:

Swallowing techniques (Brush & Camp, 1998b)
Learning key names (Brush & Camp, 1998a)
Learning name–face associations (Carruth, 1997)
Procedures for using external memory aids (Stevens, O'Hanlon, & Camp, 1993)
Learning names of objects (Moffat, 1989)

The success of SR makes sense from a theoretical perspective. Clients learn information with little effort and improve with practice without necessarily remembering that they have previously performed the task. SR is a shaping procedure that is heavily dependent upon nondeclarative memory (Schacter, 1992). As discussed earlier, nondeclarative memory does not require conscious recollection of an experience. Researchers (e.g., Brush & Camp, 1998a, 1998b) suggest that because the learning is error-free, clients do not have difficulty with remembering error responses. (See the description of errorless learning in this chapter.)

Use of Priming

Patients with severe memory impairments exhibit normal repetition priming effects. This means that they have the same likelihood of recalling previously encountered information, given partial cues, as individuals without memory impairments; however, they fail to recall the event itself during

BOX 6.1. SR Therapy Sequence to Teach Swallowing Procedures

Goal

The goal of the program was to teach an 86-year-old man with dementia who was living in a long-term care facility to implement a swallowing technique. All sessions occurred during mealtimes.

Treatment Sessions 1 and 2

At the beginning of the meal, a cue card was introduced that told the patient to take a sip of liquid after swallowing each bit of food. The therapist read the card and then asked the client, "What do you do after you swallow your food?" The client responded correctly and then was instructed to take a sip of liquid. Using the SR technique, the therapist asked the client to recall information on the card and carry out behavior at increasingly longer intervals of time (1, 2, 4, 8, and 16 minutes) without making any errors. During this process, the cue card was faded. The SR training fit naturally into the eating pauses during the meal.

Treatment Sessions 3–13

The client remembered the sequence and would only be asked, "What should you do after swallowing food?" when he made an error and put the next bite of food into his mouth without first taking a sip of liquid. He always responded correctly to the SR training provided after the error response. The client was able to remember to implement the swallowing technique with 95% follow-through and one verbal reminder during each meal.

Note. From Brush and Camp (1998b). Copyright 1998 by Haworth Press. Adapted by permission.

---

which they first encountered the information. Several researchers capitalized on this preserved learning and developed a memory intervention technique called the *method of vanishing cues* (Glisky, Schacter, & Tulving, 1986a). This faded cueing technique can be used to teach complex knowledge or behaviors that might be used in everyday life. The patient is first provided with enough information to make a correct response, and then parts of the information are gradually withdrawn across learning trials, so the patient receives fewer and fewer cues.

The primary body of research evaluating the method of vanishing cues employed it to teach computer vocabulary and procedures (Glisky & Schacter, 1988; Glisky, Schacter, & Tulving, 1986a, 1986b). This series of studies demonstrated that persons with memory impairments could learn: computer vocabulary and retain it for 6 weeks; to write and edit simple programs; to implement disk storage and retrieval operations, with 1-month retention; and basic data entry skills, with 9-month retention. The

Box 6.2. SR Therapy Protocol to Teach a Name

1. The client is told that he or she will be given practice remembering things and that the first item to be practiced is the therapist's name. "My name is _____. What is my name? That's right, I am glad you remembered."

2. There is a brief interval and the clinician says, "Now let's practice again. What is my name?"

3. If the client remembers the name, the clinician proceeds to the next longer interval (Step 4). If the response is incorrect, the clinician repeats the interval again. If the client cannot correctly remember for three consecutive initial intervals, therapy is terminated and the clinician tries again at a later date.

4. The third interval lasts about 10 seconds and is filled by saying, "Good. I will give you more chances to practice this as I'm working with you today. Let's try again. What is my name?"

5. If the correct answer, the clinician proceeds to Step 6. If an incorrect response is given, the clinician immediately provides the client with the correct answer and goes back to Step 2.

6. The fourth interval lasts about 20 seconds and is filled by saying, "Good, you are remembering my name very well, and you are remembering after a longer period of time. That's the idea—for you to be able to remember for longer and longer times so you will always remember it. I'll be asking my name every once in a while just to give you practice. What is my name?"

7. If the correct answer is given, the clinician proceeds to Step 8. Each time an incorrect response is given, the clinician says, "Actually, my name is   . What is my name?" This allows the client to finish a trial with success. Then the clinician asks for the information, using the last time interval where there was successful recall.

8. The clinician continues to ask the client to recall his or her name after increasingly longer intervals (2 minutes, 4 minutes, 8 minutes, 16 minutes, etc.).

Note. From Brush and Camp (1998a). Copyright 1998 by Haworth Press. Adapted by permission.

---

tasks in all the studies were very specific and did not require problem solving. The researchers consistently noted that clients were slow to acquire the information.

The following is an example of how the method of vanishing cues can be implemented to teach emergency orientation information. An example of target information is this address:

123 Elk Ridge Drive

A card or a computer program lists the information. The full information is presented on the initial trial and shown to the client for a lengthy period of time (e.g., 10–15 seconds). The first letter of corresponding target is then presented, with blanks indicating number of missing letters. Whenever the client fails to produce the target response within 10–15 seconds, the next letter is added.

Trial 1 presentation

123 Elk Ridge Drive

(10 seconds with no response from client)
1_ _ _ _ _ _ _ _ _ _ _ _ _ _
(10 seconds with no response from client)
12_ _ _ _ _ _ _ _ _ _ _ _ _
(10 seconds with no response from client)
123 _ _ _ _ _ _ _ _ _ _ _ _
(10 seconds with no response from client)
123 E _ _ _ _ _ _ _ _ _ _ _
(10 seconds with no response from client)
123 El_ _ _ _ _ _ _ _ _ _
(Client gives correct response)

On subsequent trials, information is contingent upon the client's performance on the previous trial. The information is presented for 10–15 seconds, accompanied by a letter fragment; the number of letters is always one less than the number that the client needed to provide the information correctly on the previous trial. In the original study teaching computer vocabulary, the computer program kept track of the subject's performance.

Wilson (1992) recommends a modification of the original technique: She suggests withholding the first letter of the to-be-recalled word until last. Clients are often able to recall the first letter spontaneously, and it also prevents clients from becoming dependent upon the provision of the first-letter prompt for recall. The first letter is a stronger recall prompt than the other letters (Glisky et al., 1986b).

There are limited reports of using repetition priming as a memory rehabilitation technique, although it has wide application for individuals with severe memory impairments who need to learn discrete information. The procedures governing practice trials and distribution of sessions have not been well explored and need further investigation.

One way to facilitate application of memory theory to memory rehabilitation practice is to combine features of priming methods with features of SR. Hunkin and colleagues (1998a) used principles of both these methodologies in their previously described study evaluating errorless learning for teaching a word-processing program. They demonstrated success for teaching a subject with a severe memory impairment to use a word processor on a microcomputer. The training provided progressively less cueing after sufficiently exposing the client to target information (principle of repetition priming), and it incorporated the errorless recall repetition used in SR. In spite of severe anterograde memory deficit, their subject learned the procedures and could perform them as quickly without instruction as he could with instructions, showing that errorless learning can be applied to learning computer skills.

Creation of Personal History

Patients with RA have a loss of memory for life events prior to their injury. They usually have concomitant deficits in learning new information. If the RA is extensive, a treatment plan will need to incorporate a method to help them relearn aspects of their personal history. As with the aforementioned techniques in this section, it will be important to take advantage of spared nondeclarative memory in order to teach essential information.

Most clients with significant RA probably will not experience any "feeling of remembering" with therapy and will continue to distinguish between those events that they actually recall and those that have been taught to them (Kapur, 1993). Either priming or expanded rehearsal practices can be used to teach discrete facts about personal history.

In addition to teaching some important facts, it can be very helpful to create an autobiography. This may take the form of a photographic life essay put together by family members, a written life history, a video composite of important people, or simple orientation pages in a memory book. Involvement of friends and family members in constructing the personal history can be therapeutic for them as well. In recommending the development of a personal history, it is critical to consider the following:

• Match the format to the client's abilities and disabilities. For example, it will be important to ask whether the client read typed labels under photographs, or whether an auditory–visual format will be more helpful.
• The client needs to have access to the history. If the history is not in a format where the client can use it whenever desired, it may not be helpful. For example, if the client does not easily use a videotape player, a videotaped history will not be effective.
• Utilize the interests, ideas, and strengths of all those producing the history—family members and friends, as well as the client him- or herself.

We have facilitated the development of personal histories that clients have reviewed countless times for months and even years. They report being comforted by having critical personal history compiled in a fashion they can easily refer to.

SUMMARY

We have begun this chapter by describing the stages of memory and associated neuroanatomical correlates. The different stages involved in remembering are closely linked and interact; they include attention, encoding, storage, and retrieval. Distinctions have also been made between different types of memory. One distinction with particular relevance to cognitive rehabilitation is the distinction between declarative (explicit) and nondeclarative (implicit) memory.

There are numerous approaches to assisting patients in managing decreased memory function. One broad category of memory interventions consists of techniques designed to improve overall memory functioning either by improving underlying processes or by teaching skills that might be utilized for a broad range of tasks and/or contexts. An example of this approach is prospective memory training, in which clients are asked to carry out specified tasks at increasingly longer intervals of time. As their ability to remember to act on an intention improves at a specific time interval, that interval is increased. Another broad category of memory interventions emphasizes improved performance on specific functional tasks. These techniques make use of spared procedural or nondeclarative memory. For example, SR is an intervention strategy in which the individual practices successfully recalling specific information (e.g., a name or procedure) over progressively longer intervals of time. The method of vanishing cues is a faded cueing technique in which the client is first provided with enough information to make a correct response, and then parts of the information are gradually withdrawn across learning trials until the patient can recall the target information with the least amount of cueing.

REFERENCES

Ahmed, S., Bierley, R., Sheikh, J. I., & Date, E. S. (2000). Post-traumatic amnesia after closed head injury: A review of the literature and some suggestions for further research. *Brain Injury, 14*(9), 765–780.

Baddeley, A. D. (1992). Implicit memory and errorless learning: A link between cognitive theory and neuropsychological rehabilitation? In L. R. Squire & N. Butters (Eds.) *Neuropsychology of memory* (2nd ed., pp. 309–313). New York: Guilford Press.

Baddeley, A. D., Wilson, B. A., Watts, F. N. (Eds.). (1995). *Handbook of memory disorders*. Chichester, England: Wiley.

Baddeley, A. D., & Warrington, E. K. (1973). Memory coding and amnesia. *Neuropsychologia, 11,* 159–165.

Brandimonte, M., Einstein, G. O., & McDaniel, M. A. (Eds.). (1996). *Prospective memory: Theory and applications*. Mahwah, NJ: Erlbaum.

Bjork, R. A. (1988). Retrieval practice and the maintenance of knowledge. In M. M.

Gruneberg, P. E. Morris, & R. N. Sykes (Eds.), *Practical aspects of memory: Current research and issues* (pp. 283–288). Chichester, England: Wiley.

Brush, J. A., & Camp, C. J. (1998a). Using spaced retrieval as an intervention during speech–language therapy. *The Clinical Gerontologist, 19*(1), 51–64.

Brush, J. A., & Camp, C. J. (1998b). Spaced retrieval during dysphagia therapy: A case study. *The Clinical Gerontologist, 19*(2), 96–99.

Carruth, E. K. (1997). The effects of singing and the spaced retrieval technique on improving face–name recognition in nursing home residents with memory loss. *Journal of Music Therapy, 34*(3), 165–186.

Cermak, L. S. (1975). Imagery as an aid to retrieval for Korsakoff patients. *Cortex, 11,* 163–169.

Cohen, N. (1984). Preserved learning capacity in amnesia: Evidence for multiple memory systems. In L. R. Squire & N. Butters (Eds.), *Neuropsychology of memory* (pp. 83–103). New York: Guilford Press.

Craik, F., & Lockhart, R. (1972). Levels of processing: A framework for memory research. *Journal of Verbal Learning and Verbal Behavior, 11,* 671–684.

Crovitz, H. F., Harvey, M. T., & Horn, R. W. (1979). Problems in the acquisition of imagery mnemonics: Three brain damaged cases. *Cortex, 15,* 225–234.

Dobbs, A. R., & Reeves, B. M. (1996). Prospective memory: More than memory. In M. Brandimonte, G. O. Einstein, & M. A. McDaniel (Eds.), *Prospective memory: Theory and applications* (pp. 199–226). Mahwah, NJ: Erlbaum.

Evans, J. J., Wilson, B. A., Schuri, U., Andrade, J., Baddeley, A. D., Bruna, O., Canavan, T., Della Salla, S., Green, R., Laaksonen, R., Lorenzi, L., & Taussik, I. (2000). A comparison of "errorless" and "trial-and-error" learning methods for teaching individuals with acquired memory deficits. *Neuropsychological Rehabilitation, 10*(1), 67–101.

Furst, C. (1986). The memory derby: Evaluating and remediating intention memory. *Cognitive Rehabilitation, 4,* 24–26.

Glisky, E. L., & Schacter, D. L. (1986). Remediation of organic memory disorders: Current status and future prospects. *Journal of Head Trauma Rehabilitation, 1,* 54–63.

Glisky, E. L., & Schacter, D. L. (1988). Long-term retention of computer learning by patients with memory disorders. *Neuropsychologia, 26,* 173–178.

Glisky, E. L., & Schacter, D. L. (1989). Extending the limits of complex learning in organic amnesia: Computer training in a vocational domain. *Neuropsychologia, 27,* 107–120.

Glisky, E. L., Schacter, D. L., & Tulving, E. (1986a). Learning and retention of computer-related vocabulary in amnesic patients: Method of vanishing cues. *Journal of Clinical and Experimental Neuropsychology, 8,* 292–312.

Glisky, E. L., Schacter, D. L., & Tulving, E. (1986b). Computer learning by memory-impaired patients: Acquisition and retention of complex knowledge. *Neuropsychologia, 24,* 313–328.

Howieson, D. B., & Lezak, M. D. (1995). Separating memory from other cognitive problems. In A. D. Baddeley, B. A. Wilson, & F. N. Watts (Eds.), *Handbook of memory disorders* (pp. 411–426). New York: Wiley.

Hunkin, N. M., Squires, E. J., Aldrich, F. K., & Parkin, A. J. (1998a). Errorless learning and the acquisition of word processing skills. *Neuropsychological Rehabilitation, 8*(4), 433–449.

Hunkin, N. M., Squires, E. J., Parkin, A. J., & Tidy, J. A. (1998b). Are the benefits of errorless learning dependent on implicit memory? *Neuropsychologia, 36*(1), 25–36.

Huppert, F., & Piercy, M. (1982). In search of the functional locus of amnesic syndromes. In L. S. Cermak (Ed.), *Human memory and amnesia* (pp. 123–137). Hillsdale, NJ: Erlbaum.

Jonides, J. (2000, February). *Working memory and the brain.* Paper presented at the International Neuropsychology Society, Denver, CO.

Kapur, N. (1993). Focal retrograde amnesia in neurological disease: A critical review. *Cortex, 29,* 217–234.

Levin, H. S., Benton, A. L., & Grossman, R. G. (1982). *Neurobehavioral consequences of closed head injury.* New York: Oxford University Press.

Markowitsch, H. J. (1998). Cognitive neuroscience of memory. *Neurocase, 4,* 429–435.

Martin, A., Wiggs, C. L., Lalonde, F. L., & Mack, C. (1994). Word retrieved to letter and semantic cues: A double dissociation in normal subjects using interference tasks. *Neuropsychologia, 32,* 1487–1494.

McClelland, J. L., & McNaughton, B. L. (1995). Why there are complementary learning systems in the hippocampus and neocortex: Insight from the success and failures of connection of models of learning and memory. *Psychological Review, 102*(3), 419–457.

McDowall, J. (1984). Processing capacity and recall in amnesic and control subjects. In L. R. Squire & N. Butters (Eds.), *Neuropsychology of memory* (pp. 63–66). New York: Guilford Press.

Miller, E. (1992). Psychological approaches to the management of memory impairments. *British Journal of Psychiatry, 160,* 1–6.

Milner, B. (1970). Memory and the medial temporal regions of the brain. In K. J. Pribram & D. E. Broadbent (Eds.), *Biological bases of memory* (pp. 29–50). New York: Academic Press.

Moffat, N. J. (1989). Home-based cognitive rehabilitation with the elderly. In L. W. Poon, D. C. Rubin, & B. A. Wilson (Eds.), *Everyday cognition in adulthood and late life* (pp. 659–680). Cambridge, England: Cambridge University Press.

Oberg, L., & Turkstra, L. S. (1998). Use of elaborative encoding to facilitate verbal learning after adolescent traumatic brain injury. *Journal of Head Trauma Rehabilitation, 13*(3), 44–62.

Patterson, M. B., & Mack, J. L. (1985). Neuropsychological analysis of a case of reduplicative paramnesia. *Journal of Clinical and Experimental Neuropsychology, 7*(1), 111–121.

Posner, M., & Petersen, S. E. (1990). The attention system of the human brain. *Annual Review of Neuroscience, 13,* 25–42.

Raskin, S. A., & Buckheit, C. (1998). *Investigation of P300 as a measure of efficacy of prospective memory.* Paper presented at the meeting of the Society for Cognitive Rehabilitation, Chicago.

Raskin, S. A., & Sohlberg, M. M. (1996). The efficacy of prospective memory training in two adults with brain injury. *Journal of Head Trauma Rehabilitation, 11*(3), 32–51.

Rebmann, M. J., & Hannon, R. (1995). Treatment of unawareness of memory deficits in adults with brain injury: Three case studies. *Rehabilitation Psychology,* 40(4), 279–287.

Schmidtke, K., & Vollmer, H. (1997). Retrograde amnesia: A study of its relation to anterograde amnesia and semantic memory deficits. *Neuropsychologia, 35*(4), 505–518.

Schacter, D. L. (1992). Understanding implicit memory. *American Psychologist, 47,* 559–569.

Schacter, D. L., & Glisky, E. L. (1986). Memory remediation: Restoration, alleviation, and the acquisition of domain-specific knowledge. In B. P. Uzzell & Y. Gorss (Eds.), *Clinical neuropsychology of intervention* (pp. 257–282). Boston: Nijhoff.

Schlund, M. W. (1999). Self awareness: Effects of feedback and review on verbal self reports and remembering following brain injury. *Brain Injury, 13*(5), 375–380.

Shimamura, A. P., & Squire, L. R. (1991). The relationship between fact and source memory: Findings from amnesic patients and normal subjects. *Psychobiology, 19,* 1–10.

Sohlberg, M. M., & Mateer, C. A. (1989). *Introduction to cognitive rehabilitation: Theory and practice.* New York: Guilford Press.

Sohlberg, M. M., Mateer, C. A., & Geyer, S. (1985). *Prospective Memory Process Training (PROMPT).* Wake Forest, NC: Lash & Associates.

Sohlberg, M. M., McLaughlin, K., Pavese, A., Heidrich, A., & Posner, M. (in press). Evaluation of attention process training and brain injury education in persons with acquired brain injury. *Journal of Clinical and Experimental Neuropsychology, 22*(1).

Sohlberg, M. M., White, O., Evans, E., & Mateer, C. A. (1992a). Background and initial case studies into the effects of prospective memory training. *Brain Injury,* 6(2), 129–138.

Sohlberg, M. M., White, O., Evans, E., & Mateer, C. A. (1992b). An investigation into the effects of prospective memory training. *Brain Injury,* 6(2), 139–154.

Squire, L. R. (1992). Declarative and nondeclarative memory: Multiple brain systems supporting learning and memory. *Journal of Cognitive Neuroscience, 4,* 232–243.

Stevens, A. B., O'Hanlon, A. M., & Camp, C. J. (1993). Strategy training in Alzheimer's disease: A case study. *The Clinical Gerontologist, 13,* 106–109.

Sturm, W., Willmes, K., Orgass, B., & Hartje, W. (1997). Do specific attention deficits need specific training? *Neuropsychological Rehabilitation, 7,* 81–103.

Tulving, E. (1966). Subjective organization and effects of repetition in multi-trial free-recall learning. *Journal of Verbal Learning and Verbal Behavior, 5,* 193–197.

Tulving, E. (1972). Episodic and semantic memory. In E. Tulving & W. Donaldson (Eds.), *Organization of memory* (pp. 381–403). New York: Academic Press.

Tulving, E., & Schacter, D. L. (1990). Priming and human memory systems. *Science,* 247, 301–306.

Wilson, B. A. (1982). Success and failure in memory training following a cerebral vascular accident. *Cortex, 18,* 581–594.

Wilson, B. A. (1986). *Rehabilitation of memory.* New York: Guilford Press.

Wilson, B. A., Baddeley, A., Evans, J. J., & Shiel, A. J. (1994). Errorless learning in the rehabilitation of memory impaired people. *Neuropsychological Rehabilitation,* 4(3), 307–326.

Wilson, B. A., & Moffat, N. (Eds.). (1992). *Clinical management of memory problems.* San Diego, CA: Singular.

Winograd, E. (1988). Some observations on prospective memory. In M. M. Gruneberg, P. E. Morris, & R. N. Sykes (Eds.), *Practical aspects of memory: Current research and issues* (Vol. 1, pp. 349–353). Chichester, England: Wiley.

APPENDIX 6.1

DATA SHEET FOR PROSPECTIVE MEMORY TRAINING

Date/ Trial #	P.M. Task	Time	Interval Activity	Outcome (correct task/ correct time*)
5/4 #1	Stand up	1 min.	Silence	+/+ Watched clock
#2	Clap hands	1 min.	Silence	+/+ "
#3	Close book	1 min.	Silence	–/+ She stood up— retroactive interference
#4	Close book	1 min.	Silence	+/+ Watched clock
#5	Blink	1 min.	Silence	+/+ "
#6	Snap fingers	1 min.	Silence	+/+ " (Three in a row, ready to move on)
#7	Tap finger	90 sec.	Silence	–/– Forgot both time and task
#8	Stamp feet	90 sec.	Silence	–/– Forgot both time and task
#9	Wink	90 sec.	Silence	+/+ Cued/15 sec. to "hold onto time and task"
5/5 #1	Open drawer	90 sec.	Silence	+/+ Cued/15 sec. to "hold onto time and task"
#2	Stick out tongue	90 sec.	Silence	+/+
#3	Point	90 sec.	Silence	+/+ Cued/30 sec. to "hold onto time and task"
#4	Nod head	90 sec.	Silence	+/+ Cued every 30 sec.
#5	Open mouth	90 sec.	Silence	+/+ Cued every 30 sec.
#6	Raise eyebrows	90 sec.	Silence	+/+ Cued every 45 sec.
#7	Smile	90 sec.	Silence	+/– Cued every 45 sec. but lost task
Several weeks later				
5/21 #1	Snap fingers	4 min.	Silence	+/+
#2	"Shiver"	4 min.	Silence	+/+
#3	Frown	4 min.	Silence	+/+ (Three in a row, ready to move on)
Several weeks later				
6/5 #1	Stand	4 min.	Easy math facts (EMF)	+/– Cued to look at watch after time elapsed
#2	Sit	4 min.	EMF	+/– "
#3	Cross legs	3 min.	EMF	+/+

---

* + or –10% of target time

7

The Use of External Aids in Cognitive Rehabilitation

EXTERNAL AIDS: A POPULAR AND POTENTIALLY EFFECTIVE TECHNIQUE

The use of external memory aids is a common rehabilitation method for managing difficulties with memory, attention, and executive functions. Several investigations have revealed external aids to be the favored mode of compensation across both nondisabled and disabled populations. Harris (1980) found that when persons without brain injury wanted to remember information, they relied on external aids (e.g., making lists). Similarly, Wilson (1991) showed that patients with acquired neurological dysfunction relied on written lists, calendars, or wall charts, rather than on internal cognitive strategies.

The somewhat limited research suggests that external aids, in addition to being popular, can be effective in mitigating a memory impairment. In a survey of the early cognitive rehabilitation literature, Glisky and Schacter (1986) concluded that external aids were superior to both drills and mnemonic strategies. Zenicus, Wesolowski, and Burke (1990) compared four memory improvement strategies—written rehearsal, verbal rehearsal, acronym formation, and memory notebook logging—in six persons with brain injury. Their findings suggested that memory notebook logging was the most effective method for increasing recall of classroom material. In a subsequent experiment, these researchers taught four persons with brain injury to utilize memory notebooks and demonstrated improved performance on homework assignments and keeping scheduled appointments (Zenicus, Wesolowski, & Burke, 1991). There are also a number of case reports demonstrating effective use of external aids to compensate for cognitive deficits following acquired brain injury (Burke, Danick, Bemis, & Durgin, 1994; Fluharty & Priddy, 1993; Kerns & Thompson, 1998; Kim,

Burke, Dowds, & George, 1999; Kim et al., 2000; Sohlberg & Mateer, 1989).

In spite of their clinical appeal, there are a number of challenges associated with teaching persons with brain injury to use external memory and organizational aids. These include associated cognitive problems, such as decreased reading or writing abilities; loss of external aids; and difficulty remembering to consult these aids. However, many of these difficulties are technical and can be addressed with systematic, effective training (Donaghy & Williams, 1998).

Training protocols describing specific methods to teach the use of external aids to individuals with acquired brain injuries are limited in the cognitive literature. Several years ago, we (Sohlberg & Mateer, 1989) outlined a three-stage behavioral training protocol. The first stage, *acquisition*, was designed to familiarize an individual with his or her memory notebook via a question-and-answer format. The second phase, *application*, involved teaching patients to record and access information in their memory notebooks. The third phase, *adaptation*, involved teaching patients to use their memory notebooks in naturalistic settings. A more recent report refines this training protocol and describes a memory journal training protocol designed to tap into typical residual cognitive strengths of persons with brain injury, including immediate attention, procedural memory, and old learning (Donaghy & Williams, 1998). It contains baseline testing, a needs assessment, five levels of training exercises, and discharge probe testing. Many of the concepts outlined in both of these protocols are expanded upon in this chapter.

The purpose of this chapter is to present a systematic method for helping clients select and implement external aids that help them compensate effectively for changes in memory, attention, and executive functions. In order to accomplish this goal, it is important to have a grounding in memory, learning, and instructional theory. The reader is encouraged to review Chapter 6, which presents theories of memory, and Chapter 9, which describes techniques to manage unawareness (a frequent challenge when teaching persons with brain injuries to use external aids). The present chapter details specific clinical principles and techniques important for the selection of compensatory strategies and external aids; it also describes clinical activities pertinent to the pretraining and training phases of therapy.*

---

*Many of the clinical protocols described in this chapter were developed with support by Grant No. H086D50012 from the U.S. Department of Education. An overview of the materials and training program is provided in Sohlberg, Todis, and Glang (1998b). Manuals were developed for educators based on the training model described in this chapter; they were written by Sohlberg, Todis, and Glang, and are available from Lash & Associates in Wake Forest, NC. Additional clinical protocols described in this chapter are from Sohlberg, Johansen, Geyer, and Hoornbeek (1994).

WHAT IS THE GOAL OF USING EXTERNAL AIDS?

Compensation versus Restitution

Most clinicians and researchers view external aids as a method to *compensate* for (vs. *restore*) reduced memory or organizational skills. Unlike attention process training, the goals of which are to reorganize underlying neural circuitry and to improve damaged cognitive functions, external aids are a means to reduce the load on memory or executive functions in order to allow a person to successfully carry out a task and circumvent the cognitive disturbance. Hence clinicians often see the process of helping clients implement external aids as teaching a set of behaviors rather than retraining a process. However, the distinction between teaching a set of skills (e.g., steps for using an electronic memory) and retraining a cognitive process (e.g., improving organizational abilities) is somewhat blurry, as both require learning and depend upon repetitive activation of associated cognitive processes.

Domain-Specific versus Generalized Use

An important distinction when a clinician is sorting out the goal of using an external aid is to determine whether it will be used to complete a specific task (or set of tasks), or whether the goal is for the external aid to be used in a variety of contexts for a variety of tasks (e.g., to compensate more globally for a memory impairment). Training the use of a memory notebook for tracking a daily schedule and logging ongoing events is a different rehabilitation activity from training someone to utilize a pill box alarm system. If the goal is to train the use of an external aid that will be used for a wide variety of tasks, the generalization and training issues will be much more complex.

Characteristics of Compensatory Behavior

Even when the goal of using external aids is viewed as purely compensatory, there are no clear theoretical foundations for implementing compensatory cognitive strategies. Although reports in the literature support the efficacy of external aids as compensatory strategies, these reports are sparse. Training the use of compensatory systems frequently causes frustration for clinicians. It is not uncommon to train a particular strategy for using an external aid in therapy and subsequently observe that the aid is not implemented consistently beyond the training period. This may in part be a result of not having an operational definition of compensation strategies for cognitive disorders.

The related field of communication disorders faces similar challenges regarding the implementation of compensation strategies. A study by

Simmons-Mackie and Damico (1997) attempted to reformulate the definition of compensatory strategies in aphasia. In order to better understand compensation as a process and its implications for strategy training, this ethnographic study used field research to analyze the naturally occurring compensation behaviors in subjects with aphasia. The study identified five characteristics of compensatory strategies, which may have implications for training cognitive strategies (for memory, attention, or executive function symptoms) as well as communication strategies. Listed below are these five characteristics:

- Compensations are purposeful and goal-oriented; they are used to compensate for a particular breakdown.
- Compensations are often preexisting or "normal" behaviors that are adapted in some way to compensate for a problem.
- Compensatory strategies appear to be employed in flexible patterns to fit a context.
- Compensations are specific to the participant.
- Many compensatory strategies are "spontaneous" rather than "trained."

Our clinical experience suggests that building upon existing strategies; tailoring strategies to individuals' needs and contexts; and providing systematic, direct training are the most promising methods for long-term use of external aids.

REVIEW OF THEORY

Teaching people to use external aids requires understanding how individuals with impaired memory can learn new procedures. Chapter 6 has outlined the different stages involved in remembering: attention, encoding, storage, and retrieval. Chapter 6 has also distinguished between two different types of long-term memory—declarative and nondeclarative learning systems. These two bodies of information guide our instructional methods.

The reader will recall that the declarative learning system is the knowledge each of us possesses. It includes knowledge about facts we have learned and ideas we have formed. It also includes knowledge about our life experiences. It is a conscious, explicit learning system. In contrast, our nondeclarative system allows us to learn procedures and certain perceptuomotor tasks without awareness of having learned them. It may be preserved in persons with brain injury. Hence, for persons with severe memory disturbances, clinicians rely upon this preserved system to teach them new procedures such as using external memory aids.

Another relevant theoretical construct discussed in Chapter 6 is prospective memory, which is thought to be an especially functional type of memory. Prospective memory—the ability to remember to act on future intentions—illustrates the interconnection of attention, memory, and executive functions. External aids may be used to manage deficits in any of these three areas. In order to remember to act on intentions, one must be able to plan (executive functions); to keep information in a storage loop that can be periodically checked in order to know when to perform the action (working memory); to recall the task (declarative memory); and to initiate the task (executive functions). These systems are vulnerable to disruption following acquired brain injury. Teaching individuals to utilize compensatory external aids allows them to compensate for deficits in prospective memory. For example, learning to utilize a daily schedule will facilitate the ability to carry out future intentions.

Understanding memory theory is important to the process of training the use of external compensatory aids. Clinicians can capitalize on intact procedural learning to teach people to utilize external aids that will compensate for deficits in episodic and prospective memory.

SELECTING AN EXTERNAL COMPENSATORY AID

The process of training an individual to use an external cognitive aid begins with the identification or development of a system matched to the individual client. Consideration of two critical elements will maximize the probability that a system will compensate for cognitive impairments and will be used beyond the training environment. The first element is for the clinician, the client, and other relevant persons to take the time to do a careful *needs assessment*. The second factor is for the clinician to have an appreciation of the available *options* for external aids. Each of these factors is addressed in this section.

Conducting a Needs Assessment

In an environment of cost containment, it is often difficult to take time to do a careful assessment of clients' needs and constraints. However, taking time for such an assessment will result in the selection of strategies or aids that can be trained with maximum efficiency and success (Donaghy & Williams, 1998; Sohlberg & Mateer, 1989). Furthermore, the type of information required for a needs assessment may be obtained by caregivers or by multiple members of a rehabilitation or school team. Rather than conducting a formal assessment, the clinician managing the selection of the aid can solicit information from relevant people in the individual's environment. The important element is to systematically evaluate the individual needs of the client.

One way to match a system to an individual is to evaluate (1) organic factors (relevant physical and cognitive functions); (2) personal factors (relevant psychosocial and environmental elements); and (3) situational factors (contexts in which use of an external aid is desirable).

Organic Factors

It is important to understand the strengths and constraints that are direct results of an acquired brain injury and that have an impact on the ability to utilize specific types of external aids. Relevant organic factors are highlighted below.

- *Cognitive/learning profile.* The system or strategy should be consistent with the client's ability to learn and remember new skills and information. For example, an individual who is densely amnesic may have difficulty learning to use a multistep, complex system. This information may be obtained from a neuropsychological or cognitive assessment.
- *Physical profile.* Significant disturbances in motor abilities or sensory functions will limit the choices of external aids. For example, paralysis or apraxia affecting hand movement may affect an individual's ability to produce legible handwriting or depress buttons on a keyboard. Mobility impairments requiring a person to use assistive devices may limit what the individual can carry (e.g., they contraindicate a heavy binder). Similarly, visual disturbances may limit a client's ability to read print in certain sizes or to decipher words on a screen. Changes in hearing acuity may render a person unable to hear a watch beep or an alarm. Information on motoric and sensory limitations may be obtained from medical charts, interview of the client and/or caregiver, or direct observation.

Personal Factors

Consideration of organic factors is critical to selecting a system that will work for an individual. It is also important to consider the following personal factors in the selection of an external aid.

- *Spontaneous use of compensation strategies.* It is often more effective to build on existing strategies than to develop and train a completely novel habit (Simmons-Mackie & Damico, 1997). Old learning is often preserved in individuals with severe memory impairment. Clinicians can capitalize on previously used systems or strategies, and can use clients' existing terminology to describe memory functioning.

It may be helpful to observe and interview clients and caregivers, to identify the clients' natural inclination for compensatory behavior. A person's experience of using organizational aids prior to injury will influence his or her behavior after injury; thus it is important to determine what types of systems or strategies (if any) the person used prior to experiencing cognitive dysfunction, as again this may provide an opportunity to build upon existing behaviors. For example, if an individual used a written day planner prior to injury, it may be wise to expand this same system to fit new circumstances.

• *Personal preference.* Making an effort to learn about a patient's personal preferences for an external aid will increase motivation and compliance to use a system. It is important to understand preferences for appearance (e.g., color, style, size); mode (e.g., electronic, paper-and-pencil, auditory); and system functions (e.g., calendar, orientation, things-to-do list).

• *Financial resources.* Available resources may limit the range of aids that are options for an individual. There is a substantial difference between the cost of a three-ring binder and that of a computerized memory system. A clinician may be influential in securing funds from an insurance carrier or other funder for a particular system by providing the necessary rationale and training plan.

• *Available support.* The level of available support in both the current environment and the projected discharge environment will also affect recommendations for an external aid. If a client has support persons who can assist with training and generalization, a more elaborate system that initially requires outside assistance may be a reasonable choice. If a client has very limited support and will essentially be alone in his or her efforts to learn to use a system, a simplified system may be preferable.

Situational Factors

We have outlined the organic and personal factors important for conducting a needs assessment. The third important task is to carefully evaluate the following situational factors that can influence a recommendation for an external aid.

• *Context.* The clinician needs to understand the context in which the cognitive problem (e.g., memory deficit) is occurring. Questions that need to be explored include these:

> Where and under what circumstances does the cognitive problem interfere with functioning?
> What are the consequences when there is a breakdown?
> Are there any contexts where the target cognitive issue is *not* a problem, and if so, why?

Basically, the clinician wants to have a clear understanding of the problem or goal that the external aid will address. For example, consider a client who is a student; the clinician and client hope to develop an external aid to increase homework completion. In order to select an appropriate aid, the clinician will want to evaluate why the student is not turning in homework. This may include determining how homework is assigned in classes, how it is filed and transported to home, how it is worked on at home, and how it is transported back to school. Such an evaluation may require talking to the student, parents, and teachers or having them fill out an observational form. To understand the context of a cognitive problem, it is necessary to complete some type of environmental assessment, either through careful interview or (if possible) through observation.

• *History.* Another situational factor that is important to the selection process is to identify what accommodations or strategies have already been tried. This is certainly more critical when the client has been seen in previous settings or received assistance prior to seeing the present clinician. It can be very helpful to determine whether other aids were attempted and why they were or were not successful.

Two examples of needs assessments are provided in the appendices. Appendix 7.1 is an example of a needs assessment that might be used for an adult client with brain injury in a rehabilitation setting. Appendix 7.2 provides an example of a needs assessment for a student with brain injury in a middle or high school setting. The important consideration is to have a systematic method for looking at the organic, personal, and situational factors described above, in order to provide the client with appropriate recommendations for an effective external compensatory aid.

Options for External Aids

There are many different options available for external compensatory aids. Several societal trends have greatly increased the number of available external aids. One trend is the "organizational revolution" that has occurred within the last 5 years. Products and techniques to save time and maximize efficiency are heavily marketed; numerous educational seminars are available to enhance careers for professionals and students by training organizational skills. This "revolution" has served to normalize and mainstream the use of compensatory systems for the nondisabled population. The second trend is the boom within the electronic and computer industries, which has further increased the range of options available to compensate for problems with attention, memory, and organizational abilities.

Guiding clients in the selection of appropriate external aids requires a clinician to be familiar with a variety of options. This includes a clear understanding of the properties and features of each device. For example, a knowledgeable clinician may anticipate that the layout of a particular keyboard is overly complex for a certain client, but that it can work optimally if seldom-used keys are covered. Parente (1998) and Kapur (1995) describe a wide range of devices helpful to the population of individuals with cognitive impairments. Some of these devices have been designed especially for individuals with disabilities, whereas others were originally developed for the nondisabled population. Parente (1998) divides external aids into integrated computer packages, which have complex scheduling and time management capabilities, and "low-tech" cognitive aids. Five categories of external aids are described below. The first four types of aids are multifunctional and may be used to compensate for a memory or organizational problem across a variety of contexts. The last category includes examples of aids that may be used to assist with specific activities.

- *Written planning systems.* These include planners, notebooks divided into sections, appointment books, and calendar systems that can be used to track daily plans and events, as well as intended and completed actions. Examples include Daytimers, Dayrunners, and Franklin Planners. Many of these written aids are available in a wide variety of formats and styles. For example, some clients are best served by a the style of Daytimer with 1 week displayed across two pages, whereas other clients may require 1 day to be displayed across two pages.
- *Electronic planners.* There are numerous electronic devices that can plan, track, and prompt someone to respond to specific information. It is important to evaluate size, price, keyboard layout, alarm features (e.g., tone, capacity for hourly/daily/monthly alarm, prealarm, associated print message), and ease of capacity for text entry and storage. There are electronic watch systems (e.g., the Casio Telememo watch) with complex data storage and reminder features that may also be useful cognitive aids for clients. Examples of companies that have manufactured a variety of electronic memory aids are Sharp and Tandy. Given the rapidly changing technology, it is important that clinicians be familiar with the current options at electronic stores.
- *Computerized systems.* The planning and alarm features available on the electronic memory aids are also available on software for personal computers. There are several integrated packages with software that can help clients record events, prompt them to carry out an action at a particular time, and provide multiple reminders. With features such as word processors, data bases, and telephone-dialing software, it is easy to develop sophisticated planning and organizational systems tailored for an individual. Kim and colleagues (1999) described the successful use of a microcomputer system for assisting a person with a closed head injury to get to scheduled appointments and take medication. The subject used a palmtop computer (Psion Series 3a), which provided visible output on a screen display. The input of schedule information for the individual user was accom-

plished by keyboard entry into an alarm application. A follow-up study (Kim et al., 2000) reviewed the experience of 12 patients with brain injury and impairments who were taught to use palmtop computers to assist with memory-dependent activities in their everyday lives. Nine subjects found the computers useful during the supervised training trials; seven of these nine continued to use the devices after the supervised trials were completed.

Another current example is the Timex Data Link Watch, which comes with a Microsoft software program that enables scheduling information to be imported from the computer to the watch alarm system. The NeuroPage provides yet another example. It is a portable paging system with a screen that can be attached to a waist belt, which uses an arrangement of micro-computers. Several articles describe successful case studies using this system (e.g., Hersch & Treadgold, 1994).

• *Auditory or visual systems.* Some clients may not be able to read and/or write, which may necessitate using purely auditory or visual symbol systems. Examples of auditory devices that can be used to help individuals track and respond to information include electronic voice organizers or voice message devices and speech compression tape recorders. Symbol systems can be individually developed using pictorial systems developed from augmentative communication devices. Clinicians, clients, and caregivers can select symbols that can be used on daily diaries or calendars.

• *Task-specific aids.* A multitude of devices that use simple technology are available to help with memory and organization for specific tasks. A sample list is provided below.

Key finders (beep responds to clapping or voice)
Car memo pads
Refrigerator pads, grocery lists
Pill box reminders
Post-It Notes or reminders written on 3 × 5 index cards
Bulletin boards with message pads and reminder notes
Spell/grammar checks, calculators
Phone dialers; electronic Rolodex
Home management systems with files for managing mail and paying bills

In summary, effective implementation of an external cognitive aid will depend heavily upon selecting a device that meets an individual's needs and accommodates any deficits. This requires conducting a needs assessment and being knowledgeable about the broad range of available devices and technology.

PRETRAINING ACTIVITIES

Adequate preparation for training a client to use an external aid is a key to successful implementation. There are three basic preparatory activities. The first is psychological; it involves making sure the clinician operates from a "mindset" conducive to training the use of an external aid. The second is to make a plan to address any client awareness issues that will affect strategy use. The third involves the clinician making sure he or she knows each of the steps and components for using a particular external aid and the contexts in which it will be used. Knowing the steps and anticipating the contexts will allow the clinician to devise an effective training protocol.

Maintaining a Constructive Mindset

Attitudes are impossible to prescribe. Clients, their families, and other caregivers all have their own sets of beliefs and attitudes, which affect their response to therapy. We clinicians also have unique sets of feelings and experiences, which influence the therapeutic nature of our service delivery. It can be helpful to examine and monitor our own beliefs and motivations, and perhaps to become more conscious of any thoughts that may enhance or detract from our therapy. Discussed below are several "beliefs" that may strengthen our therapy.

Adopting a New Habit Takes Time

Even without problems in learning and memory, most individuals require repetition and repeated opportunities for implementing a strategy before it becomes routine. It can be helpful for us as therapists to recall a past personal goal that involved establishing a new habit or routine (e.g., an exercise or home organizational goal). Most people do not reach a goal in a smooth fashion with increased and sustained implementation over time. They may experience success during the initial period, when they have increased motivation and support, and then exhibit a waxing and waning of implementation depending upon the circumstances. Individuals with brain injury are no different. Too often, because of the way we therapists write clinical goals, we feel forced to plan for clients to adopt a new system or strategy after a relatively brief explanation and exposure. We then feel defeated when the systems are not used. Alternatively, it can be helpful to plan for an acquisition period and expect periods of failed strategy use, which may require "booster shots" from us or from other caregivers. Having realistic expectations may prevent us from prematurely abandoning an external aid that has good potential to be effective. It also helps families and other people involved in supporting clients to expect inconsistency and to plan for an occasional review of procedures.

Patience Is Needed in Partnering with Caregivers

There are usually good reasons why colleagues and caregivers do not follow through with therapy goals. We clinicians know that training the use of an external aid requires involving people who interact with our clients in different settings. This in turn requires us to coordinate our efforts. For example, we may ask colleagues or other caregivers to take data relevant to a client's implementing an external aid, or to give specific types of prompting to assist with generalized use of the aid. It can be frustrating when a program is dependent upon others who do not carry out agreed-upon tasks. This frustration may lead us clinicians to label these other individuals as "noncompliant." Deciding a priori that most people will do what they can to assist us can be a very therapeutic attitude. Often people do not follow through with agreed-upon tasks because of extenuating circumstances, or the tasks do not make sense or have the same meaning to them as they may to us. Checking to make sure that the training tasks still work with the individuals' schedules and with their visions for the clients may lead to modifications that will increase follow-through. Acknowledging that follow-through is likely to be inconsistent, due to the unexpected disruptions that always occur in people's lives, may prevent us as clinicians from feeling discouraged or blaming—reactions that can inhibit the therapeutic process. Chapter 13 details strategies to promote collaborative partnerships with families and caregivers.

Like Everyone, Clients Need Reinforcement

Learning to use an external aid when a client has a cognitive impairment is a lofty ambition and can be a frustrating experience. As we clinicians set goals with our clients for how and when they will use their aids, it can be helpful to build in reinforcement. For example, perhaps a logical clinical goal is for a client to follow a daily therapy schedule independently. This may not be inherently motivating to a client even if he or she wants to learn to compensate for a memory impairment. Writing a schedule that includes chosen activities (e.g., scheduling to view a favorite TV show or making a social phone call) may be more reinforcing to following a daily schedule than searching for the time and location of the next therapy appointment.

Evaluating Awareness Issues

Lack of awareness or diminished insight into residual cognitive problems is a common consequence of acquired brain injury. It can be difficult to introduce a compensatory memory aid to an individual who is not aware of his or her memory problem. Certain clients must have an adequate level of awareness in order to use a particular type of system. Although they may learn the procedures to implement a memory aid, they are unlikely to adopt the use of the aid beyond the training context due to limitations in awareness and insight. For these clients, it may be important to work on awareness prior to or in conjunction with training the use of an external aid. Chapter 9 describes awareness management techniques.

Some clients display significantly impaired insight into their memory or executive function impairments, but can still adopt external aids without needing awareness intervention. These clients tend not to question "why" they are doing something, but can learn procedures or routines if they are given lots of repetition and support (Sohlberg, Mateer, Penkman, Glang, & Todis, 1998a). It is as if the lack of insight prevents them from contemplating the necessity of routines that are taught to them. Awareness deficits in these clients are usually due to damage to prefrontal brain structures and may coexist with passivity and lack of initiation. The external aids that are selected may thus need to be associated with specific prompts or cued by the environment.

Breaking Use of an External Aid into Component Parts and Anticipating the Contexts in Which it Will be Used

Delineating Each Component

Before beginning instruction, it is very important to conduct an analysis of the skills involved in successfully using a system or strategy. This is accomplished by identifying all the components the client must complete in order for the aid to be used effectively. In some cases, it can be helpful to generate the steps with the client. The steps will need to be individualized for the client and for the particular external aid. Two different task analyses for using a homework chart are listed below. Task Analysis 1 is for a client who knows how to fill out a homework chart but needs reminders to do it in a complete fashion. Task Analysis 2 is for a client who needs to learn how to fill out the chart and has more significant organizational difficulties.

Task Analysis 1 (4 training steps)
1. Open notebook when teacher gives assignment.
2. Write down the assignment that is given.
3. Write down the due date for the assignment.
4. Store any papers relevant to the assignment in the proper section.

Task Analysis 2 (10 training steps)
1. Bring notebook to class.
2. Open notebook to homework section when teacher gives assignment.

3. Find line for current day.
4. Write down in assignment on that line.
5. Read assignment and make sure it makes sense.
6. Find due date column.
7. Write down correct due date.
8. Have teacher initial line where assignment is written.
9. File papers relevant to the assignment in the proper section.
10. Close notebook and return it to backpack.

The task of filling out a homework chart is divided up into different subcomponents, based on the needs of each individual student. The task components will form the basis for the training protocol. It is better to err by writing down too many components than by not writing down enough. Once a clinician observes that a component is performed automatically, it does not need to be reviewed or supported. As described in the next section, performance data to guide treatment can be collected for each of the steps.

As a further example, two distinct task analyses are given for teaching a client to review a daily schedule in an electronic memory. Several steps are combined in the first task analysis, whereas they need to be trained separately in the second analysis.

Task Analysis 1 (4 training steps)
1. Push red power button.
2. Move arrow to "c" for calendar and press "enter."
3. Move arrow key to correct date and press "enter."
4. Review daily schedule.

Task Analysis 2 (6 training steps)
1. Push red power button.
2. Move arrow to "c" for calendar.
3. Press "enter."
4. Move arrow key to correct date.
5. Press "enter."
6. Review daily schedule.

Listing the Contexts

After the use of the external aid is broken down into component parts, it can be helpful to anticipate the environments and contexts in which the aid will be used. Once the client can carry out the steps for using the aid, making sure that it is used in the appropriate contexts will be the challenge. Understanding the contexts requires talking with the client and/or other caregivers. Listed below are examples of the types of contexts that might be identified for the external aids described in the task analyses above.

Possible contexts for using homework chart

- Client will use homework chart in her math and history classes, recording any assignments given.
- Client will use homework chart for all seven classes and record "nothing" when there is no homework.

Possible contexts for accessing daily schedule in an electronic memory

- Client will access daily schedule when the alarm cues him, four times each day.
- Client will access daily schedule when he gets to his work station before he turns on computer.
- Client will access daily schedule following breakfast, lunch and dinner.

TRAINING METHODS

Advances in behavioral and cognitive research have greatly improved our understanding of how individuals with damaged neurological systems learn new behaviors. Our challenge is to translate this knowledge into practice. For example, the fact that individuals with memory impairments caused by brain trauma or infection often have relatively spared procedural memory (vs. declarative memory) holds important implications for training new behaviors (Donaghy & Williams, 1998). We now know that even very amnesic individuals can be trained to complete a highly routinized set of steps independently (e.g., operating a computer) by tapping into residual procedural memory (Glisky, 1995).

Effective Instructional Techniques

Behavioral, cognitive, and instructional theories have initiated lines of inquiry that can guide therapists' training methods when they are implementing the use of compensatory aids. The research suggests that by attending to and successfully monitoring clinical behaviors, clinicians can successfully train even individuals with dense amnesia to employ such aids. We begin this section by describing two lines of research that offer prototypes for instructing individuals with brain injuries. The first prototype uses prescribed training methods to successfully teach academic skills, and the second uses training methods to improve clients' performance on functional everyday activities. Both draw heavily from the applied behavioral literature, specifically the literature on direct instruction (Engelman & Carnine, 1982).

Teaching Academic Skills

Glang, Singer, Cooley, and Tish (1992) described three case studies in which direct instruction techniques were successfully used to teach students with brain injuries who participated in a 6-week tutoring program. With about 12 hours of instruction, all three subjects showed significant academic progress in either reading/language, math, or keyboarding. The authors based their training on the foundation of the direct instruction approach, which holds that all students can learn if instructional communications are presented logically, unambiguously, and clearly. It uses task analysis, modeling/shaping, and reinforcement of appropriate responses, as well as continuous assessment. These are the same features that clinicians need to implement when training individuals with brain injuries to use compensatory aids. Specific elements of this type of training are listed below (Glang et al., 1992). This list is an excellent reminder of what clinicians need to do when training persons with cognitive dysfunction to use memory or organizational aids.

1. All component skills need to be pretaught.
2. Teaching examples need to be carefully selected, so that clients can generalize to untaught examples; examples need to be sequenced so that they can build on prior learning.
3. Instructional wording is consistent and clear to decrease confusion.
4. Systematic corrections are built into instruction to provide immediate practice with difficult tasks
5. Sufficient practice is provided to ensure mastery at each step in the learning process.
6. Cumulative review of all skills ensures integration of new skills with previously learned information.
7. Clients need to be kept engaged through high response and success rates, as well as rapid instructional pacing.

Case examples of how some of these key features can be implemented in a training protocol are provided at the end of this chapter.

Teaching Functional Skills

In a unique study, Mozzani and Bailey (1996) demonstrated that patient outcome scores are more likely to increase when rehabilitation therapists work on outcome-related activities and use effective instructional techniques. They worked with six rehabilitation clinicians whose clients were not making progress on their hospital's measure of functional independence. The therapists were trained on 14 specific instructional elements concerned with task selection, prompting, reinforcement, and managing client behavior. They were also given feedback on their performance. Results showed clear improvements in outcome measures for the patients assigned to the therapists who received the training. Examples of the teaching skills addressed in the study are provided below; again, this is an excellent list of important clinical behaviors when one is teaching the use of compensatory aids.

1. Clear cueing: Instructions need to specify the required behavior clearly, using few words and no more than one verb.
2. Patient attention to therapist: Patient needs to look at therapist when cue is given.
3. Use of a task analysis: There needs to be a written list of the components of the task being taught.
4. Treatment consistency: The same steps need to be followed across sessions when the same task is being trained.
5. Systematic prompting that fades over time: Therapist should systematically move from higher to lower levels of support (e.g., from physical to verbal prompts).
6. Practicing: Patient needs to practice the target skill multiple times.
7. Reinforcement: Correct responding needs to be reinforced within 3 seconds.
8. Behavior management: Therapist should be following relevant behavior management procedure if specified for client.
9. Arousal level: Patient should be awake and able to respond without physical prompting.
10. Task relevance: Task should be relevant to outcome measure.
11. Data: Therapist needs to collect patient response/performance data throughout therapy session.

A comparison of this list with the one for the Glang and colleagues (1992) protocol suggests important overlap. Both of these research groups evaluated instructional methods for persons with acquired brain injury, and both protocols emphasize the importance of task analysis, sufficient practice, and effective correction and prompting procedures. Given their relevance to training the use of external memory aids, specific discussions of "errorless" correction techniques and of prompting are provided below.

Errorless Instruction

As discussed in detail in Chapter 6, there is a growing body of research suggesting that persons with severe memory deficits due to brain injury learn new skills more efficiently and effectively when teaching methods are "errorless" (e.g., Baddeley & Wilson, 1994; Evans et al., 2000; Hunkin, Squires, Aldrich, & Parkin, 1998a; Hunkin, Squires, Parkin, & Tidy, 1998b; Squires, Hunkin, & Parkin, 1997; Wilson, Baddeley, Evans, & Shiel, 1994). The literature suggests that if these clients are prevented from committing errors during the initial learning process, they will learn more quickly and be less likely to repeat their errors.

In spite of mounting experimental support, errorless instruction is not widely implemented in current rehabilitation practices. Many clinicians train and instruct their patients using a traditional "test-and-correct" or "trial-and-error" method. For example, they may observe a client performing a target task such as referring to a memory book, and only provide prompting when the client becomes lost and commits an error. As reviewed in Chapter 6, having clients "guess" at answers and then supplying them with correct information may result in their forming memories for the self-generated error responses rather than the clinician-generated corrected responses. Errorless instruction prevents clients from making errors by providing systematic modeling and guidance in the initial acquisition phase.

Prompting

There are various methods to provide prompting to clients as they learn the steps or actions associated with utilizing a compensatory external aid. The goal of prompting is usually to provide just the right amount of help that will facilitate active recall of correct responses and avoid error responses. As clients learn tasks, prompting can be decreased. Riley and Heaton (2000) provide guidelines for the selection of prompting methods and the subsequent fading of cues in work with persons who have memory impairments. Their research results encourage clinicians to consider the difficulty of the tasks and the memory abilities and disabilities of the clients. Results from their study comparing two methods of fading cues when teaching general knowledge to individuals with a history of brain injury suggest the following general guidelines for selecting prompting methods:

- Rapid fading of cues is more effective for those clients with better memories.
- Rapid fading of cues is more effective for learning simpler tasks.
- Gradual fading of cues is more effective for those clients with more severe memory impairments.
- Gradual fading of cues is more effective for learning more complex tasks.

It is helpful to work from a cueing hierarchy, in order to systematically provide decreasing levels of prompting (Mozzoni & Bailey, 1996). A cueing hierarchy helps standardize prompting methods across clinicians and caregivers. Consistency in prompting allows clinicians to be objective in documenting client performance. An example of a cueing hierarchy that may be utilized when one is training the steps to use an external aid is provided below. (More levels of cueing could be described, depending upon the patient population.)

- *Full cue.* This level provides the most direct instruction on how to do a task. It may involve modeling or physical prompts. Full cues provide an overt demonstration on the part of the clinician. An example is for the clinician actually to write in a schedule entry and then to have the client copy it. This level of prompting is provided during the initial phase of instruction.

- *Specific questioning cue.* At this cueing level, the therapist poses a question that facilitates self-monitoring. In other words, the clinician asks a question whose answer represents what the client should be doing. For example, a clinician may ask, "How will you remember our appointment time next week?" in order to prompt the client to look at his or her calendar.

- *Opportunity cue.* This level represents the most minimal, nonverbal level of prompting. It is the act of providing the client with a clear opportunity to refer to or use an external aid without making any overt suggestion. Examples of opportunity cues include expectant pauses or raised eyebrows that give the client a chance to realize he or she may want to do something.

Carefully planned, systematic prompting may allow a person with a severe memory impairment to learn to use a compensatory system. One case study described the results of rehabilitation efforts with a subject who exhibited dense amnesia following status epilepticus after a motor vehicle accident. A comprehensive system of external cueing adopted across rehabilitation disciplines resulted in improved function. The researchers suggested that the patient's increased independent generalization of strategies was due to the consistent external cueing, which exploited the subject's preserved procedural memory (Kime, Lamb, & Wilson, 1996).

Clarity of Instruction

It is important to explain the procedures involved in using an external aid clearly and concisely (Glang et al., 1992). In general, more words are not necessarily better. A recent project (Sohlberg, Roth, & McLaughlin, 2001) observed speech–language pathologists in clinical settings working with people with brain injuries. Of note was the very low number of patient responses that were elicited during a session. Therapists tended to provide lots of "education" with verbal instruction, but very little practice in "doing" a skill. Providing clear instructions with ample demonstration, and then allowing clients to practice the skill until they can perform it independently, are critical. This type of instructional training can be sandwiched between more conversational interactions where the clinician connects with the client and builds the relationship.

Monitoring Clients' Progress

Ongoing monitoring of clients' progress is an important part of training. Selecting and training the use of compensatory aids are cyclical rather than linear processes. Compensatory systems and programs need to be consistently updated and modified to reflect changes in clients' needs and environments. Methods to assess the effectiveness of an aid for a client include direct observation and interview. Clients, family members, or other caregivers may do the monitoring and report information to the clinician. The critical factor is to have a plan for ongoing monitoring. That plan will need to include the following:

- A determination of what is being assessed (how will the clinician know if the aid is or is not working?)
- A monitoring system with a plan for data collection
- A method to modify instruction as needed, based on the information gathered

Several examples of a scoresheet that enables a clinician to document client performance while implementing effective instructional techniques are provided in Appendices 7.3 through 7.5. (Appendix 7.3 is the blank scoresheet; Appendices 7.4 and 7.5 are two filled-in examples.)

Self-Monitoring for Clinicians

The literature and the clinical experience of many therapists responsible for teaching individuals with memory impairments new information or procedures underscore the importance of systematic training. A checklist that clinicians can use to monitor their own training efforts or to educate new therapists is provided in Box 7.1. It incorporates the effective instructional procedures reviewed throughout this chapter.

CASE EXAMPLES

Case Example 1

Sara was a 41-year-old female hospitalized for viral encephalitis. After a 3-week course of acute care, she was transferred to the hospital's inpatient rehabilitation unit.

BOX 7.1. Training Checklist

Task Selection/Pretraining

__ I have collaborated with the client and significant others when conducting a needs assessment, and have based my recommendations on this needs assessment.

__ I have broken the strategy or use of the aid into component parts (task analysis).

__ I have a method for recording the client's performance on each of the component skills, and a systematic method for documenting level of cueing.

__ I understand the context(s) in which the client will be using the aid and what types of supports may be available.

__ I have a plan for how training can be reinforcing for the client.

Task Presentation

__ I have demonstrated or modeled the step(s) taught during the initial acquisition phase; I am using errorless instruction.

__ I have provided clear, concise instructions.

__ I have recorded data on the client's performance and on my prompting.

__ I have provided sufficient practice until the client can do the target step(s) independently.

__ As the client has mastered step(s), I have linked them to other steps until the client can do the sequence independently.

__ I have provided practice with all of the different types of situations/contexts in which the client will need to use the aid.

__ I have incorporated family members/other caregivers into my planning and training.

__ I have a plan for ongoing monitoring of strategy or use of the aid, which includes a determination of what to assess, as well as a method for collecting and acting upon performance or outcome data.

Neuropsychological evaluation documented a severe anterograde memory disturbance. Sara was unable to learn new information or remember events from day to day. A needs assessment was completed with the goal of selecting an appropriate compensatory memory aid. The needs assessment encouraged her clinicians to select a simple external aid that utilized a writing–reading modality. In addition to her memory impairment, Sara exhibited significant problems in attention and executive functions. Her reading, writing, and language skills appeared intact. Sara had limited awareness of her deficits, but was very compliant in following clinician requests. As part of the needs assessment, it was discovered that Sara had utilized a particular type of daily planner prior to her illness. This planner was retrieved from her home to be implemented in the hospital. The first function to be trained was following a daily schedule. The daily schedule included her therapy regimen and a visitor schedule, which her mother helped to coordinate. The following was the task analysis used to teach Sara initial use of her daily planner. The speech–language pathologist and Sara's husband worked to make sure that the next day's schedule of therapies and visitors was entered into the planner.

Steps for using planner
1. Notice that watch beeps.
2. Look at date on watch and say it out loud.
3. Open planner to the correct day.
4. Make sure plastic marker is on that day.
5. Look at time on watch.
6. Look at time on planner and say corresponding event out loud.
7. If you are not where planner says to be, ask someone to help you get there.

A protocol with these seven steps was created. The therapist trained Sara in the sequence of steps using errorless instruction, in which steps were modeled until she could do them independently. The cueing hierarchy (see "Prompting," above) was utilized to document level of cueing. As Sara mastered a step, it was linked to the next step in a forward chaining procedure. A written reminder of these steps was typed and taped to the outside of the planner. Sara referred to this list if she got confused about a step. In a training session, she would practice the target steps an average of 30 to 40 times. After 10 sessions she could complete all seven steps, although on occasion she would refer to the written reminder list. However, if there was no watch beep to prompt her to get started, she did not start the routine. Also, if someone were to ask Sara to *describe* the steps for using her planner (declarative memory), she would say she did not know; once she heard the watch beep, however, she would start the sequence and do it in an automatic fashion (procedural memory).

This protocol depended upon Sara's being with someone who could help her following Step 7—determining where she should go. Due to her severe amnesic disturbance and difficulties with problem solving, she was not able to figure out where to go on her own or how to find her visitor if the visitor was not there. It was decided that training her in the routes for going to her different therapies would be too time-consuming, since she would eventually be going home, and that for her it was reasonable that she would need assistance.

After Sara mastered this protocol, it was expanded to teach her to make a note about what she was doing at the time of the watch beep on the opposing page in the planner. This gave her diary information about what she had done during the day. Prior to this, her therapists and husband had made the diary entries. The diary function was trained in the same manner described above. When Sara had mastered this function, she was trained to make entries into the planner, again using this same approach.

The speech–language pathologist made up a training book with the basic principles for expanding Sara's planner and teaching her to use it. She was going to be receiving outpatient therapies, and the plan was for her husband to have a way to communicate with the new therapist about how to support and monitor the use of the planner.

Case Example 2

Miles was an eighth grader who had returned to school after a traumatic brain injury received in a motor vehicle accident. He had been out of school for 6 months; during that time, he had received cognitive rehabilitation and home tutoring. When he returned to school, he was made eligible for special education services. He seemed to perform adequately on assignments in class, but demonstrated significant trouble with turning in homework, which was causing him to fail his classes. A meeting with the special education teacher, several of his classroom teachers, Miles, and his parents was held to discuss his homework problem.

During that meeting, it was decided that Miles would probably benefit from some type of compensatory aid to help him track his homework. However, when the special education teacher was filling out the needs assessment, she found it difficult to select a strategy because it was not clear why Miles was having such difficulty with his homework. His parents felt that they helped him with some homework, but thought that maybe not all of the assignments were getting home. Miles said he did not know what why he had so many zeros for homework. In order to select a helpful strategy, the team members decided they needed to determine the cause of the breakdown. They devised a parent information form for the parents to fill out. This form would allow the teachers and Miles to see whether his problem was due to difficulty with keeping track of the assignment, initiating homework, completing the homework, or keeping track of completed work and turning it in. After several weeks of the parents' completing the information form, it became clear that Miles was not turning in homework because he did not return his completed assignments. This allowed the school team to devise a homework return strategy. First, Miles selected a new school notebook with pockets. Then the team members made up the following steps for Miles to follow:

Homework return strategy
1. As soon as it is finished, put completed homework in front notebook pocket.
2. Put notebook in backpack.
3. Have parents initial tag on notebook.
4. As soon as you get into class, put homework in designated place. (In math, there was a basket; in social studies, there was a box; English homework was supposed to be kept on top of the desk until it was collected.)
5. Ask teacher to initial tag on notebook.

(When Miles had had his parents and teachers initial his tag for 10 consecutive days, his parents agreed to buy him a CD of his choice.)

Miles's special education teacher had him role-play each of these steps, using errorless instructional procedures. At first they just practiced the steps to be completed at home, using mock homework, while the teacher role-played being his parents. Then they practiced the steps for returning homework in math class, then social studies, and then English. The teacher had Miles's parents and his classroom teachers begin by giving him specific questioning cues. Eventually he was able to follow the steps independently. A monitoring system was set up whereby the special education teacher received a weekly homework report from the classroom teachers. After Miles got his first CD reward, he became inconsistent about using the strategy, so he and the special education teacher did several more practice sessions.

SUMMARY

This chapter describes methods for teaching individuals to implement compensatory aids successfully and independently. It is an ambitious goal to expect a person with disordered learning and/or organizational abilities to adopt a new habit such as using an external aid. The first important step is to conduct a needs assessment, which involves careful collaboration with the client and relevant persons in the client's environment to determine strengths, barriers, and contexts for using an aid. The needs assessment will help identify options for compensatory aids that are consistent with the client's individual profile. Once an appropriate system or external aid is selected, effective instructional strategies are implemented that will allow a client with severe to mild memory deficits or executive function impairments to adopt compensatory habits.

Three notable strengths of most persons with severe memory impairments are the preservation of immediate memory or attentional abilities, procedural memory, and old learning. Clinicians can capitalize on these abilities to teach clients to implement external compensatory aids. The adoption of theoretically sound instructional methods based on applied behavioral methodology has furthered cognitive rehabilitation efforts. This chapter discusses important clinical practices such as errorless instruction, guided practice, and systematic prompting, as well as the monitoring of strategy use.

Effective training is labor- and time-intensive. However, as noted by Tate (1997) and echoed by Donaghy and Williams (1998), the clinical practices appear quite reasonable when one considers the efforts required for the rehabilitation of physical impairments. Training persons with brain injuries to use compensatory techniques is a necessary and critical tool for managing changes in memory, attention, and executive functions.

REFERENCES

Baddeley, A. D., & Wilson, B. (1994). When implicit learning fails: Amnesia and the problem of error elimination. *Neuropsychologia, 32*(1), 53–68.

Burke, J. M., Danick, J. A., Bemis, B., & Durgin, C. J. (1994). A process approach to memory book training for neurological patients. *Brain Injury, 8*(1), 71–81.

Donaghy, S., & Williams, W. (1998). A new protocol for training severely impaired patients in the usage of memory journals. *Brain Injury, 12*(12), 1061–1070.

Engelman, S. E., & Carnine, D. W. (1982). *Theory of instruction: Principles and Applications.* New York: Irvington.

Evans, J. J., Wilson, B. A., Schuri, U., Andrade, J., Baddeley, A. D., Bruna, O., Canavan, T., Della Salla, S., Green, R., Laaksonen, R., Lorenzi, L., & Taussik, I. (2000). A comparison of "errorless" and "trial-and-error" learning methods for teaching individuals with acquired memory deficits. *Neuropsychological Rehabilitation, 10*(1), 67–101.

Fluharty, G., & Priddy, D. (1993). Case study: Methods of increasing client acceptance of a memory book. *Brain Injury, 7*(1), 83–88.

Glang, A., Singer, G., Cooley, E., & Tish, N. (1992). Tailoring direct instruction techniques for use with elementary students with brain injury. *Journal of Head Trauma Rehabilitation, 7*(4), 93–108.

Glisky, E. L. (1995). Acquisition and transfer of word processing skills by an amnesic patient. *Neuropsychological Rehabilitation, 5,* 299–318.

Glisky, E. L., & Schacter, D. L. (1986). Remediation of organic memory disorders: Current status and future prospects. *Journal of Head Trauma Rehabilitation, 1*(3), 54–63.

Harris, J. (1980). Memory aids people use: Two interview studies. *Memory and Cognition, 8,* 31–38.

Hersch, N., & Treadgold, L. (1994). NeuroPage: The rehabilitation of memory dysfunction by prosthetic memory and cueing. *Neuropsychological Rehabilitation, 4,* 187–197.

Hunkin, N. M., Squires, E. J., Aldrich, F. K., & Parkin, A. J. (1998a). Errorless learning and the acquisition of word processing skills. *Neuropsychological Rehabilitation, 8*(4), 443–449.

Hunkin, N. M., Squires, E. J., Parkin, A. J., & Tidy, J. A. (1998b). Are the benefits of errorless learning dependent on implicit memory? *Neuropsychologia, 36*(1), 25–36.

Kapur, N. (1995). Memory aids in the rehabilitation of memory disordered patients. In A. D. Baddeley, B. A. Wilson, & F. N. Watts (Eds.), *Handbook of memory disorders* (pp. 534–556). Chichester, England: Wiley.

Kerns, K. A., & Thompson, J. (1998). Implementation of a compensatory memory system in a school age child with severe memory impairment. *Pediatric Rehabilitation, 2*(2), 77–87.

Kim, H. J., Burke, D. T., Dowds, M. D., & George, J. (1999). Utility of a microcomputer as an external memory aid for a memory impaired head injury patient during in-patient rehabilitation. *Brain Injury, 13*(2), 147–150.

Kim, H. J., Burke, D. T., Dowds, M. M., Robinson Boone, K. A., & Park, G. J. (2000).

Electronic memory aids for outpatients with brain injury: Follow-up findings. *Brain Injury, 14*(2), 187–196.

Kime, S. K., Lamb, D. G., & Wilson, B. A. (1996). Use of a comprehensive programme of external cueing to enhance procedural memory in a patient with dense amnesia. *Brain Injury, 10*(1), 17–25.

Mozzoni, M. P., & Bailey, J. S. (1996). Improving training methods in brain injury rehabilitation. *Journal of Head Trauma Rehabilitation, 11*(1), 1–17.

Parente, R. (1998, October). *Memory aids/memory notebook.* Paper presented at the 17th Annual Symposium of the Brain Injury Association, New Orleans, LA.

Riley, G. A., & Heaton, S. (2000). Guidelines for the selection of a method of fading cues. *Neuropsychological Rehabilitation, 10*(2), 133–149.

Schacter, D. L., & Glisky, E. L. (1986). Memory remediation: restoration, alleviation and the acquisition of domain-specific knowledge. In B. P. Uzzell & Y. Gross (Eds.), *Clinical neuropsychology of intervention* (pp. 257–282). Boston: Nijhoff.

Simmons-Mackie, N. N., & Damico, J. S. (1997). Reformulating the definition of compensatory strategies in aphasia. *Aphasiology, 11*(8), 761–781.

Sohlberg, M. M., Johansen, A., Geyer, S., & Hoornbeek, S. (1994). *A manual for teaching patients to use compensatory memory systems.* Puyallup, WA: Association for Neuropsychological Research and Development.

Sohlberg, M. M., & Mateer, C. A. (1989). Training use of compensatory memory books: A three state behavioral approach. *Journal of Clinical and Experimental Neuropsychology, 11*, 871–891.

Sohlberg, M. M., Mateer, C. A., Penkman, L., Glang, A., & Todis, B. (1998). Awareness intervention: Who needs it? *Journal of Head Trauma Rehabilitation, 13*(5), 62–78.

Sohlberg, M. M., Roth, K., & McLaughlin, K. (2001). *Observation of SLPS: Is there a relationship between practice and theory?* Manuscript in preparation.

Sohlberg, M. M., Todis, B., & Glang, A. (1998b). SCEMA: A team-based approach to serving secondary students with executive dysfunction following brain injury. *Aphasiology, 12*(12), 1047–1092.

Squires, E. J., Hunkin, N. M., & Parkin, A. J. (1997). Errorless learning of novel associations in amnesia. *Neuropsychologia, 35*(8), 1103–1111.

Tate, R. L. (1997). Beyond one-bun, two-shoe: Recent advances in the psychological rehabilitation of memory disorders after acquired brain injury. *Brain Injury, 11*, 907–918.

Wilson, B. A. (1991). Long-term prognosis of patients with severe memory disorders. *Neuropsychological Rehabilitation, 1*, 117–134.

Wilson, B. A., Baddeley, A. D., Evans, E., & Shiel, A. (1994). Errorless learning in the rehabilitation of memory impaired people. *Neuropsychological Rehabilitation, 4*, 307–326.

Zenicus, A., Wesolowski, M. D., & Burke, W. H. (1990). A comparison of four memory strategies with traumatically brain injured clients. *Brain Injury, 4*, 33–38.

Zenicus, A., Wesolowski, M. D., & Burke, W. H. (1991). Memory notebook training with traumatically brain-injured clients. *Brain Injury, 5*, 321–325.

SELECTED MEMORY AID RESOURCES

The external aids referred to in this chapter are representative of current options; they are by no means the only ones available in the current market. There are many other such devices, and they constantly change. Our intention has been merely to provide some examples.

Dayrunners: Dayrunners Inc. Consumer Inquiries, 1-800-635-5544.
Daytimers: Available in most office supply stores.
Franklin Planner: The Mead Corporation, 1-937-865-6800.
Casio, Tandy, and Sharp electronic devices: Available in most electronic retail outlets.
Timex Data Link Watch: United States, 1-800-367-8463; Canada, 1-800-263-0981; United Kingdom, +44-171-630-8180; Internet, data.link@timex. com.
NeuroPage: Interactive Proactive Mnemonic Systems, 6657 Camelia Drive, San Jose, CA.
Psion Series 3a: Psion PLC, London.

APPENDIX 7.1

NEEDS ASSESSMENT FOR EXTERNAL
COGNITIVE AIDS (ADULT CLIENT)

Client's Name _____ Date _____

Clinician's Name _____

I. COGNITIVE PROFILE

Check the areas that are of concern. For those areas that are checked, describe the nature of the impairment underneath type of memory.

__ Episodic memory (ability to remember daily events and personal experiences)

_____

__ Semantic memory (ability to remember facts and knowledge-based information)

_____

__ Prospective memory (ability to initiate a planned future action at a specific time)

_____

__ Procedural memory (ability to learn procedures or steps—may be learning without awareness)

_____

__ Retrograde amnesia (pattern of loss of memory for events prior to injury)

_____

__ New learning (ability/rate of learning new information)

_____

__ Decreased attention

_____

__ Limitations in executive functions (e.g., initiation, planning, organization, etc.)

_____

__ Reduced reasoning/problem solving

_____

__ Language problems affecting ability to read, write, or type entries

_____

II. PHYSICAL PROFILE

__ Visual problems affecting ability to read, write, or type entries

_____

__ Motoric difficulties affecting ability to write in, manipulate, or carry system

_____

__ Auditory problems affecting ability to hear alarms or watch beeps

_____

III. PERSONAL FACTORS

A. *Current or Past Use of Memory/Organizational Aids (Check all that apply)*

__ No systems used	__ Notes to self
__ Calendar in the home	__ Wore a watch
__ Datebook system	__ Elaborate organizational system
__ Spouse/partner keeps track of things	__ Other _____

Comments: _____

B. *Level of Acceptance/Awareness of Memory Impairment (Check best description)*

__ Has limited understanding or awareness of impairment (awareness deficit due to organic brain damage)

__ Exhibits significant psychological denial (difficulty accepting disability)

__ Can state knowledge of impairment but does not think aids are necessary

__ Openly discusses memory problem but inconsistent in using compensation strategies

__ Appears willing to learn and use aids

C. *Client Preferences for a Memory System*

1. Appearance (color, style, size) _____._____

_____

2. Types of functions (e.g., calendar, things to do list, budget planner, etc.)

_____

3. Mode (electronic, written, auditory, pictorial) _____

_____

D. Financial Resources

__ Insurance (or other third-party payer willing to pay)
__ Personal funds available to purchase system of choice
__ Funds available for system up to ____ dollars
__ No funds available

E. Available Support

__ Patient would need to be able to utilize systems independently due to lack of available support
__ Family/staff/significant others able and willing to be trained but will require structured program
__ Persons to be involved with patient will vary; will need to provide description of system, procedures for using it, and methods for providing assistance

IV. SITUATIONAL FACTORS

Context: Describe goal of external aid

_____

When and where would it be used?

_____

Functions of systems—external aid system will need to provide the following functions:

__ Autobiographical information (personal history, orientation sheets, photos, fact sheets, etc.)
__ Daily schedule
__ Calendar
__ Things to do
__ Daily diary/events log
__ Specific journal (e.g., anger log)
__ Therapy goals
__ Other _____

Recommendations: _____
_____
_____
_____

APPENDIX 7.2

NEEDS ASSESSMENT FOR EXTERNAL
COGNITIVE AIDS (STUDENT CLIENT)

Student's Name _____ Date _____

Name of Person Completing Form _____

A. LEARNING AND MEMORY PROFILE

Check and describe any areas of concern:

__ Remembering daily events and personal experiences

_____

__ Learning new information

_____

__ Starting and following through with a planned activity at a specific time

_____

__ Loss of memory for events before injury

_____

__ Organizing materials and actions to get a task done

_____

__ Understanding oral and/or written directions

_____

__ Paying attention and staying focused

_____

__ Ignoring distractors

_____

__ Reasoning and problem solving

_____

__ Other

_____

Describe academic strengths _____

_____

_____

B. OTHER COGNITIVE AND PHYSICAL ABILITIES

Check and describe any areas of concern:

__ Language problems affecting ability to read, write, or type
__ Visual problems affecting ability to read, write, or type
__ Hearing problems affecting ability to understand others or use tape recorder
__ Motor difficulties affecting ability to write in, manipulate, or carry system

C. HOME AND SCHOOL CONTEXTS

1. Who is available at school to teach the student to use a compensatory system?

_____

_____

2. Are there others at school who can monitor and reinforce system use?

_____

_____

3. Who might be available at home to monitor and reinforce system use?

_____

_____

D. STUDENT PREFERENCES

1. Appearance (e.g., color, style, size) _____

2. Types of functions (e.g., calendar, homework list, phone list) _____

_____

3. Mode (electronic, written, auditory, picture-based) _____

_____

E. WHAT ACCOMMODATIONS HAVE BEEN TRIED?

Managing assignments
__ Help finding assignments
__ System for tracking assignments (provided by home, not school)
__ Reminders to record assignments (how often?)
__ Help putting assignments where your child can find them in notebook
__ Reminders to turn in assignments (how often?)

Doing homework
   __ Reminders to get started on homework (how often?)
   __ Reminders, encouragement to keep working (how often?)
   __ Help with homework

Organization
   __ Help setting up organizational system for assignments and materials
   __ Reminders to keep assignments and materials organized (how often?)
   __ Help keeping materials organized
   __ Other accommodations for recording, tracking, completing, turning in
      assignments

Remedial help
   __ Review of basic math, reading, spelling, writing skills—who provides?

_____

For those checked, describe and indicate how effective you think the accommodation is.

If any of the accommodations above have been tried but are not currently used, please explain.

Use of school organizational aids (Check all that apply)
__ Uses an electronic or written organizational system __ Wears a watch
__ Asks friends or family for needed information   __ Homework list
__ Writes notes to self   __ Other _____

If your child used any of these aids in the past but is currently not using them, please indicate which ones and explain why they are no longer used.

F. RECOMMENDATIONS: _____

_____

_____

_____

APPENDIX 7.3

SCORESHEET FOR PRACTICE TRIALS

Name _____

Type of Memory System _____

Target Function _____

Cueing Hierarchy
1. Opportunity Cue
2. Specific Questioning Cue
3. Full Cue

To fill out scoresheet: List component steps for using an aid. For each trial, document the trial number and date. Record accuracy (+/-) and the level of cueing needed for patient to complete each step. Record any relevant observations in the appropriate box on the "Comments" row.

Date											
Trial #											
STEPS											
COMMENTS											

SUMMARY
TOTALS:

APPENDIX 7.4

EXAMPLE OF COMPLETED SCORESHEET FOR PRACTICE TRIALS

Name __PM__

Type of Memory System __pill box with alarm__

Target Function __daily independent use of pill box__

To fill out scoresheet: List component steps for using an aid. For each trial, document the trial number and date. Record accuracy (+/-) and the level of cueing needed for patient to complete each step. Record any relevant observations in the "Comments" row.

Cueing Hierarchy
1. Opportunity Cue
2. Specific Questioning Cue
3. Full Cue

Date	10/11	10/11	10/11	10/11	10/11	10/11	10/11	10/11	10/11	10/11	
Trial #	1	2	3	4	5	6	7	8	9	10	
STEPS											
Acknowledge alarm	3	3	2	1	1	1	1	1	1	1	
Look at date display	3	3	2	1	1	1	1	1	1	1	
Find today's box	3	/	/	/	3	2	2	1	1	1	
Open box	3	/	/	/	/	/	/	/	3	2	
Take pill	3	/	/	/	/	/	/	/	3	1	
COMMENTS	demon-strated steps			did steps 1 and 2 indep.				remembers model; mastered steps 1–3		just needs practice	
SUMMARY TOTALS:											

228

APPENDIX 7.5

EXAMPLE OF COMPLETED SCORESHEET FOR PRACTICE TRIALS

Name _T. C._

Type of Memory System _Memory book_

Target Function _Write in diary after each meal_

Cueing Hierarchy
1. Opportunity Cue
2. Specific Questioning Cue
3. Full Cue

To fill out scoresheet: List component steps for using an aid. For each trial, document the trial number and date. Record accuracy (+/-) and the level of cueing needed for patient to complete each step. Record any relevant observations in the appropriate box on the "Comments" row.

Date	5/4	5/4	5/4	5/4	5/4	5/5	5/5	5/5	5/5	5/5	
Trial #	1	2	3	4	5	1	2	3	4	5	
STEPS											
Takes book to meal	role play 1	1	1	1	1	1	1	1	1	1	
Opens book to diary section	1	1	1	1	1	1	1	1	1	1	
Looks at wall calendar	1	1	1	1	1	1	1	1	1	1	
Finds correct date in diary	2	2	2	1	1	2	2	1	1	1	
Writes entry	2	2	2	2	2	2	1	2	1	1	
Checks that entry is complete	2	2	2	2	2	2	2	2	2	1	
COMMENTS	remembered steps taught earlier in week	prompt = "how can you remember?"	today"							Got it!	

SUMMARY TOTALS:

8

Management of Dysexecutive Symptoms

It is well established that the abilities involved in planning, initiating, and regulating behavior are dependent upon the functions of the frontal lobes and their widespread connections throughout the central nervous system. For individuals with acquired brain injury, damage to these brain networks, and the associated dysexecutive symptoms, do more to determine the extent of community reintegration than does damage to any other cognitive system. This chapter begins with a review of frontal lobe functioning and a presentation of a clinically relevant executive function model. The remainder of the chapter presents four approaches to managing dysexecutive symptoms: environmental/ecological management, training task-specific routines, training the selection and execution of cognitive plans, and self-instructional therapies.

THE FRONTAL LOBES

Neuroanatomical Considerations

The human frontal lobes are unique. They are very large structures and constitute approximately 30% of the total cortical surface (Goldman-Rakic, 1984). Phylogenetically, as one moves up the animal chain, an increasing proportion of the cortex is devoted to the prefrontal structures. Thus primates have more prefrontal cortex than dogs, dogs have more than cats, and cats have more than rodents. This region of the frontal lobes is the most recently developed part of the brain evolutionarily and is the latest to develop in a maturing individual. The relatively massive growth of the prefrontal cortex is considered responsible for human beings' superior mental capacity (Stuss & Benson, 1986).

There has been an increasing appreciation of the frontal lobes as part of an extensive brain network system with robust afferent and efferent connections throughout the central nervous system. They represent the most highly interconnected regions of the brain, with rich reciprocal connections to temporal, parietal, and occipital cortices. These connections transmit high-level auditory, somatosensory, and visual information to the frontal lobes. The frontal lobes also have strong connections with limbic structures (e.g., the hippocampus and amygdala), which are involved in learning, memory, and emotional processing (Kaufer & Lewis, 1999).

Executive functions have been localized to the prefrontal and frontal brain regions; however, the precise neural mechanisms underlying these processes are not fully understood. Mesulam (1990) asserts that cognitive abilities are generated from interconnected neural grids that are both localized and distributed. The prefrontal lobes' widespread connections to cortical and subcortical regions serve to organize behavior by activating, inhibiting, and integrating ideomotor and sensorimotor activity. In other words, the frontal lobes act as an executive branch of the brain that controls the function of subservient neural systems involved in goal-directed behavior. Hence the prefrontal regions' dense interconnections with other brain regions and their independence from sensorimotor activities explain the disruption of complex functions seen in patients with frontal lobe damage (Mesulam, 1990). Elsewhere, we (Sohlberg, Mateer, & Stuss, 1993) describe a clinically useful framework of frontal lobe functions, based on the premise that there is a hierarchy of interrelated independent functions. We describe sensation and basic knowledge as the lowest part of the hierarchy, executive functions as the middle component, and self-reflectiveness as the highest component. Each of the three components is associated with particular neuroanatomical connections.

Although most cognitive processes seem to be represented throughout the prefrontal cortex unevenly, there is some lateralization of functions to specific hemispheres. For example, episodic retrieval tasks activate the right prefrontal lobe while semantic retrieval and encoding activate the left prefrontal lobe (Grady, 1999). Some researchers, however, suggest that different regions of the frontal lobes are associated with specific abilities. For example, lateral frontal lobe lesions tend to result in initiation disorders, whereas damage to the orbital region is associated with disinhibition or impulsivity (Stuss & Benson, 1986). Clinically, it is more often the case that both areas are disrupted, although one type of behavioral symptom may predominate.

The location of the frontal lobes in the skull renders them susceptible to damage in the event of a closed head injury. When the head strikes an object, such as a windshield, the brain is thrust forward against surrounding bony protrusions. Figure 8.1 shows how the orbital regions of the frontal lobe are situated against bony, ridged processes and stiff membranes.

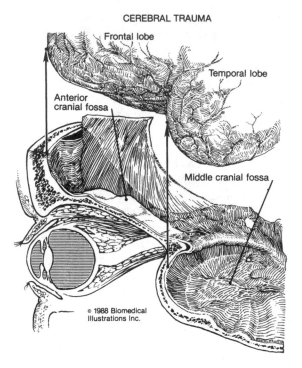

FIGURE 8.1. Schematic pull-away illustrating the position of the orbital and anterior frontal regions and the anterior temporal lobe relative to bony processes. Copyright 1988 by Biomedical Illustrations, Inc. Reprinted by permission.

Figure 8.2 shows the tendency for traumatic brain injury to result in damage to the orbital, frontal, and temporal regions. The frontal lobes are further prone to damage because they receive blood supply in part from the middle cerebral artery, a common site of stroke (see Chapter 2). Given the propensity for damage, it is critical for clinicians to be aware of the different cognitive and behavioral manifestations of frontal lobe pathology.

Frontal Lobe Functions

Through their widespread connectivity, the frontal lobes are integral to a variety of cognitive, behavioral, and emotional functions. Central to this chapter is their importance in executive functions. We know that the frontal lobes are responsible for coordinating and actualizing the activities involved in cognitive processing, but they are not necessarily responsible for primary cognitive functions. For example, frontal lobe damage does not interfere with the memory stage directing storage of information, but it does

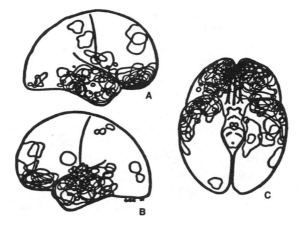

FIGURE 8.2. Drawing of contusions after traumatic brain injury, based on 40 consecutive cases. Depicts the tendency for maximum pathology in the orbital frontal and temporal regions. From Courville (1937). Copyright 1937 by Pacific Publishers. Reprinted by permission.

affect other processes related to memory, such as attention, organization of information, temporal tagging, and self-monitoring. Executive functions supported by the frontal lobes include goal identification, planning and organizing behavior to achieve goals, and monitoring goal directed activity (Mateer, 1997; Shallice & Burgess, 1991). A clinical model of executive functions is described below.

The frontal lobes are important in several aspects of attention that are related to executive functions. Working memory and alternating and divided attention, described in Chapter 5, appear to be dependent upon frontal systems (as well as nonfrontal brain systems). The frontal lobes are also critical for creativity, cognitive flexibility, and problem solving. Patients with dysexecutive syndromes may display a rigid and concrete thinking style and may experience difficulty generating fluent and novel thoughts. In addition to their role in cognition, the frontal lobes are further involved in regulating mood and emotion. Behavioral and personality changes are often ascribed to frontal lobe dysfunction. Patients with frontal lobe dysfunction may exhibit a blunt or flat effect. They can often experience more swings in their mood; they can be quick to respond with anger or irritability; and they are often less sensitive to the feelings or perspectives of those around them (Prigatano, 1991).

A number of different models have been described to capture the concept of executive functions. Most of the models are derived from analyzing the symptoms associated with frontal lobe impairment or damage to frontal lobe circuitry. One model that has important clinical relevance for persons with acquired brain injury is Norman and Shallice's (1986) model of a supervisory system. They suggest that routine and nonroutine activities operate differently and involve distinct cognitive processes. For example, frontal systems are often not activated to complete overlearned or automatic tasks (e.g., dressing, making coffee), but are heavily employed in nonroutine activities (e.g., a new work task or managing a change in schedule). They describe several components (e.g., contention scheduling and the supervisory attention system) that are activated when task success cannot rely on routine, habitual behavior. For example, contention scheduling allows a person to prioritize the order of completing competing tasks (e.g., making a sandwich when the phone rings) and the supervisory attention system would be called into play when there was no known solution to a specific task (e.g., not knowing how to operate a new microwave oven). Executive functions may be considered those abilities that are required to complete goal-directed activity that is not overlearned, automatic, and routine.

The evaluation of frontal lobe functions is a frustrating, yet critical, clinical endeavor. Although symptoms caused by damage to this region are difficult to identify, their adverse effects on people's lives are very clear. Damage to frontal brain systems has devastating consequences for social competency, the ability to manage daily tasks, and the skills required to maintain employment (Lezak, 1995).

There are several reasons why the functions of the frontal lobes remain somewhat elusive to clinicians and researchers. One perplexing characteristic of frontal damage is that seemingly opposite symptoms are often manifested in the same individual. For example, a patient may display difficulty with initiation characterized by an inability to start activities independently without external prompting, while also displaying impulsivity characterized by inappropriate verbal comments and "acting before thinking." Another somewhat baffling characteristic is the fact that many frontal lobe symptoms are seen in noninjured individuals, making it difficult to discern what is "normal" and what is "disordered." Difficulty with planning, organization, absent-mindedness, impulsivity, and the myriad other symptoms related to frontal lobe damage are widely displayed in individuals without brain damage. A further challenge in trying to pin down frontal lobe symptoms stems from the fact that these impairments can coexist with normal or even high IQ test scores. It is often only by interviewing individuals familiar with a client that a clinician can identify and document frontal lobe symptoms (Varney & Menefee, 1993). The extensive connections between the frontal lobes and other brain regions as well as the involvement of a variety of cognitive processes in executive functions account for the complexity in trying to understand these functions.

A CLINICAL MODEL OF EXECUTIVE FUNCTIONS

Mateer (1999) offers a model of executive functions that incorporates neuroanatomically and cognitively based theories of frontal lobe functioning. She conceptualizes different domains of executive functions with high clinical relevance. An extension of these domains and possible neuroanatomical correlates are described below; these constitute a clinical model of executive functions. Note that several of the components (initiation, response inhibition, task persistence, and generative thinking) are critical for handling nonroutine or novel situations, as described in Norman and Shallice's (1986) model.

• *Initiation and drive (starting behavior).* In order to respond to information or intentions, a cognitive system must be activated. Damage to the medial frontal lobe can lead to apathy and inability to initiate behavior voluntarily. The anterior cingulate is a structure thought to be important for initiation (Duffy & Campbell, 1994).

• *Response inhibition (stopping behavior).* The ability to inhibit automatic or prepotent response tendencies is critical for flexible goal-directed behavior. Frontal lobe damage can alter a person's ability to act independently of internal drives and external stimuli. Common problems produced when response inhibition is impaired include impulsive responding, stimulus-boundedness (overresponding to environmental stimuli and acting reflexively when a stimulus is produced), and perseveration (getting stuck on one response and not being able to shift to a new response set). The orbitofrontal cortex is associated with the ability to control response tendencies (Dempster, 1993).

• *Task persistence (maintaining behavior).* The ability to maintain attention and persist until task completion is a critical executive function. It relies on intact working memory. Problems with task persistence are evident when an individual discontinues a task prior to completion. Task persistence is heavily reliant on response inhibition.

• *Organization (organizing actions and thoughts).* The frontal cortex is involved in controlling how information is organized and sequenced. It functions to avoid responding to nonessential information by clearing it out from working memory. It further assists in the processes required to retrieve and sequence information in an organized fashion. These abilities are specifically related to the dorsolateral convexity (Stuss & Benson, 1986). Goal identification, planning, and time sense are functionally related to organization.

• *Generative thinking (creativity, fluency, cognitive flexibility).* The ability to generate solutions to a problem and think in a flexible manner is critical to solving problems. Frontal lobe damage can cause rigid, narrow thinking; such individuals may experience difficulty understanding perspectives different from their own. A common dysexecutive symptom is an inability to generate novel ideas. These abilities are typically related to lesions in the parasagittal frontal lobe region.

• *Awareness (monitoring and modifying one's own behavior).* The capacity for insight into one's own actions and feelings, and for incorporating environmental feedback to modify behavior, is critical for successful functioning. Self-awareness is highly reliant on prefrontal brain systems and the interaction between frontal and right parietal regions (Damasio, 1994). The ability to detect and respond to errors requires awareness. Awareness of memory and attention difficulties provides motivation for individuals to adopt compensatory strategies.

These six categories, which are summarized in Table 8.1, capture the broad array of cognitive and behavioral disorders that may occur as part of a dysexecutive syndrome. The different categories are related and interdependent. An individual may present with a distinct problem in one category, such as an initiation disorder. Alternatively, an individual may have compromises in multiple areas (e.g., reduced initiation and disinhibition). Table 8.2 illustrates the application of the clinical model with two real-world examples of compromised executive functions. The first column represents a client with communication difficulties. The second column represents a client who is unable to shop for groceries independently.

Chapters 5 and 6 review models of attention and memory, and this chapter focuses on executive functions. A review of these models and the relevant theoretical concepts highlights the overlap among attention, memory, and executive functions (see Figure 8.3). Perhaps the best example of the interdependence of these systems lies within the domain of working memory, which is a cornerstone system involved in all three systems. Having models to conceptualize each of the areas, and an appreciation of their complex interplay, allows a clinician to assess and manage the associated impairments appropriately.

ASSESSMENT OF EXECUTIVE FUNCTIONS

We have acknowledged the difficulty in evaluating dysexecutive syndromes. Formal cognitive assessments typically use standardized psychometric tests that provide explicit instructions and a rigid structure, which direct client behavior. Such structure may provide enough cues to allow clients with dysexecutive syndromes to perform well, and thus may mask executive function impairment. Chapter 4 describes tests that tend to be most sensitive to dysexecutive symptoms. These include measures of working memory and attention, fluency, and problem solving. In addition, it is critical to interview the client and others close to the client about possible

TABLE 8.1. Clinical Model of Executive Functions

Domain	Functions covered
Initiation and drive	Starting behavior
Response inhibition	Stopping behavior
Task persistence	Maintaining behavior
Organization	Sequencing and timing behavior
Generative thinking	Creativity, fluency, problem-solving skills
Awareness	Self-evaluation and insight

TABLE 8.2. Application of Executive Function Model to Functional Activities

Domain of executive function model	Dysexecutive syndrome applied to communication disorder	Dysexecutive syndrome applied to grocery shopping
Initiation and drive	Does not initiate conversation; exhibits flat affect with limited expression	Does not initiate going to grocery store even when refrigerator is empty
Response inhibition	Makes inappropriate comments; does not wait for turn in conversation	Impulsive shopping; buys unnecessary items that look appealing during the shopping excursion
Task persistence	Loses interest in conversation; cannot maintain topic	Does not get all the items on the list
Organization	Poor verbal organization; jumps from topic to topic; seems to talk "around a subject" and not get to the main idea	Does not make a grocery list; does not use aisle headings to shop in an organized manner; inefficient use of time when gathering groceries
Generative thinking	Unable to generate conversation; seems to have little to say; has difficulty responding to open-ended questions	If desired item is not available, cannot generate appropriate substitute
Awareness	Seemingly unaware of communication deficits; does not seem to notice if others are not interested in topic	Is not aware that getting groceries is an area of concern

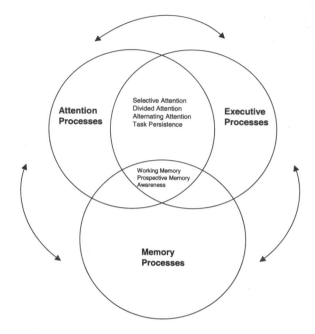

FIGURE 8.3. Illustration of the interdependence of attention, memory, and executive processes.

changes in behavior and personality that are difficult to measure out of context. Observation of behavior in naturalistic settings, using tasks that place demands on frontal lobe abilities, is perhaps the most revealing assessment approach (although it is not possible in every treatment setting).

Observational Methods

When one is observing a client completing naturalistic tasks as a means to assess executive functions, it is important to use a taxonomy of executive behaviors. The Profile of the Executive Control System (PRO-EX; Braswell et al., 1993) provides seven scales delineating key executive abilities (see the PRO-EX summary sheet in Appendix 8.1). These scales include Goal Selection, Planning/Sequencing, Initiation, Execution, Timesense, Awareness of Deficits, and Self-Monitoring. The clinician interviews significant others and observes the client performing multistep activities in several settings (e.g., a cooking task and a money management task). On the basis of this information, he or she rates the client's performance, using the behavioral descriptors for each of the seven areas. Ideally, it is helpful to have two clinicians (or a clinician plus the client and/or caregiver) fill out the rating scale, so that interrater reliability can be checked.

The Executive Function Route-Finding Task (EFRT; Boyd, Sautter, Bailey, Echols, & Douglas, 1987; Lezak, 1993) combines features of naturalistic observation and standardized assessment to evaluate possible dysexecutive symptoms. Route finding is highly dependent on the integration of information and requires initiation, planning, and organizational skills, making it a useful assessment task. When developing this task, the authors observed dozens of patients' route-finding behavior. They gave patients open-ended instructions indicating that they were to locate a particular office on the hospital campus in as efficient manner as possible. The authors noted four distinct approaches to this task: "wandering aimlessly" (nondirected walking around, with patients hoping that they would see the location); "trial and error" (guessing about the location and using a gradual process of elimination); "step by step" (asking for information limited to the next closest location); and "strategy use" (obtaining a map or written directions). The EFRT rates performance on the following parameters: (1) Task Understanding, (2) Incorporation of Information Seeking, (3) Retaining Directions, (4) Error Detection, (5) Error Correction, and (6) On-Task Behavior. Types of cueing are recorded that are particularly useful for documenting level of support required to carry out an executive task. They document nonspecific cues, which are used to remind the patient to self-monitor (e.g., "What should you do now?"), and specific cues, which provide information about how actually to execute a task (e.g., "It might be helpful to write that down"). The EFRT is provided in Appendix 8.2.

For a review of other assessment practices, including standardized tests, observational methods, and interview protocols sensitive to frontal lobe dysfunction, the reader is referred to Chapter 4.

Questionnaires

Several questionnaires are available that elucidate the effects of dysexecutive symptoms on daily functioning. The Dysexecutive Questionnaire (DEX) is part of the Behavioural Assessment of Dysexecutive Syndrome (Burgess, Alderman, Wilson, Evans, & Emslie, 1996). It contains 20 questions describing problems related to decreased attention and executive control that commonly occur following brain injury. The respondent rates each problem on a frequency of occurrence scale. There are "self" and "other" rating forms. The DEX generates a raw score ranging from 0 to 80, with a higher score reflecting greater deficits in executive function.

The Brock Adaptive Functioning Questionnaire (BAFQ; Dywan & Segalowitz, 1996) is another instrument that can provide a measure of adaptive functioning, which is difficult to quantify psychometrically. It contains 68 questions that were developed through clinical practice and with the help of community volunteers who had sustained brain injuries and their families. Questions are divided into five behavior domains:

Planning, Initiation, Attention/Memory, Arousal/Inhibition, and Social Monitoring. There are forms for both significant others and clients. A pilot study evaluating this tool showed that a frontally generated electrophysiological response elicited during a simple attention task was strongly predictive of family and patient responses on the Planning and Initiation scales (Dywan & Segalowitz, 1996). The scoring also provides an index of awareness by computing the difference between client and significant other ratings. Sample questions from the BAFQ are provided in Appendix 8.3.

One potential shortcoming of questionnaires is that they only indicate individuals' perceptions of functioning on the specific questionnaire items. The questionnaire may not contain items relevant to actual changes in an individual's functioning. Sohlberg, McLaughlin, Pavese, Heidrich, and Posner (2000) found that the use of structured interviews was necessary to determine how cognitive impairments affected subjects' functioning. For example, several subjects indicated no changes in their abilities following cognitive treatment as measured by standardized questionnaires, but when interviewed, clients spontaneously offered concrete examples such as "I can watch a whole movie," "I can drive and listen to the radio," and "I can remember phone numbers." These examples of daily functioning were not items on the questionnaires. Combining structured interviews with standard questionnaires may reveal the most information about adaptive functioning. See Chapter 13 for a discussion of effective interviewing techniques.

MANAGEMENT APPROACHES

Dysexecutive symptoms may be addressed via a broad variety of clinical approaches. Mateer (1997) raises a key issue that needs to be considered in planning any type of cognitive treatment. She asks whether rehabilitation specialists should look globally at a client's level of functioning and try to improve abilities in particular settings (i.e., use a wholly "functional" approach), or whether they should attempt to understand and improve the functioning in the various cognitive processes contributing to changes in ability, in the hope that this will lead to more generalized improvement across a multitude of settings. The former approach (sometimes termed a *top-down* approach) is likely to affect a targeted behavior, while the latter approach (a *bottom-up* approach) is more likely to result in generalization, if it is within the abilities of the client (Levine et al., 2000). Different patient profiles call for different remediation approaches.

Effective management of dysexecutive symptoms requires the clinician to be proficient in approaches on both ends of the functional versus process-oriented continuum, as well as in approaches that have features of both types of therapies. For example, in some cases, it will be advantageous to address environmental, external determiners of a client's behavior (a more functional approach). Chapter 11 describes the appropriateness of environmental management therapies to establish external situational controls over behavior. If a client is having difficulty with agitation (a potential frontal lobe symptom), reduction of stimulation in the environment may be the preferred initial management approach. In other cases, it may be more efficient to remediate cognitive processes responsible for decreased executive functions. An example of this is providing high-level attention process training (described in Chapter 5) to address difficulties in maintaining and switching attention, which are often impaired after frontal lobe damage. An example of a therapy approach that uses functional *and* process-oriented therapy principles is teaching a self-regulation strategy such as pacing to manage a problem in sustained attention or task persistence (also described in Chapter 5). This requires a functional analysis of when and where the problem is occurring, as well as an accommodation of processing difficulties in order to teach strategy use until it becomes automatic.

Selection of a therapy approach will depend upon the following variables:

- Time since injury
- Severity of dysexecutive symptoms
- Co-occurrence of other cognitive deficits
- Client's level of awareness
- Rehabilitation priorities of client, family, and staff
- Support available in the "discharge environment"

The reader is referred to Table 8.3 for a list of therapies described in other chapters within this text that may also be used to manage dysexecutive functions.

Therapeutic Rapport

Developing a therapeutic relationship with a client is essential to assisting with the management of dysexecutive symptoms, regardless of the specific therapy approach that is utilized. Brain damage may result in diminished motivation and initiation, as well as problems with behavioral control—all of which increase the importance of establishing a therapeutic rapport that will enhance cooperation. Based on a review of the available literature, Ducharme (1999) summarizes several interaction skills that may help clinicians develop a therapeutic alliance and a milieu conducive to therapy:

TABLE 8.3. Therapies Described in Other Chapters That Also Address Dysexecutive Symptoms

Therapy	Description of therapy	Chapter
Attention process training	A process-oriented therapy directed at improving sustained, alternating, and divided attention. May be helpful in improving difficulty with task persistence, holding on to information, and manipulating information.	5
Selecting and training use of external aids	Set of procedures and principles for facilitating the selection and implementation of compensatory aids, such as electronic memories or planning books. May be helpful for difficulties with planning and organization, in addition to providing external prompts to remember specific strategies.	7
Awareness intervention	Therapies for managing decreased awareness of deficits. May focus on enhancing an individual's level of awareness, or may help caregiver to manage an awareness problem.	9
Prospective memory training	A process-oriented therapy that extends the amount of time an individual can hold on to and initiate an intended action. May address problems with organization and initiation.	6
Behavioral intervention	Approaches to increase desired behavior and extinguish undesired behavior, which draw upon principles of behavior analysis. Often used to address behavior problems due to disinhibition and perseveration.	11

1. A clinician should choose discussion topics that help develop a therapeutic alliance. Statements need to be sincere and reflect the clinician's actual feelings. This includes statements related to the following:
   • Topics of client interest or individual expertise
   • Development of a partnership between client and clinician to work collaboratively on rehabilitation goals
   • Empathy, with an emphasis on understanding of the challenges experienced by the client
   • Progress that the client is displaying
2. When a client perseverates on a situation that is upsetting, the clinician can provide subtle redirection by diverting attention to other topics or events and then reinforcing responses to the more adaptive topics.
3. The clinician should use body language that facilitates communication.
   • Physical posture needs to be open and receptive. When talking to a

client, the clinician should stand or sit at an angle rather than face to face and thus avoid encroaching on the client's personal space.
- Eye contact needs to demonstrate respect and concern.
- Tone of voice needs to be sincere and caring but not condescending.

The development of a therapeutic relationship based on empathy, respect, and trust will increase the likelihood that clients will cooperate with treatment and benefit from services (Horvath & Luborsky, 1993). This therapeutic alliance is particularly important in work with individuals who have frontal pathology and the resulting dysexecutive symptoms.

The remainder of this chapter reviews four broad therapeutic approaches useful for managing dysexecutive symptoms. The first two approaches are environmental support and teaching task-specific routines. They focus on factors external to the client and capitalize on automatic responding. The second two approaches, training the selection and execution of cognitive plans and self-instructional therapies, attempt to improve internally generated, cognitive behavioral responses.

Environmental Management

Environmental management is a critical approach for managing dysexecutive symptoms. We use *environmental management* as a catch-all term for a wide variety of clinical considerations that can mitigate the effects of dysexecutive syndromes. The goal is to set up a client's environment or external world to circumvent or prevent problems that might arise due to impairments in initiation and self-regulation. We suggest two categories of environmental management:

- Organization of physical space
- Manipulation of physiological factors

Organization of Physical Space

Facilitating the organization of a client's physical space can effectively reduce the load on executive function abilities. The notion is to set up the environment to take on the role of the damaged frontal lobes. This environmental modification approach has been discussed in Chapter 5 as a way to address attention deficits; it includes such recommendations as setting up filing systems and message centers. Systematic evaluation of clients' living space is critical for identifying environmental modifications that will help circumvent and prevent problems related to reduced initiation and self-regulation. Listed below are examples of environmental modifications we have utilized in our clinical practice. Certainly the selection of organizational approaches will be dependent upon input from the client and family or other caregivers. The establishment of these environmental modifications usually requires assistance from a rehabilitation professional, including systematic training and prompts for all affected persons living in the environment.

- Labeling cupboard contents
- Using large bulletin boards with separate labeled sections for different types of information
- Designating kitchen shelves (or refrigerator shelves) for specific types of foods
- Establishing a designated place for clutter—only items that are not critical can go in this bin
- Establishing clutter-free zones in specific work spaces, such as desks
- Setting up bill-paying systems
- Using large family planning calendars
- Putting a family message center on the refrigerator
- Setting up file cabinets with labeled folders for home management tasks

An extension of organizing the physical space is to post prompts or cues to increase adaptive behavior that compensates for dysexecutive symptoms. Written reminders or cues can be posted for an infinite variety of home management tasks. Examples include the following:

- Reminders of what to take to school or work each day, posted by the front door (e.g., keys, wallet, lunch, bus card)
- Grooming routine, posted on the bathroom mirror
- Menus for specific meals, posted on the refrigerator
- Before-going-to-bed (or morning-rising) routine, posted on the bedroom closet door (e.g., turn off lights, turn down heat, set alarm, take medication)
- Reminders of operating procedures for laundry machines, dishwasher, computer, and the like, posted next to those appliances.
- Conversation prompts such as photo albums, placed at suitable locations
- Schedules to help with time management, placed wherever necessary

Again, effectively modifying the environment is dependent upon a careful assessment of the client's living situation and must introduce modifications that will work for those people living in the environment. Family members or other caregivers, if supported in their efforts to observe when and where problems occur, will often identify helpful solutions. Environmental manipulation is a collaborative effort among therapists, clients, and relevant caregivers. See Chapter 13 for methods to encourage collaboration.

Manipulation of Physiological Factors

Brain injury often has a negative impact on physiological factors that regulate internal states and ultimately affect performance. When a person is physically uncomfortable or physiologically compromised, cognitive impairments become more disruptive, particularly executive function impairments. Ducharme (1999) calls this class of conditions *ecological factors*, and describes the first three items on the following list of ecological variables that should be considered in assisting individuals with executive function impairments:

- *Nutrition.* Nutrition affects performance. It can be helpful to limit behavior-altering substances such as caffeine, and to assist clients in regulating food and water intake. Dehydration and fluctuating blood sugar can affect cognitive performance.
- *Sleep hygiene.* Sleep disturbance is a common sequela of brain injury. Behavioral strategies and relaxation training can be used to improve sleep patterns. Sleep deprivation increases dysexecutive symptoms.
- *Activity level.* Changes in neurological functioning can make it difficult to handle the effects of over- or understimulation. Helping individuals set up schedules that allow them to pace themselves and to eliminate extra stimulation is important. Setting up therapy schedules to take advantage of clients' most effective time of day, building in rest times, and counseling persons to return to work part-time are all examples of helping people to regulate activity levels. Difficulties with initiation, organization, impulsivity, and task persistence may be minimized by attending to a client's activity level.
- *Medication monitoring.* Being able to identify a client's medications, monitoring when they are taken, and documenting suspected cognitive side effects can be very helpful to the prescribing physicians. Following brain injury, the manner in which medications are metabolized often changes, and responses to dosing may be very different than for a person without a brain injury. In addition, a common problem for individuals with dysexecutive symptoms is taking medications as prescribed. Training clients to use external memory aids is an effective method to increase independence in this area (see Chapter 7).

Teaching Task-Specific Routines

The goal of task-specific routines, the second broad approach to managing dysexecutive symptoms, is to teach an affected individual a behavior or set of behaviors that is adaptive for a *specific* setting. Once the skill has been trained, the client should be able to initiate and maintain the new behavior(s) independently, albeit in an automatic response mode.

Often the first step in teaching task-specific routines is task modification. Changing the nature of a difficult task can be helpful in mitigating executive function impairments. For instance, simplifying meal preparation and using dishes with three or less ingredients may allow someone with significant impairment to prepare his or her own meal independently. Modifying a task or activity can also be helpful for managing a communication problem, for example, disruptive arguing in group therapy. Specifically, the group therapy session can be set up to avoid the topics that trigger arguments, thereby preventing the client's disinhibition from interfering with the group process. When the occurrence of dysexecutive symptoms is consistent and can be predicted to interfere with the execution of a task or particular set of tasks, clinicians can analyze the tasks and experiment with different modifications. Manipulating the conditions under which the task is performed can result in effective compensation for problems with executive functions.

Once a task has been appropriately modified, a task routine can be generated and subsequently taught to increase the independence of persons with even severe dysexecutive syndromes. The assumption is that some clients cannot complete a variety of action plans in different settings due to dysexecutive symptoms such as stimulus-boundedness, perseveration, extreme impulsivity, lack of initiation, and limited awareness (Mateer, 1997). With such clients, it may not be realistic to teach a broad, flexible approach for completing multistep tasks; however, they may be able to learn a particular sequence of steps. Examples of routines that can be taught include the following:

- Grooming
- Dressing
- Riding the bus
- Washing the dishes
- Housecleaning chores
- Writing letters
- Playing solitaire
- Doing laundry
- Writing e-mail
- Making phone calls
- Hobbies involving sequential tasks, such as gardening or painting
- Operating the TV or stereo

Training task-specific routines incorporates many features of behavioral programming, described in Chapter 11. Discussions of behavioral techniques are often limited to interventions for behavioral disturbances rather than for learning impairments. However, cognitive programming draws upon principles of behavioral intervention (Sohlberg & Raskin, 1996). For example, Chapter 7 describes skills training for teaching clients to use external compensatory aids to manage cognitive impairments. The procedures and principles described in that chapter rely heavily on behavioral programming.

A number of researchers describe the utility of teaching task-specific routines to persons challenged by dysexecutive syndromes (Burke, Zenicus, Wesolowski, & Doubleday, 1991; Martelli, 1999). The important features for successful instruction of task-specific routines are similar to those for training an individual to utilize a compensatory cognitive aid (see Chapter 7). They include the following:

1. Writing a task analysis, in which the routine is broken into single, logically sequenced steps
2. Developing and implementing a checklist that makes each of the steps in the routine very explicit, so that the client can judge when each step is completed
3. Providing sufficient practice for each step, using errorless learning
4. Making sure that reinforcement and motivation to succeed at the task are embedded in the training

Martelli (1999) incorporates each of the four components into a clinical model for teaching task routines. He encourages clinicians to implement what he calls the "three P's"—*plan, practice,* and *promote therapeutic attitudes.* The task analysis and checklist are developed during the planning stage. Each of the routines listed earlier can be described as a sequence of discrete steps with a place to check off each step when it is completed. Task analysis checklists serve to mitigate fatigue and limit the cognitive energy required on the part of the client to plan, sequence, and execute multistep procedures. Training clients to follow task analysis checklists helps reestablish everyday functional routines.

Once a task analysis checklist is developed, most clients will require intensive practice in carrying out the steps. Sufficient practice is necessary to make the steps become habitual and automatic. Practice needs to be carried out in the same context as the training.

There are several ways to build in reinforcement for working on task routines, which is another key component of training. Clinicians can reinforce clients' efforts to complete routines by empowering them and using internal motivation, as well as by providing external reinforcers. We (Sohlberg & Mateer, 1989) encourage the initial selection of routines that are highly motivating to a client. Examples of routines that some of our clients have been motivated to learn include using the computer to correspond via e-mail, preparing favorite recipes, and operating video equipment to view movies. However, for some clients with severe initiation problems and little internal drive, identifying routines that are reinforcing is very difficult. Whenever possible, it is useful to increase the involvement and investment of clients and significant others by facilitating their input in the selection of the routines and the delineation of the steps.

Martelli (1999) uses a structured protocol to determine reinforcers that can be coupled with completing routines. He has clients identify highly reinforcing events, and designs a formal behavioral contingency program that allows points earned by completing task routines to be exchanged for rewards. A client, clinician, and family can collaborate on identifying the rewards by generating a list of enjoyable stimuli or events in the following categories: eating, watching TV/videos, traveling/visiting/leisure, intimacy, and home activities/games.

In his case report, Martelli (1999) presents impressive outcome data on using task analyses and checklists to complete home routines (including morning grooming, leisure activities, and meal preparation), coupled with a reward contingency plan, for a client who had suffered an anterior communicating artery aneurysm with a resulting dysexecutive syndrome. The client's decreased initiation was of great concern. Data showed a proliferation in the number of activities performed, from an average of about 10 per week to the agreed-upon quota of 50 per week following training. The author did note that although the client became semiautonomous in completing routines, he required a booster training session if there was a change in the environment (e.g., a holiday schedule). Occasional support was needed even after routines had become automatic.

Training the Selection and Execution of Cognitive Plans

The aforementioned PRO-EX (see Appendix 8.1) assesses a number of components critical to the selection and execution of cognitive plans, including goal selection, planning/sequencing, initiation, execution, and sense of time. This section describes exercises designed to improve functioning in these areas. The underlying belief motivating these exercises is that practice will lead to an improvement of the specific executive functions targeted in these tasks, or at least will improve ability on related tasks in the same domain. This is in contrast to task-specific routines, which seek to instill automatic responding for very specific procedures without an expectation of generalization. The exercises in this section require instructing clients to identify cues about when to implement the behavior (Hart & Jacobs, 1993). A major challenge is to help clients override premorbid automatic responses to situations, as well as to help them manage the interfering effects of impairments in initiation, prospective memory, and impulsivity that so often accompany acquired brain injury. Generalization from the training environment to naturalistic contexts requires careful and systematic planning (Sohlberg & Raskin, 1996).

There is not sufficient research as yet to indicate whether practice on such exercises may actually be domain-specific (i.e., improvement occurs on tasks with similar features, and there is no corresponding changes in underlying cognitive functioning), or whether improvement occurs because the exercises facilitate an improvement in the associated executive functions required to perform that task. Chapter 10 describes a variety of exercises for teaching communication and social skills—an arena greatly affected by dysexecutive syndromes. When these exercises result in improved communication (e.g., increased initiation of conversation), it is unclear whether this is due to the adoption of a new behavior or whether there has been improvement in the neurological processes related to initiation.

Planning Scenarios

Therapy can provide practice planning by giving a client repeated opportunities to plan activities. Therapy of this type usually progresses from hypothetical planning to actually carrying out a planned activity. The therapist provides sample situations that the patient uses to devise a planning scheme. Initially, the patient writes or indicates the steps and tasks involved in planning an activity or event; gradually, he or she is provided with the opportunity and resources to carry out the plan. Certainly, the clinician needs to be creative in providing opportunities that address a client's particular problems with planning. For example, any of the following may be a therapy objective when planning scenarios are used:

- Increasing accuracy in listing the essential steps involved in a multicomponent task (e.g., improving the client's knowledge of critical task components)
- Increasing the accuracy of sequencing (the client may know all the steps but have difficulty ordering them correctly)
- Improving organization or efficiency in planning (e.g., improving the client's ability to group similar tasks, teaching the client a systematic strategy for completing planning tasks)

Examples of therapy tasks that might be used to achieve these objectives include the following:

- Planning hypothetical activities such as a barbecue, a "graduation" event for another rehabilitation client, a fund-raising project, a recreational activity, or any event with possible meaning to the client whose complexity can be appropriately adjusted

- Planning the order of therapy tasks for the next session or series of sessions
- Arranging for refreshments or activities as part of a group therapy project
- Planning tasks that can be implemented with the family or other caregivers

Descriptive or quantitative data can be kept in a log that lists the particular components being addressed.

Errand Completion Tasks

Errand completion tasks can be arranged to address planning, sequencing, initiation, and execution. The client is given errands either within the treatment facility or within the community, depending upon the constraints and opportunities inherent in the specific setting. The client may be practicing completing tasks using specific compensatory strategies (e.g., following notes on a "to-do" list) or may be working on specific components of initiation, planning, or organization. The goal of the activity should be explicit, so that the client can focus on the target ability. Therapy activities move from easier to harder errands as clients improve. Examples of errand completion tasks are as follows:

Concrete hospital-based tasks
- Going to the gift shop to determine hours of operation
- Going to the cafeteria to identify the lunch special
- Going to the hospital information desk to get a "patient comment" card

Concrete community-based tasks
- Finding out the price of a hamburger at a fast-food restaurant
- Obtaining a business card from a local company
- Buying a postcard stamp
- Getting a bus schedule
- Finding out the Saturday hours at a designated business
- Getting income tax forms from the post office

Abstract community-based tasks requiring planning
- Obtaining something free
- Getting something printed
- Finding out the steps to get a passport

The data collection on the errand completion tasks will depend completely upon the clinician's objective. If the goal is to have the client use

compensatory strategies (e.g., write down errands on a "to-do" list and refer to it), then performance data relevant to using the system will be kept.
If the goal of the errand completion task is to have the client remain focused and complete the task, then performance data relevant to time
needed to complete the errand and/or prompts required to keep the client
on task may be recorded.

Planning and errand completion activities may be modified for a high-
functioning client in order to improve flexibility or the ability to repair or
take corrective action. Tasks may be generated that force the client to
change a plan. For example, maybe the client will be sent to a designated
place that has been relocated. Perhaps after a client has planned a social
event, the clinician may reveal that the guest of honor is sick, or that someone is allergic to the refreshments that have been ordered. The client may
be given practice generating alternative solutions for the planning or errand completion task.

Time Management Tasks

Many clients with dysexecutive symptoms benefit from practice in regulating their behavior according to time constraints. An important component
of time management is the ability to gauge the passage of time accurately.
This can be practiced in either a single-task format (without distractions)
or a dual-task format (with intervening distractions). The client is told to
keep track of a specified number of minutes and to inform the therapist
when the target amount of time has elapsed. In the intervening time period,
the client can either do therapy activities (distractor paradigm) or simply
sit quietly (nondistractor format). This is similar to the prospective memory training described in Chapter 6. The data collection protocol for prospective memory training can be adapted for time estimation.

As an extension of the planning or errand completion activities, clients
can be given structured worksheets (or use their external aids) and practice
scheduling their therapy activities. As their scheduling and planning abilities improve, they can practice following their schedules. Even a significantly impaired client can learn to follow a therapy agenda, track time,
and cue the therapist when it is time to switch activities. The idea is to turn
the responsibility for managing therapy activities over to the client. If we
clinicians continually direct clients in what they are to do, we do not assist
them in improving their executive functions. This activity can be extended
to naturalistic tasks outside the therapy setting. See Appendix 8.4 for an
example of a scheduling worksheet that includes space for planning a
schedule and a chart for evaluating scheduling performance.

The tasks described in this section are designed to give clients practice
in the selection and execution of cognitive plans. We know of no experimental research measuring the outcome of this type of therapy, however.
Giving clients practice with planning and organization is a widespread

clinical practice and makes good intuitive clinical sense, but it greatly needs to be a focus of future research. Anecdotally, from our own experience, improvement using these methods depends minimally upon clients' receiving sufficient practice in targeted aspects of the planning or execution process (e.g., time estimation). This requires that clinicians do the following:

- Clearly define the objectives of the specific planning or goal completion activity.
- Make sure clients understand the objectives and are provided with sufficient support to engage in the activity (support can be withdrawn as clients improve).
- Measure or describe performance, in order to be able to determine progress or areas in need of further intervention.
- Design a sufficient number of tasks or a hierarchy to allow sufficient practice on target skills.
- Have a method for measuring generalization of executive skills.

Metacognitive Strategies/Self-Instructional Training

A fourth approach to managing impairments in executive functions is to teach clients to use *self-instructional* or *metacognitive* routines. Clients are taught to regulate their behavior via self-talk. The foundation of this approach lies in the early work of Vygotsky and Luria, who suggested that volitional behavior originates not in mental acts but rather is mediated by inner speech. Luria (1982) postulated that a child's external speech serves to regulate his or her behavior and is eventually transformed into the adult regulative practice of internal self-talk. He further hypothesized that the frontal lobes are integral to inner speech processes, and that dysexecutive syndromes characterized by poor self-regulation (i.e., impulsivity, perseveration, reduced planning, and deficient problem solving) result when there is damage to frontal systems. Luria's writings led cognitive and developmental psychologists to apply verbal self-instruction and self-regulation techniques to the remediation of planning and problem-solving deficits and impulsivity in children and adults.*

Cognitive rehabilitation using self-instructional techniques has been modeled after successes by developmental psychologists in teaching children with impulsivity disorders to regulate their behavior. For example, Meichenbaum and Goodman (1971) reported success in training five young subjects with poor self-control to use self-instruction. First, the experimenter modeled verbal self-instruction and error correction while completing a task.

---

*Special thanks to Rosannah Hayden for organizing the background information on self-instructional training.

This component included (1) asking questions about the task demands; (2) providing answers to the questions via cognitive rehearsal and planning; (3) talking to oneself about steps in the process, to provide self-guidance during task completion; and (4) self-reinforcement upon task completion. This was followed by coaching the subjects to perform the verbal self-instruction elements that had been modeled. The subjects then implemented the self-instruction procedures aloud without coaching. This was subsequently faded to a whisper, and finally self-instruction was performed covertly. The tasks that were used included complex problem-solving tasks. Results showed improvement on neuropsychological tests of planning and problem solving, which were maintained at a 1-month follow-up. No changes were measured in terms of classroom behavior.

Over the past 20 years, cognitive rehabilitation professionals have made increasing use of such pioneering research in verbal self-instruction. Self-instructional training using elements of Meichenbaum's techniques has been successfully employed in the remediation of attention deficits (Webster & Scott, 1983), verbal memory impairment (Lawson & Rice, 1989), motor impersistence (Stuss, Delgado, & Guzman, 1987), and executive impairments (Alderman, Fry & Youngson, 1995; Cicerone & Giacino, 1992; Cicerone & Wood, 1986; Duke, Weathers, Caldwell, & Novack, 1992; Levine et al., 2000; von Cramon & Matthes-von Cramon, 1994) in individuals with brain injuries.

Cicerone and Giacino (1992) outline a clear treatment program for remediation of planning and error utilization deficits in six patients with brain injuries. They emphasize that the goal of self-regulatory therapy is not to train a specific task, but to guide the internalization of self-regulation processes. Training consisted of having subjects verbalize actions before and during performance on training tasks. The training involved three phases: overt verbalization (talking out loud), whispering, and covert verbalization (inner talk). Training consisted of between 10 and 20 hours of verbal self-instruction training over a period of 5–9 weeks. Results of their experiment indicated significant error reduction in five of the six subjects as a result of verbal mediation training. Two of the subjects received generalization instruction, where they were given practice using the self-regulation techniques on real-life problems as well as the treatment tasks. These two subjects demonstrated spontaneous use of self-regulation strategies. Cicerone and Giacino assert that verbal self-instruction can be effective in remediating planning deficits and impairments in other executive processes.

A case study described by von Cramon and Matthes-von Cramon (1994) further illustrates the application of faded self-instruction to remediate executive function impairments. They trained a 33-year-old physician to apply systematic analysis, problem solving, decision making, and solution evaluation in order to work in a limited capacity as a pathologist.

He had sustained a severe bilateral frontal trauma 9 years previously. He exhibited preserved intellect with a moderate dysexecutive syndrome, which was characterized by impairments in awareness, ability to shift tasks, and interpersonal skills (all of which affected his ability to work productively as a pathologist).

Part of the training was to teach the client a problem-solving procedure that consisted of three "headings" written on a flip chart. The first heading was "Problem Identification and Analysis." The client tended to approach problems rigidly and commit himself to a solution too early. He was explicitly instructed to look systematically for all the information available when conducting macroscopic and microscopic evaluations. The second heading was "Generation of Hypotheses and Decision Making." He was taught how to separate relevant from irrelevant information and to test the pros and cons of his diagnoses. The third heading was "Evaluation of a Solution." The client was taught to give a rating for how certain he was about every diagnosis; only with high certainty levels was he allowed to write up a pathology report. For cases with low certainty scores, he was taught to discuss the cases with his superiors. In accordance with self-instruction techniques, rules were at first guided externally by the therapist, followed by overt self-instruction ("thinking aloud") and then by gradual substitution of internal self-talk.

After 12 months of intensive therapy, the subject went from 40% to 100% accuracy in his job task of interpreting pathological reports. His problem-solving ability improved slightly, as measured on a timed errand task, and his awareness of problem areas improved, as measured by greater agreement between the patient's and therapist's ratings on the Patient Competency Rating Scale (see Chapter 9). However, the researchers noted that although the subject was able to perform professional duties successfully, and the training helped him end a cycle of drifting from job to job, the gains were hyperspecific; transfer of learning did not occur. He only improved on those tasks that were directly trained via the self-instruction techniques. In contrast to Cicerone and Giacino (1992), von Cramon and Matthes-von Cramon (1994) advocate using self-instructional training to teach task-specific skills.

Verbal self-instruction may also be applied to help a client learn a specific metacognitive strategy. Lawson and Rice (1989) trained an adolescent male to improve reading comprehension by working on executive processes. They taught him to implement a series of self-monitoring steps associated with the acronym WSTC. W refers to asking, "What am I supposed to be doing?"; S refers to "Select a strategy"; T refers to "Try the strategy"; and C refers to "Check the strategy." These steps were put on cue cards that could eventually be faded. The subject was taught to use the steps in completion of English, math, and geography homework assignments that involved memorization. The four WSTC steps promote defining a goal

TABLE 8.4. Examples of Self-Instruction Used to Help Manage Impulsivity, Reduced Planning and Organization, Difficulty Shifting Tasks, and Poor Problem Solving

Metacognitive strategy taught using an acronym such as WSTC: "What should I be doing?"; "Select a strategy"; "Try the strategy"; "Check the strategy" (see, e.g., Lawson & Rice, 1989).

Self-monitoring: Providing external feedback on errors and successes, with clients recording errors and comparing performance across trials. Can have clients verbalize impressions. May rely on external feedback to recognize errors (see, e.g., Cicerone & Giacino, 1992).

Verbal mediation: Verbalizing each step of a multistep task as it is completed (e.g., "First, I'll select a recipe; now I'll get out all the ingredients; now I'll read the recipe all the way through aloud; now I'm putting in the flour . . . ")(see, e.g., Cicerone & Giacino, 1992).

Problem-solving process: Problem identification and analysis; generating possible hypotheses with supporting evidence; evaluating the solution (sec, e.g., van Cramon & Matthes-van Cramon, 1994).

Task completion process—goal management training (GMT): Stop!; define main task; list steps; learn steps; execute task; check (Levine et al., 2000).

(orienting the client to a task), selecting and implementing a strategy, and self-monitoring the outcome. Results showed improved performance on relevant neuropsychological tests and reading tests. More importantly, however, implementation of the metacognitive strategy was observed beyond the training on tasks that required memorization.

Principles of self-instruction may also be applied to teaching individuals to self-monitor. Consistent practice and support for evaluating one's performance can result in improved error recognition and correction. Chapter 9 describes the effectiveness of prediction and behavioral logging in improving awareness. Cicerone and Giacino (1992) applied these principles in their therapy approach to improving planning and error recognition in a number of subjects with planning and self-monitoring deficits. Teaching two clients to predict their performance on a problem-solving task resulted in one of the subjects' applying the prediction strategy to improve time management and interpersonal communications. The client learned to anticipate the effects of behaviors. A third subject was taught a formal error-monitoring procedure. Whenever the client made a mistake, his attention was immediately drawn to his error; he was helped to keep a record of errors and to systematically compare his responses on subsequent trials. The error-monitoring routine was transferred from the problem-solving training task to a clerical task, although the client continued to require external support and prompts. Self-instructional techniques (overt verbalization faded to inner self-talk) can thus be implemented to teach clients to anticipate and monitor their behavior.

Recently a group of researchers assessed the effects of a task completion procedure, *goal management training* (GMT), for managing deficits in executive functions (Levine et al., 2000). This report is unique because the intervention is based on a theoretical model of goal management deficits following frontal system damage (Duncan, 1986), and because it is one of the very few executive function interventions that has been experimentally evaluated. GMT trains patients in five stages:

1. Asking themselves, "What am I doing?" (STOP)
2. Defining the "main task" (DEFINE)
3. Listing the steps (LIST)
4. Asking themselves whether they know the steps (LEARN)
5. Executing the task (DO IT)
6. Asking, "Am I doing what I planned to do?" (CHECK)

Clients are trained to deliberately consider each of the stages while completing multistep tasks. The GMT protocol thus targets parameters relevant to selecting goals and defining the target task, partitioning the task into subgoals, holding on to the steps as the task is being completed, and monitoring task outcome. Results of the experimental evaluation suggested that patients with brain injury who were randomly assigned to the GMT group improved on everyday paper-and-pencil goal management tasks carried out in a laboratory setting. Training effects appeared generalizable, as improvement extended to a task that was not included in the training regimen (Levine et al., 2000). In the same report, the authors provide a case study documenting the success of GMT on improved meal preparation abilities in a postencephalitic patient. This included anecdotal report of generalization to activities beyond the targeted meal preparation.

A review of the research encourages training clients with dysexecutive syndromes in the use of metacognitive strategies. For some clients, this approach may be limited to helping them initiate behavior, plan, and solve problems while performing specific trained tasks. For other clients, self-instruction may improve underlying executive processes directly and help them use inner speech to regulate their functioning. In our experience, this approach will be most useful for clients who have some awareness and insight into deficits and who feel motivated to address their problems. Levine and colleagues (2000) note that the success of GMT depends on patients' insight into their own goal management deficits, and that those persons with intact awareness and motivation are more likely to benefit from the training than those with denial or unawareness. Individuals with varying degrees of awareness deficits will require varying amounts of clinician structure and support to transfer use of strategies or self-instruction to their day-to-day functioning. Persons with severe amnesia or severely compromised executive functions may not be able to internalize self-instructional strategies and may be best served by learning task specific routines. Thus the location and extent of brain lesions may determine clients' potential to benefit from self-instruction. For example, patients with substantial left frontal brain damage may not be able to use verbal mediation (Luria, Pribram, & Homskaya, 1964).

The components of metacognitive/self-instructional training are summarized below and followed by a case example from our clinical practice.

1. Identify the tasks or problems where the executive function impairments interfere (e.g., specific vocational tasks, home management tasks). Select activities that will improve the client's daily functioning, even if training effects are hyperspecific and do not generalize beyond the training tasks.
2. Identify the nature of the executive dysfunction (e.g., impulsivity, perseverative responding, lack of planning, poor problem solving, lack of error detection, etc.).
3. Design a self-instructional procedure or choose a metacognitive strategy that will assist with that issue (see Table 8.4).
4. Model doing the task, using each step or stage in the self-instructional procedure.
5. Have client practice doing the task while saying the self-instructional elements aloud.
6. Provide cue cards when helpful, in order to give the client prompts to use the self-instructional strategy.
7. When the client can independently perform the task using the self-instructional procedures, have the client perform the task while whispering self-instruction. Give lots of practice.
8. Fade whispering to inner speech.
9. Decide whether self-instructional procedures can be generalized to other tasks, and if so, begin using the same procedures to provide practice on other types of tasks.
10. If generalization looks possible, have the client keep a log of times when he or she used self-instruction and/or when self-instruction might have been useful even if the client did not remember to implement it.

Case Example of Self-Instructional Training

Jeff was a 30-year-old male who had received a brain injury 1 year prior in an industrial accident. On cognitive testing, Jeff demonstrated mild impairments in attention and new learning, as well as moderate executive function impairments characterized by impulsive responding and a disorganized approach to problem solving. Although he was living independently, his family was concerned about his poor nutrition, hygiene, and finances, due to problems with cooking, shopping, and household management. In addition to formal testing, Jeff was observed in his apartment doing some cooking and cleaning chores. He and his family were interviewed about their perceptions of what went awry when tasks were not successful (e.g., dinner burned) and what occurred when tasks were successful (e.g., he paid bills on time).

Results of cognitive testing and interviews suggested that Jeff tended to begin tasks without any planning, and that when he got into trouble he was not an effective problem solver. When he was successful, it was usually because there was some time between intention to do the task and initiation of the task, or because someone provided a prompt for doing the task. He appeared to have some awareness about his difficulties (e.g., "being a bad cook"), but limited awareness about the underlying reasons for his problems. He was also motivated to improve.

In a collaborative effort, the clinician and Jeff brainstormed "things you can tell yourself so you will think before acting." The clinician described the WSTC technique, which Jeff liked, and they made slight modifications of the wording in order to reflect Jeff's own words. They made cue cards with the four steps. He and the clinician practiced implementing each of the steps on a computer program that required problem solving, so Jeff could learn the steps. Initially, the clinician modeled the steps. She said, "OK, in Step 1 I ask, 'What should I be doing?' I'm doing the Problem Solver computer program. In Step 2 I select a strategy—I select reading each instruction aloud twice before I touch the keyboard." She continued with the other two steps, and then had Jeff practice while he said the four steps aloud. Each time she encouraged him to choose different strategies so he could practice generating ideas. After he was able to apply the WSTC technique to the computer program, which was a very structured task, they began practicing on some cooking tasks. In three sessions, Jeff was able to implement the strategy independently while whispering. He did continue to report making impulsive cooking errors.

The clinician was not in a setting where she could accompany Jeff at home to do the training, and he was quite resistant to involving family members as cotrainers. Jeff agreed to use the written cue cards during some preset cooking tasks and report on the outcome. It took several reminders to get follow-through, and with a phone cueing system, Jeff eventually did the home task. He reported that it was quite useful. It also became apparent to Jeff and the clinician that he really only needed the first step ("What should I be doing?") in order to control his impulsivity. If he simply took a bit of time before task initiation to think about what he was going to do, he was able to prevent errors. For example, he noted how doing this prompted him to get out all of the ingredients for cooking, instead of getting halfway through and needing to do a preparation activity (e.g., slicing the ham when an omelet was already cooking).

During the month of training, there was no initial generalization to untrained activities (i.e., to noncooking tasks). The clinician then began interviewing Jeff each week about other activities when he experienced difficulty that might have been avoided by using his self-instructional techniques. After generating ideas about when he could have used the techniques but had not thought of them (e.g., packing for a visit and forgetting his medication; doing a home repair task and not having necessary tools), he began to report instances of when he successfully used the WSTC for other activities. Although he continued to display significant dys-executive symptoms, his family noted that he completed more home management tasks successfully without impulsive responding. Jeff continued to ask for support to use the self-instructional techniques.

SUMMARY

This chapter has begun by discussing the role of the frontal lobes in medi-ating goal-directed behavior. It reminds the reader that the frontal lobes are involved in a variety of cognitive, behavioral, and emotional functions. Among the most devastating problems following frontal lobe damage are dysexecutive syndromes, which are characterized by changes in the ability to initiate, maintain, and inhibit behavioral responding, as well as to orga-nize thoughts and behaviors, generate ideas, and possess self-awareness. Even minor damage to executive functions can cause extreme disruption in independent functioning.

This chapter discusses four different approaches to managing dys-executive symptoms: environmental/ecological management, training task-specific routines, training selection and execution of cognitive plans, and metacognitive/self-instructional training. Evaluation of the environment and of characteristics inherent in the tasks required of clients often reveals ways to modify supporting contexts in order to circumvent disruption from dysexecutive symptoms. Individuals with severe impairments in exec-utive functions may benefit from training in individually tailored, highly repetitive, and prescribed task routines for everyday activities such as grooming. Training in the selection and execution of cognitive plans offers clients systematic practice with planning and organizational skills while carrying out functional activities. Self-instructional training refers to the process of using "self-talk" messages or deliberately following specific task completion routines to regulate behavior and successfully complete goal-directed activities.

REFERENCES

Alderman, N., Fry, R. K., & Youngson, H. A. (1995). Improvement of self-monitor-ing skills, reduction of behavior disturbance and the dysexecutive syndrome: Comparison of response cost and a new programme of self monitoring training. *Neuropsychological Rehabilitation, 5,* 193–221.

Boyd, T. M., Sautter, S., Bailey, M. B., Echols, L. D., & Douglas, J. W. (1987, February). *Reliability and validity of a measure of everyday problem solving.* Paper presented at the annual meeting of the International Neuropsychological Society, Washington, DC.

Braswell, D., Hartry, A., Hoornbeek, S., Johansen, A., Johnson, L., Schultz, J., & Sohlberg, M. M. (1993). *Profile of the Executive Control System.* Wake Forest, NC: Lash & Associates.

Burgess, P. W., Alderman, N., Wilson, B. A., Evans, J. J., & Emslie, H. C. (1996). The Dysexecutive Questionnaire (DEX). In B. A. Wilson, N. Alderman, P. W. Burgess, H. C. Emslie, & J. J. Evans (Eds.), *Behavioural assessment of the Dysexecutive Syndrome.* Burry, St. Edmunds, England: Thames Valley Test Company.

Burke, W. H., Zencius, A. H., Wesolowski, M. D., & Doubleday, F. (1991). Improving operative function disorders in brain injured clients. *Brain Injury, 5*(3), 241–252.

Cicerone, K. D., & Giacino, J. T. (1992). Remediation of executive function deficits after traumatic brain injury. *Neurorehabilitation, 2,* 73–83.

Cicerone, K. D., & Wood, J. C. (1986). Planning disorder after closed head injury: A case study. *Archives of Physical Medicine and Rehabilitation, 68,* 111–115.

Courville, C. B. (1937). *Pathology of the central nervous system, Part 4.* Mountain View, CA: Pacific.

Damasio, A. R. (1994). *Descartes' error: Emotion, reason, and the human brain.* New York: Putnam.

Dempster, F. N. (1993). Resistance to interference: Developmental changes in a basic processing mechanism. In M. L. Howe & R. Pasnak (Eds.), *Emerging themes in cognitive development* (pp. 3–27). New York: Springer-Verlag.

Ducharme, J. M. (1999). A conceptual model for treatment of externalizing behaviour in acquired brain injury. *Brain Injury, 13*(9), 645–668.

Duke, L. W., Weathers, S. L., Caldwell, S. G., Novack, T. A. (1992). Cognitive rehabilitation after head trauma. In C. J. Long & L. K. Ross (Eds.), *Handbook of head trauma* (165–190). New York: Plenum Press.

Duffy, J. D., & Campbell, J. J. (1994). The regional prefrontal syndromes: A theoretical and clinical overview. *Journal of Neuropsychiatry, 6,* 379–387.

Duncan, J. (1986). Disorganization of behavior after frontal lobe damage. *Cognitive Neuropsychology, 3,* 271–290.

Dywan, J., & Segalowitz, S. J. (1996). Self and family ratings of adaptive behavior after traumatic brain injury: Psychometric scores and frontally generated ERPs. *Journal of Head Trauma Rehabilitation, 11*(2), 79–95.

Goldman-Rakic, P. S. (1984). The frontal lobes: Uncharted provinces of the brain. *Trends in Neurosciences, 7,* 425–429.

Grady, C. (1999). Neuroimaging and activation of the frontal lobes. In B. L. Miller & J. L. Cummings (Eds.), *The human frontal lobes: Functions and disorders* (pp. 196–230). New York: Guilford Press.

Hart, T., & Jacobs, H. E. (1993). Rehabilitation and management of behavioral disturbances following frontal lobe injury. *Journal of Head Trauma Rehabilitation, 8*(1), 1–12.

Horvath, A. O., & Luborsky, L. (1993). The role of therapeutic alliance in psychotherapy. *Journal of Consulting and Clinical Psychology, 61,* 561–573.

Kaufer, D., & Lewis, D. (1999). Frontal lobe anatomy and cortical connectivity. In B. L. Miller & J. L. Cummings (Eds.), *The human frontal lobes: Functions and disorders* (pp. 27–41). New York: Guilford Press.

Lawson, M. J., & Rice, D. N. (1989). Effects of training in use of executive strategies on a verbal memory problem resulting from closed head injury. *Journal of Clinical and Experimental Neuropsychology, 6*, 842–854.

Levine, B., Robertson, I. H., Clare, L., Carter, G., Hong, J., Wilson, B. A., Duncan, J., & Stuss, D. T. (2000). Rehabilitation of executive functioning: An experimental-clinical validation of goal management training. *Journal of the International Neuropsychological Society, 6*, 299–312.

Lezak, M. (1985). *Neuropsychological assessment* (3rd ed.). New York: Oxford University Press.

Lezak, M. (1993). Newer contributions to the neuropsychological assessment of executive functions. *Journal of Head Trauma Rehabilitation, 8*, 24–31.

Luria, A. R. (1982). *Language and cognition.* Washington, DC: Winston.

Luria, A. R., Pribram, K. H., & Homskaya, E. D. (1964). An experimental analysis of the behavioral disturbance produced by a left frontal arachnoidal endothelioma. *Neuropsychologia, 2*, 257–280.

Martelli, M. (1999, December). Protocol for increasing initiation, decreasing adynamia. *HeadsUp: RSS Newsletter,* pp. 2, 9.

Mateer, C. A. (1997). Rehabilitation of individuals with frontal lobe impairment. In J. Leon-Carrion (Ed.), *Neuropsychological rehabilitation: Fundamentals, innovations and directions* (pp. 285–300). Delray Beach, FL: GR Press/St. Lucie Press.

Mateer, C. A. (1999). The rehabilitation of executive disorders. In D. T. Stuss, G. Winocur & I. Robertson (Eds.), *Cognitive neurorehabilitation* (pp. 314–332). Cambridge, England. Cambridge University Press.

Meichenbaum, D. H., & Goodman, J. (1971). Training impulsive children to talk to themselves: A means of developing self-control. *Journal of Abnormal Psychology, 77*, 115–126.

Mesulam, M. (1990). Large-scale neurocognitive networks and distributed processing for attention, language and memory. *Annals of Neurology, 28*, 115–126.

Norman, D. A., & Shallice, T. (1986). Attention to action: Willed and automatic control of behavior. In R. J. Davidson, G. E. Schwarts, & D. Shapiro (Eds.), *Consciousness and self-regulation: Advances in research and therapy* (pp. 1–18). New York: Plenum Press.

O'Neill, R. E., Horner, R. H., & Albin, R. W. (1990). *Functional analysis of problem behavior: A practical assessment guide.* Sycamore, IL: Sycamore Press.

Prigatano, G. (1991). Disturbances of self-awareness of deficit after traumatic brain injury. In G. P. Prigatano & D. L. Schacter (Eds.), *Awareness of deficit after brain injury: Clinical and theoretical perspectives.* New York: Oxford University Press.

Shallice, T., & Burgess, P. W. (1991). Higher-order cognitive impairments and frontal-lobe lesions in man. In H. S. Levin, H. M. Eisenberg, & A. L. Benton (Eds.), *Frontal lobe function and dysfunction* (pp. 125–138). Oxford: Oxford University Press

Sohlberg, M. M., & Mateer, C. A. (1989). *Introduction to cognitive rehabilitation: Theory and practice.* New York: Guilford Press.

Sohlberg, M. M., Mateer, C. A., & Stuss, D. T. (1993). Contemporary approaches to the management of executive control dysfunction. *Journal of Head Trauma Rehabilitation, 8*(1), 45–58.

Sohlberg, M. M., McLaughlin, K. A., Pavese, A., Heidrich, A., & Posner, M. (2000). Attention process training and brain injury education in persons with acquired brain injury. *Journal of Clinical and Experimental Neuropsychology, 22*(1), 656–676.

Sohlberg, M. M., & Raskin, S. (1996). Principles of generalization applied to attention and memory interventions. *Journal of Head Trauma Rehabilitation, 11*(2), 65–78.

Stuss, D., & Benson, F. (1986). *The frontal lobes.* New York: Raven Press.

Varney, N. R., & Menefee, L. (1993). Psychosocial and executive deficits following closed head injury: Implications for orbital frontal cortex. *Journal of Head Trauma Rehabilitation, 8*(1), 32–44.

von Cramon, D. Y., & Matthes-von Cramon, G. (1994). Back to work with a chronic dysexecutive syndrome?: A case report. *Neuropsychological Rehabilitation, 4,* 399–417.

Webster, J. S., & Scott, R. R. (1983). The effects of self-instructional training on attentional deficits following head injury. *Clinical Neuropsychology, 5,* 69–74.

APPENDIX 8.1

SUMMARY SHEET FROM THE PROFILE
OF THE EXECUTIVE CONTROL SYSTEM (PRO-EX)

Name _____

Evaluator _____

Date of 1st Measurement _____

Date of 2nd Measurement _____

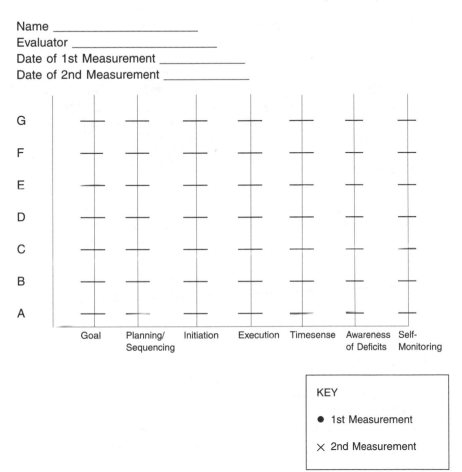

APPENDIX 8.2

WOODROW WILSON REHABILITATION
CENTER EXECUTIVE FUNCTION ROUTE-FINDING TASK (EFRT)

Client's name _____ Date of evaluation: _____
Disability ____/____/____ Examiner _____

Instructions: "I am going to give you an exercise that involves your finding an unfamiliar office, _____. How you do this is up to you. I will go with you but cannot answer questions about how to find _____. I want you to do this exercise as quickly and efficiently as possible. Before you begin, I would like you to tell me what I have asked you to do."

I. Task Understanding

1. Failure to grasp nature of task despite several elaborations.
2. Faulty understanding of important element requiring specific or explanatory cuing and elaboration (e.g., "How am I supposed to know where it is?").
3. Distorts peripheral detail requiring slight clarification or a nonspecific cue (e.g., "Can you tell me where it is?").
4. Shows a clear grasp or asks for clarification appropriately (e.g., "Can I get someone to take me there?"). Initiates task spontaneously.

II. Incorporation of Information Seeking

1. Aimless wandering.
2. Follows a hunch without gathering information first (unless shows prior knowledge of destination) or exhaustive door-to-door search.
3. Gathers information before commencing search, but without appraisal of information source.
4. Shows judgment in use of information sources (e.g., selects staff over clients; clarifies confusing directions; verifies information with another person).

III. Retaining Directions (functional memory)

1. Continual forgetting of directions or name of destination and failure to use suggested means of compensating (e.g., note taking) unless cued repeatedly.
2. Needs repeated nonspecific cuing or provision of concrete strategy for coping with memory deficits.
3. Forgets detail(s) but compensates after nonspecific cue (e.g., "How might you keep yourself from forgetting the destination?").
4. Paraphrasing or clarification sufficient for remembering, or spontaneous compensation (e.g., note taking).

IV. Error Detection (self-monitoring)

1. Continued errors without self-detection even after repeated examiner cues.
2. Some spontaneous awareness of errors, but more instances of cuing required.
3. Some cuing required, but more instances of spontaneous error detection shown.
4. Verifies correctness independently when appropriate; may exploit incidental information (e.g., signs) to prevent errors.

V. Error Correction (troubleshooting)

1. Helpless or perseverative behavior.
2. Inefficient strategy (e.g., returns to original information source).
3. Seeks help immediately once aware of error.
4. Reasons efficiently (e.g., looks for signs; considers where he or she may have erred in following directions to self-correct independently).

VI. On-Task Behavior

1. Must be held to task in ongoing fashion (e.g., distractible, stimulus-bound).
2. Digression from task requiring cues to redirect attention to task needed.
3. Incidental behaviors (e.g., small talk) interfere with efficiency.
4. Any incidental behaviors (e.g., waving to a friend) do not hinder performance observably.

Contributory Problems

Emotional
__ Indifference, lack of effort
__ Frustration, intolerance
__ Self-criticism, depression
__ Defensiveness
__ Thought disturbance
__ Euphoria, mania
__ Other

Interpersonal
__ Self-consciousness, shyness
__ Social skills
__ Setting context for requested information
__ Flirting
__ Interrupting
__ Other

Communication
__ Speech reception
__ Expressive speech
__ Reading ability
__ Writing ability
__ Other

Perceptual
__ Visual acuity
__ Auditory acuity
__ Right/left confusion
__ Neglect
__ Other visuospatial problem

_____   _____

_____   _____
_____   _____

Motor
Manual limitations
Ambulation
Other comments: _____

_____

_____

_____

Evaluation of Overall Independence

	Client's rating	Examiner rating	Overall
Extensive cuing required	___	___	___
Appreciable cuing required (specific cues or several nonspecific cues)	___	___	___
Occasional nonspecific cuing required	___	___	___
Independent of cuing	___	___	___

SCORING SUMMARY

Task Understanding	1	2	3	4
Information Seeking	1	2	3	4
Retraining Directions	1	2	3	4
Error Detection	1	2	3	4
Error Correction	1	2	3	4
On-Task Behavior	1	2	3	4

Overall average _____

Rules for Cuing

1. When to cue
   a. *A nonspecific cue* is given when client deviates from path approaching goal (not necessarily most direct) and passes up a subsequent opportunity for correction (e.g., sign, staff person, office doorway that might lead to information, path leading toward goal).
   b. *A specific cue* is given following a nonspecific cue after client fails to attempt correction or passes another opportunity for correction in doing so.
2. Nature of cues
   a. *A nonspecific cue* alerts the client to monitor performance (i.e., "Tell me what you need to do now").
   b. *A specific cue* provides information on how to execute the task.

THE BROCK ADAPTIVE FUNCTIONING QUESTIONNAIRE (BAFQ): SAMPLE ITEMS FROM FIVE SCALES

Planning
When you have several tasks to do, do you organize them in an efficient way?

Initiation
Do you have trouble getting started on a project unless someone helps you get going?

Attention/Memory
Are you likely to forget that you have left the stove or kettle on?

Arousal/Inhibition
Do you feel as though you get much too excited about things?

Social Monitoring
Can you tell when someone is feeling overtired or worried?

_____/_____/_____/_____/_____

Hardly ever   Rarely   Sometimes   Often   Almost always

These sample items are from the self-report version. The family report version differs only in that the pronouns "he/she" are substituted where appropriate. Each scale consists of a number of questions related to a specific behavioral domain.

Note. From Dywan and Segalowitz (1996). Reprinted by permission.

APPENDIX 8.4

SCHEDULING WORKSHEET

Date: _____
Time slot: _____
Tasks: _____

_____
_____
_____
_____

Plan

Time: Task   _/_/_ Completed _____
                                                                        Time

____ _____

Time: Task   _/_/_ Completed _____
                                                                         Time

____ _____

Time: Task   _/_/_ Completed _____
                                                                         Time

____ _____

Time: Task   _/_/_ Completed _____
                                                                         Time

____ _____

Time: Task   _/_/_ Completed _____
                                                                         Time

____ _____

Scheduling Performance Chart

Date	Hours planned	Time to plan	Ability to stay within schedule	Repair

268

9

The Assessment and Management of Unawareness

Unawareness, a common result of acquired brain injury, produces significant barriers to recovery. Individuals who have limited understanding of the nature, degree, and/or impact of their impairments may be resistant to therapy or reluctant learners of compensatory behaviors to lessen their handicaps. The prevalence of unawareness following brain damage, coupled with the problems produced when an individual does not recognize his or her difficulties, has encouraged researchers and clinicians to expand their knowledge of this complex and uniquely human phenomenon.

Awareness disorders possess a certain allure, due to the fascinating interplay among neurological, psychosocial, and cognitive factors. Successful management requires clinicians to merge behavioral, psychotherapy, and neurorehabilitation traditions. For example, the management of a psychological denial may require focused counseling, while the treatment of an organically based unawareness may suggest a combination of cognitive awareness exercises and behavioral logs. Before we begin our clinical discussion, we must recognize the field's infantile understanding of awareness. An attempt to address the clinical syndrome of unawareness could be considered premature. However, as modeled by Damasio (1994), it is through working with patients who have damaged awareness as a result of neurological trauma or disease that we extend our knowledge of this incredible ability and disability. These patients illustrate the complex interplay between cognition and emotion and serve as a reminder of the rich integration of the human neuronal networks. That said, this chapter humbly begins with a discussion of definitional issues related to unawareness. The remainder of the chapter presents a clinical framework for assessing and managing problems of unawareness of self based on our current state of knowledge.

269

CONCEPTUAL FRAMEWORKS

Numerous conceptual frameworks attempt to capture the phenomenon of unawareness. The various descriptions reflect its complexity and the existence of multiple types of awareness disorders. Purely theoretical classifications can be grouped into two broad categories, depending upon whether the emphasis is on psychodynamic or neuropsychological factors. In addition to these categories, we consider several clinical models in this section.

Psychodynamic Theories

Psychological theories emphasize the role of emotion, personality, and context in limited awareness. Perhaps the most widely cited psychological theory is Weinstein and Kahn's (1955) description of unawareness following brain damage as an adaptive technique to make sense of newly acquired symptoms. For example, mistaking a hemiplegic limb for another person's body part may be interpreted as a need to explain and make sense of the nonfunctional limb. These researchers introduced motivational factors as responsible for awareness problems.

Other psychological theories view unawareness as a method to spare individuals the pain of acknowledging impairments (Crosson et al., 1989). Examples of psychological denial are thought to include blocking unpleasant thoughts or repressing memories. Today, we recognize that most clinical syndromes following brain injury that include unawareness have at least some biological origin in addition to psychological factors.

Neuropsychological Theories

Neuropsychological theories attempt to account for unawareness stemming from direct brain injury (vs. psychologically mediated awareness difficulties or denial). Several theories differentiate disturbances in self-awareness from disturbances in perceptions of changes in physical, sensory, or language abilities. Stuss (1991) distinguishes higher-level disorders of self-awareness from lower-level focal unawareness such as left-sided neglect. He describes self-awareness as the highest brain function, housed in the prefrontal brain region. Self-awareness is the capacity for self-reflection; it utilizes and interacts with other brain processes so that individuals can function adaptively in their environments by incorporating past and ongoing information. Self-awareness is thus related to judgment and insight (Stuss & Benson, 1986). Stuss (1991) suggests that the prefrontal lobes interact with posterior and basal brain regions, which play a role in knowledge about specific sensory and perceptual abilities. When there is damage to posterior and basal brain regions, specific behavioral disturbances of unawareness can occur. For example, parietal lesions may produce unawareness of a hemiplegic limb, or damage to the supramarginal gyrus may produce unawareness for aphasic errors. Hence Stuss makes an important distinction between generalized unawareness about self and so-called *behavioral awareness disorders* such as neglect and aphasia, which tend to be related to specific functional systems.

McGlynn and Schacter (1989) also differentiate a supraordinate awareness system that analyzes and monitors information from lower-order cognitive systems. They have termed the supraordinate system a *conscious awareness system*, and suggest that damage to this system produces global unawareness of self. If lower-order cognitive subsystems are damaged, they become disconnected from the conscious awareness system; the individual then displays domain-specific unawareness, such as unawareness for only memory or unawareness of hemiplegia. In a related theory, Berti, Ladavas, and Della Corte (1996) also describe the possibility for domain-specific and generalized unawareness in their conceptualization of a higher-order awareness process that interacts with subordinate cognitive, perceptual, and sensory subsystems.

Prigatano (1991) argues that self-awareness is an emergent brain function dependent upon both cognitive and affective states. His work suggests that patients who show impairments of self-awareness have disturbances in both affective and cognitive domains. Damasio's (1994) analysis of two decades of clinical and experimental work supports the view that awareness depends upon several brain systems working in concert across many levels of neuronal organization. He notes that both "high-level" (e.g., prefrontal) and "low-level" (e.g., hypothalamus) brain centers cooperate in the execution of awareness.

Stuss (1991) integrates the awareness literature by proposing that damage to posterior areas (such as the right parietal region, plus its connections) and to left-hemisphere language centers results in altered knowledge or facts about self. This knowledge is no longer transmitted to the frontal lobes for self-reflecting. Unawareness will be specific to the functional system that has been damaged (e.g., the language comprehension center). In a case where there is damage to the prefrontal region, there is a disorder of self-awareness, but knowledge or facts about functioning often remain intact. Patients have difficulty with using knowledge about their own functioning and with monitoring their behavior. Prigatano (1991) reminds clinicians to assess both affective and cognitive dysfunction as sources of unawareness.

Summary of Theories

The majority of investigators recognize that unawareness is a common consequence of focal or diffuse brain damage that alters the functioning of the systems necessary for intact awareness. They differentiate these types of organically based unawareness from more psychologically mediated problems related to denial. We have noted the critical nature of the frontal lobes for successful self-awareness, as well as the role of posterior and subcortical structures in specific unawareness deficits (Damasio, 1994; Stuss, 1991). Figure 9.1 illustrates the roles of these sets of structures. Awareness disturbances observed in people who have progressive dementia, traumatic brain injury, and schizophrenia all suggest involvement of the frontal lobes. In contrast, lesion sites in the right hemisphere, particularly the parietal region, are responsible for changes in specific types of awareness for sensory, motor, and language deficits—for example, unawareness of a paralyzed limb (Biach, Valler, Perani, Papagano, & Berti, 1986) or inattention to the left side of space (Weinstein & Friedland, 1977). Focal lesions in the left temporal lobe have been associated with unawareness of disordered speech (Lebrun, 1987). This chapter focuses on the assessment and treatment of deficits in self-awareness, as opposed to discrete types of unawareness (for sensory, motor, or language deficits).

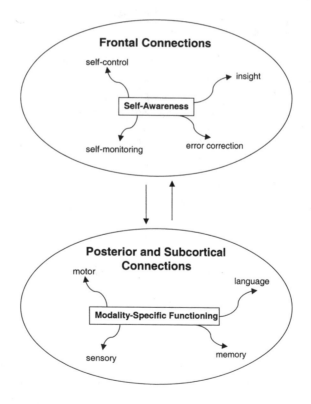

FIGURE 9.1. Neural connections involved in awareness.

Clinical Models of Unawareness

Several clinical models of awareness have been proposed to conceptualize problems with awareness and to guide assessment and treatment. These models attempt to identify possible sources of unawareness, which can then be matched to specific interventions. Three clinical models are described below.

Crosson and colleagues (1989) distinguish three types of awareness that can be impaired following brain injury. The first type is *intellectual awareness*, which is a patient's ability to understand that a particular function is impaired. It is knowledge of a deficit. They describe a second type of awareness, termed *emergent awareness*, as the ability to recognize a problem when it is actually occurring. The third type is *anticipatory awareness*, which is the ability to anticipate that a problem will occur as a result of some deficit. Patients may have disruption in one or all of these types of awareness. Intellectual, emergent, and anticipatory awareness are viewed as constituting a hierarchy, with intellectual awareness as the foundation and basis for the other two types of awareness. These authors acknowledge *psychological denial* as a potential additional barrier to awareness.

Langer and Padrone (1992) also present a tripartite model to conceptualize unawareness. They describe three sources of awareness problems. Like Crosson and colleagues (1989), they describe a basic level of awareness, which they call *information*. An individual may have difficulty at this level because information has not been provided, or because the person is unable to remember or understand the information. A second level of awareness is termed *implication*. Problems at this level suggest that the person has the information about deficits, but is not able to understand the implications or consequences of the information. The third source of unawareness in this model is *psychological denial*: The person has the information and could potentially be aware of its implications, but ignores the information to lessen the emotional pain.

Giacino and Cicerone's (1998) observations on the results obtained from a clinically derived, structured interview again reveal potential factors contributing to unawareness. They describe three varieties of limited awareness. The first type is *unawareness due to cognitive impairments*, particularly memory and reasoning deficits. The second type is *unawareness due to psychological reactions* or denial of deficits. The third variety of unawareness is a *dense inability to recognize areas of deficit functioning*, directly due to organic brain damage. These authors emphasize the complexity of unawareness and acknowledge the likelihood of multiple sources of unawareness.

Table 9.1 summarizes the clinical models of unawareness, which clearly have several common themes. One theme is the recognition of knowledge as the most basic level of awareness. When an individual does

TABLE 9.1. Clinical Models of Unawareness

Sources of unawareness (Langer & Padrone, 1992)	Types of awareness (Crosson et al., 1989)	Varieties of awareness deficits (Giacino & Cicerone, 1998)
1. Lack of information	1. Intellectual awareness	1. Cognitive impairments
2. Absence of implication	2. Emergent awareness	2. Psychological reactions
3. Denial	3. Anticipatory awareness	3. Pure, dense unawareness
	4. Lack of denial	

not have information about changes in functioning, he or she will have difficulty accommodating impairments. The lack of knowledge may be due to a cognitive impairment (e.g., a memory deficit) that prohibits an individual from remembering information about his or her brain injury (Giacino & Cicerone, 1998). Alternatively, an individual may not have information because it was never provided, or because it was not given at a time or in a manner for it to be successfully processed. Some individuals may not have had the opportunity to experience the impact of their deficits due to being hospitalized.

Clinical models also recognize a type of unawareness caused by difficulty applying information to real-world contexts. For example, a person may acknowledge the existence of a memory impairment, but may not understand the utility of using a compensatory memory book. Difficulty with abstraction, reasoning, or judgment, which is common with frontal brain injury, may produce this problem. Another obvious theme running through the research is the dichotomy between neuropsychological unawareness and psychological denial. We understand that damage to parts of the brain responsible for integrating information about ourselves produces an organically based unawareness. We also recognize an emotionally based unawareness produced by a psychological reaction to changed functioning.

Understanding the varieties of unawareness is critical for identifying the source(s) of an awareness problem, so that one can match the intervention to the type of unawareness. For example, if the primary source of an awareness problem is psychological denial, it may not be therapeutic to provide education on the nature of deficits until the individual is ready. Alternatively, if the source of unawareness is lack of information, brain injury education may be the recommended place to start awareness intervention.

A review of the theoretical and clinical awareness literature reveals a number of important characteristics of awareness disorders. These are summarized below.

• There are various types of unawareness. The causes of unawareness are complex. There are usually multiple sources, although often a primary and a secondary source can be identified (Giacino & Cicerone, 1998).

- Sources of unawareness include cognitive impairments affecting awareness, psychological reactions, and damage to brain regions directly responsible for awareness (Crosson et al., 1989; McGlynn & Schacter, 1989; Stuss, 1991).
- Disorders of awareness can be present with normal intellectual and sensory functioning. It is possible to have significantly compromised unawareness without concomitant changes in other cognitive functions. This is due to the fact that frontal brain systems are critical to awareness and may be selectively impaired (Stuss, 1991).
- Knowledge is distinct from other aspects of awareness. There is a dissociation among having correct information, using that information, and understanding the consequences of that information (Crosson et al., 1989; Langer & Padrone, 1992; Stuss, 1991).
- Awareness is intertwined with executive functions, including planning, self-monitoring, and behavioral control. These abilities share neural networks involving the frontal lobes (Stuss, 1991).
- It may be helpful to match intervention to the primary source of an awareness problem.
- Some types of unawareness are less amenable than others to intervention. Some researchers believe that psychological denial is harder to manage than a cognitively based unawareness problem (Fordyce & Roueche, 1986; Giacino & Cicerone, 1998).

MEASUREMENT OF AWARENESS

The measurement of awareness is difficult. One reason is that awareness cannot be measured directly, but must be inferred. Awareness is an attribute of feeling or knowing that has both psychological and behavioral correlates (Sohlberg, Mateer, Penkman, Glang, & Todis, 1998b). Assessing the nature or severity of an awareness deficit requires identifying these correlates. The three most common methods for measuring awareness are to (1) analyze clients' verbal descriptions of their functioning, (2) compare clients' reports with other persons' reports, and (3) compare clients' prediction of their performance with their actual performance. Additional techniques include analysis of error detection and correction, and observation of client behavior. Each of these is briefly reviewed.

Clients' Verbal Description of Functioning

One frequent indicator of awareness is to evaluate clients' verbal reports regarding their level of functioning. This may be elicited via interviews or by spontaneous observation. A researcher or clinician makes a judgment about an individual's level of awareness, based upon the evaluator's perception of the "accuracy" of the client's reporting.

One potential problem with using a client's report as an index of awareness is the potential mismatch between verbal report and actual knowledge. For example, a client may have awareness about impaired functioning, but may not report it out of fear of losing a freedom such as driving.

Examples of using clients' reports as an indicator of awareness are provided in a number of different awareness intervention studies (Beardmore, Tate, & Liddle, 1999; Deluca, 1992; Langer & Padrone, 1992). These studies describe improvements in awareness when subjects either verbally acknowledge impairments or "correctly" answer questions regarding level of functioning. Despite such verbal reports, it is difficult to know clients' true beliefs about their abilities and disabilities. Clinically, listening to how a client describes ability and disability remains a common method for evaluating awareness.

Comparison of Clients' and Other Persons' Reports

Comparison of clients' responses on questionnaires that probe functional levels with the responses of others (e.g., family members, clinicians) is a very common strategy to measure awareness. The notion is that a family member or health professional will provide a more objective perception of functioning against which to compare a client's self-appraisal.

Several questionnaires have been developed for these purposes. Fordyce and Roueche (1986) introduced the Patient Competency Rating Scale (PCRS) as a tool to compare clients' ratings of ability with those of staff and family members. A 5-point Likert scale is used to rate a client's level of difficulty in performing 30 different behavioral tasks. The patient and other each make judgments about how the patient would perform the tasks, but the actual tasks are not implemented. Several different scoring options for the PCRS have been proposed, depending upon the research questions (Prigatano & Altman, 1990; Roueche & Fordyce, 1987). Other scales that may be used to compare client and family impressions of functioning include the Dysexecutive Questionnaire (DEX; Burgess, Alderman, Wilson, Evans, & Emslie, 1996) and the Brock Adaptive Functioning Questionnaire (BAFQ; Dywan & Segalowitz, 1996), both of which are described in Chapter 8.

Another questionnaire approach is the Self-Awareness of Deficits Interview (Fleming, Strong, & Ashton, 1996; see Appendix 9.1). This is a structured interview designed to obtain both qualitative and quantitative data on the status of self-awareness of deficits. It questions the client in three areas: self-awareness of deficits, self-awareness of functional implications of deficits, and the ability to set realistic goals. Responses are rated by the interviewer on a 4-point scale. Prior to administering the interview, the interviewer obtains information from relatives and from staff members who have a close association with the client, in order to appreciate the client's current level of functioning.

A relatively new interview approach has been proposed by Giacino and Cicerone (1998). They advocate using a structured interview that begins with open-ended questions about a patient's difficulties, followed by more specific questioning on perceptions of how certain the patient is that a particular ability is intact or impaired. The confidence rating is the unique part of this interview. Giacino and Cicerone propose that having patients state a belief, and rate on a 5-point scale how certain they are that they do not have a problem, provides important direction for therapy. They suggest that patients whose convictions are malleable may have a better prognostic profile and may be more responsive to education.

A study completed by Tepper, Beatty, and Dejong (1996) suggested a particular pattern of discrepancy between self and other for persons with brain injury. They found that the least amount of agreement between clients and families was in the area of home integration. They suggest that the change in a person's roles within the family causes dissatisfaction, which in turn may be responsible for discrepant reporting. There was relatively high agreement in the domains of motor, cognitive, and social functions.

Several reports in the literature encourage caution when family or staff reports are used as a basis for evaluating client awareness (Cavello, Kay, & Ezrachi, 1992; Fleming et al., 1996). Because families are under much stress, they do not always respond consistently; they may also have specific biases, depending upon the characteristics of an individual family system. Similarly, clinicians may rely on stereotypical views of patient performance, which are influenced by differing sociodemographic factors between clinicians and patients (Cavello et al., 1992). It is also important to keep in mind that clinicians may have unrealistic expectations for patients. For example, if a client is in a medical or clinical setting and has not yet had a chance to experience changes in abilities, it may be reasonable for the client not to acknowledge any changes in abilities. Unlike a broken leg, cognitive impairments are not physically painful and are only evident upon a client's trying tasks that reveal a deficit.

Using comparisons between clients' and others' perceptions to measure awareness also assumes that family and staff perceptions would change over time if clients' awareness were to improve. A pilot study challenges this assumption, however: It showed that caregivers did not change their awareness ratings even when the client behaviors that they had identified as indicative of lack of awareness had improved (Sohlberg et al., 1998b). The caregivers acknowledged the improved behavior that had been targeted, but did not change their awareness ratings. Caregiver perceptions may not always be amenable to change.

Comparison of Clients' Predicted versus Actual Performance

Another strategy for examining self-awareness is to compare discrepancies between clients' predicted and actual performance on discrete tasks. For example, Sunderland (1990) showed a weak relationship between how individuals with brain injuries rated their general memory ability and how they actually performed on specific memory tasks. Similarly, Allen and Ruff (1990) compared subjects' performance on neuropsychological tests to their self-ratings of real-world functioning, and found only a limited relationship. Schlund (1999) suggests that if clinicians use comparisons generated from analyzing performance on real-life tasks that are meaningful to clients, they may circumvent some of these measurement problems.

Comparison of predicted performance and behavior has been used in several studies, both as a measure of awareness and as the actual intervention approach. Schacter, Glisky, and McGlynn (1990) implemented an awareness training program in which a client predicted his recall performance for word lists and future actions. The client was given feedback on his performance, which was compared to his predictions. Results showed that the client's rating of general memory ability became more accurate with the treatment, although the predictions of his own performance were inconsistent. Rebmann and Hannon (1995) measured three subjects' awareness by comparing predicted memory test scores to actual scores. An awareness training program, involving estimating performance followed by the provision of feedback on actual performance, was implemented. Clients were reinforced for accuracy of prediction. In this study, differences between the predicted and actual test scores decreased over time.

Error Correction

A relatively new method of evaluating awareness is to analyze clients' ability to detect and correct their own errors (Hart, Giovannetti, Montgomery, & Schwartz, 1998). Although there has only been one empirical investigation of this method with persons who have acquired brain injury, Hart and colleagues' (1998) study offers a reliable methodology to code naturally occurring errors according to whether subjects correct their errors and whether they have awareness of errors. The researchers manipulated the difficulty level of a functional task, gift wrapping, in order to observe subjects' responses to errors. They suggest that this error response coding methodology may be applied to any number of behavioral tasks.

Behavioral Observation

Many clinicians take a behavioral perspective in evaluating clients' level of awareness. They infer level of awareness from the degree to which an individual will utilize compensatory strategies to accommodate for impairments and the degree to which clients cooperate with therapy regimens. They may look for naturally occurring or spontaneous use of strategies, or may elicit opportunities for clients to use a strategy (e.g., they change an appointment time and observe whether a client writes down the information).

Summary of Measurement Methods

Five different methods to measure awareness have been described above: clients' own descriptions of abilities and disabilities; comparison of clients' and others' perceptions of the clients' functioning; comparison of clients' predicted versus actual performance; error correction; and behavioral observations of clients' use of compensatory strategies. Each method has its own advantages and disadvantages. The measurement challenges in trying to evaluate awareness are substantial; it is thus important to look at awareness from a number of different perspectives, in order to appreciate the nature and degree of a deficit. A process for systematically assessing awareness in a multidimensional fashion is described in the next section.

A SYSTEMATIC PROCESS FOR ASSESSING AWARENESS

This section describes a systematic, based on the field's current level of understanding for evaluating awareness by addressing five assessment questions. The process of attempting to answer these five questions should provide the information about the nature and severity of a client's awareness deficit that a clinician needs in order to plan intervention. This process employs most of the measurement strategies described in the preceding section. We begin by presenting the five questions; this is followed by a review of the sources for answering these questions.

Assessment Questions

- *Question 1. What is an individual's knowledge or understanding of strengths and deficits?* This question focuses on assessing an individual's knowledge about his or her neurological problem and residual strengths and impairments—regardless of the individual's behavior. The clinician is interested in knowing what the person understands intellectually about changes in functioning, but not whether he or she can apply or incorporate this information. As we have noted above in discussing clinical models of awareness, knowledge is the most basic level of awareness (Crosson et al., 1989; Langer & Padrone, 1992).
- *Question 2. If there is decreased awareness, to what degree is it psychoemotional denial versus organically based unawareness?* Awareness

issues are complex; it can be very difficult to sort out psychological reactions from neuropsychological symptoms. Clinicians often try to tease out what is an attempt to minimize the loss and spare oneself the emotional pain from what is unawareness due to brain damage in a region that provides accurate self-appraisal. We have noted clinically that emotional reactions to changes in abilities *and* organic brain damage frequently interact to contribute to an awareness problem. Often the relative contribution of each source may change over the course of recovery. Commonly, an individual initially exhibits an organically based denial in the acute phase, which is followed by the emergence of a psychological defense mechanism as he or she recovers (Prigatano & Klonoff, 1998).

• *Question 3. If an individual demonstrates significant unawareness, is it generalized or modality-specific, and does it accompany other cognitive impairments?* Some models of awareness differentiate between global unawareness and unawareness for specific types of deficits (Giacino & Cicerone, 1998; McGlynn & Schacter, 1989). A clinician will want to discern whether an individual seems to be unaware of all neuropsychological deficits or just specific changes, (e.g., a left-sided neglect). It helps to know whether an individual can appreciate changes in physical functioning such as an ataxic gait, but is unaware of changes in personality of behavior.

• *Question 4. Does the client demonstrate behaviors, conscious or unconscious, suggesting accommodation to changes in functioning?* Verbal report and behavioral actions may reveal different types of information. Some patients may not have the declarative knowledge or insight (see Question 1) that functioning has changed, but they will evidence behaviors that compensate for deficits. This is more often the case for compensatory behaviors that are ritualized or part of an established behavioral routine. Similarly, some may not admit verbally to having a problem, but behave in ways demonstrating that they know their functioning has changed. The early literature indicated that clients needed to have knowledge about their own limitations before implementing compensatory strategies (e.g., Crosson et al., 1989), but recently we have begun to recognize that for a subset of patients knowledge and behavior may not be hierarchically organized (Sohlberg et al., 1998b).

• *Question 5. What are the consequences of deficits in unawareness?* This question is extremely important. We need to know how an awareness deficit affects an individual and those in the individual's community. Is decreased awareness a problem because the client will not use a memory book or perhaps engages in activities that are dangerous? Alternatively, is it a problem only because a caretaker is annoyed when the individual talks about future plans that are very unrealistic? The impact of an awareness deficit on an individual's life will be a major determiner of the direction of intervention.

Sources for Answering the Assessment Questions

How can clinicians effectively answer these five assessment questions? Four different sources of information clarify responses to these questions; each is described below.

Source 1. Medical History and Cognitive Testing

The patient's medical history and specific profile of strengths and weaknesses will provide important information relevant to awareness. As discussed earlier, the neuroanatomical correlates of self-awareness are in the prefrontal cortex (Stuss, 1991). Results from cognitive testing or neuroimaging can provide information about damage to relevant brain regions that may indicate an awareness disorder. Similarly, performance on neuropsychological tests that measure abilities commonly tied to a region associated with awareness, such as executive functions, divergent thinking, reasoning, and judgment, may point to the presence of awareness disorders. In addition, cognitive impairments may be the primary source of an awareness deficit. For example, memory impairment may prevent an individual from remembering information pertinent to an injury, and its effects or a reasoning impairment may prevent understanding the consequences of a deficit.

Medical history and cognitive profile may be particularly helpful in responding to Questions 2 and 3. Question 2 encourages clinicians to identify the relative contribution of psychological denial versus organically based unawareness. Objective findings of brain damage, and a profile of cognitive impairments that includes memory and executive function impairments, may suggest an organically based disorder. Question 3 requires ascertaining whether an individual's unawareness is global or modality-specific. Again, identifying the regions of damage may reveal helpful information. For example, damage to the prefrontal regions is more likely to produce disturbances in self-perception of one's social behavior, whereas damage to the parietal region can produce a lack of awareness of sensory or motor deficits.

Source 2. Awareness Questionnaires, Rating Scales, and Interviews

Interview and comparison of clients' and others' responses on questionnaires of functioning may be very revealing about the nature of an awareness deficit. This topic has been discussed in detail in the section on measurement of awareness. The responses obtained from interviews and questionnaires can be particularly useful for answering questions regarding a client's knowledge about changes in functioning (Question 1), the degree to which the client compensates for impairments (Question 4), and the barriers in quality of life caused by awareness problems (Question 5). Hence it will be important that questionnaires and/or interviews provide information in these domains.

A clinician's knowledge and experience in interviewing techniques are critical for obtaining information on awareness. For example, knowing how to move from open-ended to more structured questioning, so that the interviewer is not feeding information to the client, requires practice. In addition, the approach to questioning and the establishment of a good rapport will determine the richness of the information obtained. For instance, an interviewer can elicit defensive responding if the client feels the interviewer is trying to force him or her to identify impairments.

Source 3. Direct Client Observation

Several different types of direct client observation can be utilized to provide information on awareness. These include (1) observing use of compensatory strategies; (2) observing performance on tasks and comparing this to predicted performance; and (3) observing response to errors. Each of these has been reviewed in the section on measurement of awareness. Observation of a client will be most useful in discerning the client's knowledge about changes in functioning (Question 1) and the degree to which the client compensates for impairments (Question 4).

Source 4. Response to Feedback

Clinicians can provide clients with feedback on test performance or on activities (such as a daily living task) and observe their response. Response to feedback may be evaluated at several different levels, including the patients' cognitive response (i.e., did they understand the feedback?), the emotional response (did they display any sentiment when given feedback?), and the behavioral response (did they incorporate the feedback?).

Response to feedback will be most useful in sorting out an organically based from a psychologically based awareness problem (Question 2). A patient who is able to acknowledge deficits when given feedback and who can modify beliefs (even temporarily) when given information about impairments is more likely to have unawareness linked to cognitive deficits that make it difficult for the individual to integrate and maintain knowledge about his or her own functioning. Hence patients with an organically based unawareness may exhibit a cautious willingness or an indifference to information about themselves, in contrast to patients with denial, who may reject or have an angry response to feedback regarding behavioral or functional limitations (Prigatano & Klonoff, 1998). A note of caution is necessary when one is using response to feedback as a means to measure awareness: For some individuals, particularly clients who are at an early stage in their recovery, denial of deficits may be functional in protecting them from confronting losses before they are emotionally well prepared. Hence a clinician needs to make a judgment about clients' readiness to receive feedback on their performance. If the clinician is unsure, referral to a clinical psychologist may be necessary.

Summary of the Assessment Process

This section has reviewed five assessment questions, as well as four relevant sources to guide the evaluation of awareness. Many of the recommended measurement tools and sources can be implemented as part of an existing cognitive or behavioral assessment protocol. For example, a family assessment can include information from the awareness questionnaires. Similarly, cognitive assessment information can be interpreted to shed light on awareness issues, in addition to examining functioning in the specific cognitive domains. An examiner can ask clients to predict their performance on some familiar activities, and can also observe the clients' responses to feedback on tasks during their evaluation process. The assessment of awareness should be a critical part of any evaluation for persons with acquired neurological impairments.

MANAGEMENT OF AWARENESS DEFICITS

The difficulty of measuring awareness contributes to the lack of awareness intervention research. Although there has been an increased focus in the literature on the phenomenon of unawareness, there is still only limited information on the effectiveness of awareness intervention strategies. This section reviews three different approaches to managing problems of unawareness. Although each of the approaches is distinct, it is not uncommon to use them all at some point in the recovery process. The three approaches are (1) an individual awareness-enhancing program, (2) caregiver training and education, and (3) procedural training and environmental support (PTES).

Individual Awareness-Enhancing Program

An individualized approach to awareness focuses on the person with the awareness problem and is aimed at increasing the individual's level of awareness. It is most appropriate for clients who (1) suffer from denial or a combination of denial and organically based unawareness, (2) have at least a rudimentary intellectual understanding that some abilities have changed as a result of an accident or disease, and (3) have sufficient cognitive capacity to integrate information and experience. It will *not* be helpful to a client who has a very dense, global unawareness with coexisting cognitive impairments.

Two approaches can be used in setting up an individual awareness-enhancing program—an educational approach and experiential exercises. These are reviewed in the following sections.

Educational Approach

One approach to increasing awareness is to provide people with the information that they lack. In our own experience, current service delivery models approach education as a supplement or "side dish" to "real" intervention. Clients and families are provided with standard handouts or verbal information as part of an interview process or as helpful tidbits they can take away from therapy. This is different from systematically targeting and measuring the outcome of education in the same way as one would deliver language therapy. Providing individuals with information they can internalize and apply needs to be individualized, systematic, and planful. Figure 9.2 depicts four educational exercises that can be employed: three more conventional tasks, and a board game format developed in recent research. These are discussed below.

Sample Educational Tasks to Increase Awareness. The most traditional approach to education is to provide clients with information about their neurological problem (e.g., brain injury) in print, on videotape, or on audiotape. This academic approach is most useful for clients who are open

| **Academic** |
| Provides clients with relevant information and a process for personalizing it. |

| **Review of Medical Records** |
| Assists clients in understanding the history of their accident or disease. |

| **Comparison of Client's and Other's Ratings** |
| Explores discrepancies and agreements between client and selected "other." |

| **Board Game Format** (Chittum et al., 1996; Zhou et al., 1996) |
| Individualized questions are developed and learned in a game context to increase knowledge and application. |

FIGURE 9.2. Sample educational exercises.

to receiving information. The challenge is to give information in a way that accommodates the clients' cognitive problems (such as reduced memory or comprehension), in a format that facilitates awareness and does not elicit a defensive reaction. One way to do this is to personalize the information. The clinician can have clients read information or view videos, and then share what does *and* does not match their own experiences. Clients can present what they have learned to others in a group, can educate their family members, or can write sequels to a reading or video. The goal is to increase the meaningfulness of information for clients. Often it is more important that they engage in the process of *seeking* information than that they learn specific facts relevant to a topic.

Another therapeutic task to educate a client about his or her situation is to review the medical records with the client. The goal here is to increase the individual's understanding that there is damage to the brain, which is responsible for some changes in functioning. Essentially, the clinician helps the client make the link between injury to the brain and changed abilities. Interpretation of the information contained in a client's medical records may become part of a personalized brain injury education notebook. Different protocols can be used, depending upon the client's level of functioning. The exercise provides a systematic review of information in a medical record that "tells the story" of what happened to the client and offers a way for the client to understand and remember the information. An example of a protocol used for this task is provided in Appendix 9.2.

A third example of an educational task is to compare ratings of others' perceptions of the client's functioning to those of the client. Discrepancies and agreements can be used as a counseling vehicle. There are many scales for rating performance in the domains of cognition, psychosocial functioning, and daily living skills; whichever ones are used at a particular facility can be adapted to this exercise. The steps in this process are (1) having a rating scale that lists different ability areas (a sample is provided in Appendix 9.3); (2) asking the client to select a person to fill it out, and facilitating this process; (3) helping the client to complete the rating scale using self-perceptions; (4) putting both sets of ratings in different colors of ink on the same protocol; and (5) exploring agreements and disagreements with the client.

An important caveat for the educational exercise just described—and, indeed, all awareness activities—is preventing a defensive reaction. The clinician does not want to force a client to admit deficits by pushing the ratings of the "more knowledgeable" other person. The clinician may instead observe, "I notice that you rated yourself as average in memory, but your mom rated that as a bigger problem area." If the client minimizes the other person's ratings, the clinician can explore what behaviors the other person may be responding to, or the clinician can just make the observation and move on. It is as important to point out areas of agreement as it is to discuss areas of discrepancy. For example, the clinician may observe, "Both you and your mom rated you 'above average' in reading ability."

A second important caveat in providing education in order to increase awareness is to monitor the emotional distress of clients. Several studies have noted the correlation between increased awareness of deficits and increased emotional distress (Godfrey, Partridge, Knight, & Bishara, 1993). Beardmore and colleagues (1999) encourage monitoring self-esteem in individuals receiving education about deficits. Results from their study (see below) suggested that those children who displayed the most limited levels of awareness often reported the highest levels of self-esteem.

Intervention Research Using an Educational Approach. Several studies have attempted to evaluate the efficacy of educating individuals about their brain injury for improving awareness. Two studies reported positive outcomes using a board game format to educate individuals about cognitive and behavioral issues following brain injury (Chittum, Johnson, Chittum, Guercio, & McMorrow, 1996; Zhou et al., 1996). In the Chittum and colleagues (1996) study, researchers used a board game (Road to Awareness) in conjunction with individualized training packages targeting information relevant to each of three subjects with acquired brain injury. Participants were given some instruction about brain injury prior to each game session. During the game, they were then asked questions about the concepts that had been reviewed. The questions included basic knowledge questions, as well as questions requiring them to demonstrate problem solving using the information and to apply the information. Results showed that all three clients increased the percentage of questions answered correctly during the game sessions, and that their performance improved on postgeneralization probes evaluating their knowledge and application in cognitive and behavioral categories.

Beardmore and colleagues (1999) evaluated education as an awareness intervention for children with acquired brain injury. They developed an interview to measure children's knowledge about brain injury. The study examined differences in interview responses between a group of children who received brain injury education and a group of children who did not receive the information. Their findings suggested that education was not successful in increasing the children's knowledge of their deficits. It should be noted, however, that the intervention consisted of only one educational session. Children with cognitive deficits will require more repetition. The authors discuss the importance of repetition and visual cues to aid children in remembering information, as well as the provision of small amounts of information and checking to make sure the information is understood and retained. Their study questions the efficacy of giving information in a one-time feedback session following neuropsychological testing or in a school planning meeting; instead, it encourages a more comprehensive educational approach.

Experiential Exercises

Experiential exercises are another approach for enhancing an individual's self-awareness. All experiential exercises have as their goal to help clients actually experience changes in their ability, in order to increase their awareness of the nature of these changes. Experiential exercises are most helpful for individuals whose awareness problems are due in part to organic brain damage and who have enough cognitive abilities to begin to link cause and effect.

A Case Illustration from the Literature. A number of methods can be used to help clients' experience and integrate knowledge about changes in functioning. Many of them facilitate clients' paying attention to or reflecting on certain behaviors or actions. Stuss (1991) provides a case illustration of a highly educated patient with right frontal lobe damage after a tumor was surgically removed. Neuropsychological testing revealed excellent cognitive abilities, but the patient had difficulty organizing and completing basic daily tasks, including grooming and getting herself to work. She exhibited significant unawareness of her difficulties. Stuss describes the following combination of methods used to increase the client's awareness, which illustrates an individual awareness-enhancing program: (1) verbal self-regulation during multistep tasks (i.e., having the patient talk to herself to guide her behavior); (2) explicit establishing of appropriate goals; (3) visual cues posted in her surroundings (e.g., "Stay on task"); and (4) role-playing exercises where she would act the part of her work supervisor and show how to deal with the problem behaviors she exhibited at work. The goal of all of these exercises was to increase the client's awareness and therefore her functional abilities. The case report suggests that the client's productivity and punctuality improved; however, there remained significant problems in self-awareness. Often the most realistic goal is not to achieve a premorbid level of awareness or functioning, but to improve abilities or skills in a specific context or set of contexts.

Sample Experiential Exercises. Depending upon the specific awareness profile of the client, various tasks or exercises can be utilized, in combination or separately, to increase awareness. In addition to verbal self-regulation, as described above in connection with the Stuss (1991) case study, we recommend the following:

- Comparison of prediction and performance
- Tracking of performance or behavior
  - Self-monitoring
  - Behavioral logs
- Goal-setting process

One experiential exercise that has already been described as a method for measuring awareness is the process of having clients compare predictions with actual performance. It has also been used as an intervention approach. As previously described, Rebmann and Hannon (1995) implemented an awareness training program involving estimating performance, followed by the provision of feedback on actual performance. Clients were reinforced for accuracy of their predictions. In this study, differences between the predicted and actual test scores decreased over time. Schlund (1999) also provided feedback and review for a client who predicted performance on recall of personal information. Results suggested that the provision of feedback on accuracy of prediction of recall ability reduced the variability between self-reports and recall performance.

This prediction–performance paradigm can be applied to a number of different tasks. The exercise can be introduced to the client as a mechanism to see where strengths and weaknesses lie, so that "time is not wasted working on things that do not need to be addressed." It is very important to include prediction tasks that are well within the individual's capability, as well as those that are likely to illustrate his or her impairments. For example, consider a case where the goal is to increase a client's awareness of memory deficits, so that he or she will be more receptive to using a compensatory system. First, the clinician and client make a list of memory-dependent activities that the client finds meaningful. Tasks can be selected that have the greatest chance of revealing critical information—the preserved and damaged aspects of memory. Tasks that are concrete, with specific performance outcomes, are the most useful. A sample list may include (1) measures of academic skills, such as reading comprehension (the client will need to be familiar with such measures and have an accurate sense of his or her ability prior to injury); (2) prediction of how many trials will be needed to learn information, such as a medication regimen or computer procedures; and/or (3) performance on memory-dependent recreational games, such as the card game Concentration. A list for a client trying to learn more about his or her executive functions may include (1) changing the oil in the car (if this was a maintenance chore the client could complete prior to injury); (2) ordering multiple items from a catalogue; and (3) meal planning.

The prediction–performance paradigm is essentially a risk-taking activity, in which clinicians partner with clients and help them reflect on their predictions and performance to facilitate their awareness of their own abilities. It should *not* be set up to prove to clients that they are impaired, or the process will fail. Selecting tasks that have a high probability of concretely illustrating strengths *and* weaknesses is the critical step. For clients who have difficulty with the abstract concept of prediction or anticipation, or for clients who are highly defensive, it may be beneficial to elicit self-evaluation *after* performance. Having clients first describe the strengths of their performance and then offer self-critiques can be therapeutic in improving awareness.

Another common method for helping clients structure their experiences so they can better understand their abilities and disabilities is to have them track their performance or behavior. Clients and clinicians jointly decide what they want to monitor, and design a protocol and a process to gather the information. Examples of tracking sheets that clients have used include sheets for monitoring performance on meal planning, getting to appointments, having materials ready for class, controlling impulsive responding, and using a memory system. Sometimes this process requires having a support person help monitor and then review the data with a client. The point is to give the client information about his or her real-world functioning in such a way that the client can learn more about what is working and not working. As in the prediction–performance exercise, it is critical to track successes as well as problems. The process should illustrate some successful behaviors, as well as highlight areas that may require some support.

Several intervention studies have described the utility of having clients track performance. Cicerone and Giacino (1992) provide data supporting the efficacy of monitoring error responses in clients with decreased awareness. They outline a process whereby a client is stopped during a task each time an error is committed. The client's attention is directed toward the error, and he or she enters a record of the error in a log. The client is assisted to compare responses on subsequent trials to the error record. Sohlberg, Glang, and Todis (1998a) suggest that tracking information can be therapeutic not only for improving awareness, but for improving the behaviors that are being monitored.

An extension of tracking performance is goal setting. A number of researchers have noted that an explicit goal-setting process—one that involves the client—can be helpful in improving awareness (Bergquist & Jacket, 1993; Stuss, 1991). Bergquist and Jacket (1993) describe a goal-setting process in which therapists play a supportive but nondirective role, and goals are developed that incorporate information in self-awareness. They discuss the importance of establishing a trusting relationship with the client and selecting goals that the client is motivated and able to pursue. They further encourage wording goals so that they are easily understood by the client and state a positive behavioral objective (e.g., "Increase using electronic memory" rather than "Decrease episodes of forgetting").

Caregiver Training and Education

It is important to understand families' or caregivers' perceptions of clients' abilities and disabilities. They will have a major influence on clients' successful functioning. The individual awareness-enhancing exercises described above have been divided into educational and experiential exercises, and their overall goal is to increase an individual client's understanding and appreciation of his or her own strengths and weaknesses. All of these exercises may also be helpful for families or caregivers of persons with acquired brain injury. Although caregivers do not share the organically based unawareness, they may experience the same types of unawareness due to psychological denial, or may lack information because it has not been given at such a time or in such a way that they could process it.

In our discussion of options for measuring awareness, we have encouraged clinicians to be cautious when using family or staff reports in evaluations of client awareness, for several reasons (Cavello et al., 1992; Fleming et al., 1996). On the other hand, caregivers provide critical information about clients' previous and current levels of functioning. They will also be the ones with the most potential to influence clients following treatment.

A study by Sohlberg and colleagues (1998a) encourages addressing caregivers' beliefs and attitudes as a part of any awareness therapy program. They examined the relationship among various indicators of awareness in three individuals with brain damage over a 9-month period. Results suggested a dissociation between behavioral and perceptual indices of awareness: Improvements in client behaviors that were selected by caregivers as indicative of decreased awareness did not result in improved awareness ratings by the same caregivers. It may be that caregivers were correct in noting that although behaviors changed (e.g., increased use of a checklist), these improvements were not associated with increased self-awareness. Alternatively, it may be that caregivers' perceptions are not easily modified, even if patients improve. It appeared that the caregivers did not link awareness with learning, but instead may have linked it with the clients' open admission of impairment. Hence, exploring caregivers' expectations about the goal of therapy (e.g., improving a behavior vs. improving insight into self) may be helpful.

It can also be beneficial to help caregivers (and fellow clinicians) understand that some people can learn to use systems or strategies without having to "own up" or describe their deficits. The desire by some caregivers to have patients acknowledge their limitations is particularly problematic in relationships with clients whose unawareness is due in part to denial or emotional reactions. Clinicians will want to teach some caregivers that confronting patients with their deficits usually leads to a polarization of ideas, with each party becoming more entrenched in his or her own position. Caregivers may benefit from tracking their responses to clients' "unawareness behaviors" and charting how the clients in turn respond to the caregivers' actions or reactions.

In short, a clinician should talk with a caregiver to determine the following:

- The caregiver's expectations for treatment
- Whether/how the client's unawareness is troublesome to the caregiver

- Whether there is an urge to have the client "admit" deficits
- Whether the caregiver could benefit from counseling not to confront the client about deficits

Procedural Training and Environmental Support

Providing PTES is important in cases where efforts to increase clients' self-awareness are likely to be unsuccessful. The goal of this approach is to maximize functioning without being concerned about whether a client acknowledges or understands his or her limitations. PTES is most appropriate for clients who exhibit severe unawareness and/or severe cognitive impairments that preclude them from responding to an individualized awareness-enhancing program (e.g., a client who has very little insight into existing impairments and whose beliefs are not malleable, even when given direct feedback). Similarly, a client who consistently appears indifferent to or nonplussed by evidence of decreased abilities may benefit the most from PTES. Examples of PTES interventions include the following:

- Training the use of a compensatory system without educating the client why he or she should use the system
- Facilitating prompts by others in the clients' environment to improve functioning
- Rearranging physical space to facilitate task completion (e.g., labeling cupboard contents)

In this approach, other individuals may be trained in specific skills or routines to increase the client's level of functioning, and/or modifications may be made to the environment to reduce the impact of the client's impairments.

PTES will be idiosyncratic for every skill or routine and for every client. The instruction principles reviewed in Chapters 6 and 7 will be critical for successful training. The clinician will be attempting to teach a routine and have the client carry it out in an automatic fashion. The idea is that the client's procedural memory (see Chapter 6) will be employed to learn a routinized task that will not require insight or self-awareness.

Summary of Intervention Approaches

This section thus far has reviewed three broad approaches to awareness intervention:

1. Setting up an individual awareness-enhancement program, which is primarily directed at improving an individual's understanding and insight into residual abilities and disabilities so that the individual can incorporate

this information into daily life decisions. This approach can use educational and/or experiential exercises.

2. Providing caregiver training and education. Clinicians should always remember to look at those individuals most affected by awareness decrements—family members and caregivers. These individuals may benefit from a structured educational approach. Also, it may be important to look at their expectations to see whether they feel the need for clients to admit deficits. Helping caregivers to focus on their own behavior or examine their own expectations and perceptions can be very useful.

3. Providing PTES. These interventions are for individuals who probably will not benefit from direct awareness intervention. In this approach, a clinician taps into implicit learning and develops procedures for using a system or strategy without addressing the client's declarative knowledge of why the systems or strategies are important. The clinician evaluates the environment to determine how best to support an individual with awareness difficulties.

Adolescents: Their Special Needs

The three major management approaches reviewed thus far are appropriate for adults, adolescents, and older children with awareness disorders. However, the special nature of adolescence warrants a bit more discussion. The major goal of adolescence is the development of an individual identity that is independent of parents, teachers, and other caregivers. Neurological impairment may cause adolescents to become more dependent at the very time when they are trying to establish their autonomy.

Adolescents exhibit the same types of unawareness described in the beginning of this chapter; however, unawareness problems are often compounded by the emancipation process that is a normal part of this developmental phase. As they strive for autonomy to make personal decisions, adolescent clients can feel particularly frustrated by adults who give them increased input and guidance. They may reject attempts to assist them in managing problems brought about by a brain injury.

The following guidelines offer reminders about what to do (and not to do) to assist adolescents with awareness disorders (Sohlberg, Todis, & Glang, 1999):

• Clinicians need to align themselves with their adolescent clients. They should not enter into power struggles or try to convince the clients that deficits exist. Forming a partnership with a young client is particularly important at this phase. The use of collaborative language, compromise, and reframing will all be important interactional skills.

• Special efforts should be made to preserve self-esteem by focusing on strengths, as well as deficits. Clinicians can avoid a problem-centered focus of therapy. For example, they can make lists of attributes that were not affected by brain injury, and provide attention for preserved abilities as well as for problems.

CASE EXAMPLE

The following case illustrates an awareness intervention program utilizing both educational and experiential exercises. Caregiver (spouse) beliefs and education were also addressed as part of the program.

Tim was a 45-year-old man who had received a moderate brain injury in a motor vehicle accident 2 years prior. He was hospitalized after a brief period of unconsciousness (less than 24 hours). A brain scan revealed no focal lesions, and the report suggested the probability of axonal shearing. Tim was an attorney at the time of the accident. When he came in for an initial interview, he recounted how he had been to multiple professionals all over the country, none of whom understood his situation and none of whom were helpful. He was very articulate and expressed significant anger at the professionals who had "failed" him and at the driver responsible for the accident.

Neuropsychological testing revealed significant impairment in attention, new learning, and executive functions. Tim said he had been unable to work since the time of his accident. He attributed most of his inability to work to reduced concentration and headaches. He did not seem to appreciate changes in memory or cognitive functioning as responsible for his reduced abilities. He stated that his goal was "to be fixed." He was very resistant to questioning regarding compensatory strategies, and stated that he was "not looking for a crutch, but a fix." An interview with his wife revealed a similar preoccupation with deficient professional care and the driver who caused the accident, in addition to a lack of appreciation for how brain damage might be responsible for Tim's cognitive changes.

The awareness assessment suggested that Tim had both an organically based unawareness of self and some psychological denial. The client appeared to lack information about his abilities and disabilities, and was unable to appreciate the implications of the information he did have (e.g., about reduced attention) for his daily functioning. It was decided that in order for him to become receptive to using some compensation strategies, he would benefit from a better understanding of his residual strengths and limitations, and an individual awareness-enhancing program was designed. It was also felt that Tim's progress would be more likely to be maintained if his wife developed a realistic appraisal of his strengths and weaknesses. It was further decided that given the client's degree of anger toward professionals, it would be important for therapy to be nondirective, supportive, and nonconfrontational.

Therapy began with an academic educational task: The clinician asked Tim and his wife to read an article about mild brain injury and to highlight those symptoms they felt Tim also experienced. Due to the client's difficulty with reading comprehension, a plan was made for his wife to read him the article. In order to establish rapport and trust, the client and his wife were also provided with supportive listening, where they were allowed to talk about their frustration with the failings of the previous professionals. The clinician did not try to defend the profession; instead, she acknowledged the couple's frustration and shared her perceptions that the optimal first step would be for them to learn more about their situation.

Tim and his wife were very interested in the contents of the article. They asked for more information. The clinician helped them put together a "fact" book. The client seemed reassured to learn that other individuals experienced the same symptoms, and that cognitive symptoms secondary to a brain injury were not the same as lowered intelligence secondary to mental retardation. Tim began independently mailing copies of this information to professionals he had seen and to family and friends. He also participated in a review of his medical record, with a focus on common symptoms of diffuse axonal injury. Because he tended to perseverate on certain themes and questions (e.g., "Will my brain ever completely heal?", "Why didn't someone give me this information earlier?"), a sheet with common questions and corresponding responses was added to the book for easy reference. Tim gradually became less aggressive in his demeanor when talking about his injury.

The fact book was progressively expanded to include a calendar and daily schedule. This was accomplished in a nondirective way by asking Tim whether the fact book would be a convenient place to put a reminder list of things he had said he wanted to do. Initially the daily schedule only contained a list of "to-do" items he had expressed interest in completing (e.g., "Mail a copy of this article to Dr. Jones"). Eventually, both he and his wife used the schedule to organize their day.

When Tim began to understand that he had changes in thinking ability (new learning, speed of processing, flexible thinking) due to his accident, the clinician began some experiential exercises with both him and his wife. Together, they developed a list of tasks Tim could complete in order to learn more about what had changed and not changed as a result of his head injury. The list included some vocational tasks involving reading law briefs, a phone meeting, and some household chores. The clinician asked the client to predict what would be easy and hard aspects of each of the tasks, and they wrote these down. Over a period of several weeks, Tim attempted the tasks. Although he did not write in the log provided for reflecting upon performance, the clinician was able to fill out the log using an interview format. They developed a list of strengths, as well as areas that required more focus. An example of a strength was "high-level vocabulary and discourse." This was drawn from the phone meeting task, where Tim recognized he had strong verbal abilities. An example of an area that required focus was "holding on to information." This was drawn from Tim's reading a law brief and not being able to carry information from one paragraph to the next.

After the list was developed, Tim ranked the areas he wanted to focus on. Being able to hold on to information that he read was his first priority, and therapy moved into teaching him a metacognitive reading comprehension strategy.

Early in the educational sessions, Tim's wife declared that she now realized how impaired the head injury had made him. She was asked to keep a log of what types of things she did that appeared to help him compensate for memory and attention problems. She was also helped to understand that he probably would need to compensate for changes in cognition for a long time. This encouraged her to begin to look at disability options for her husband, and together they began to think about some "home business" opportunities that they could pursue together.

In summary, over a 3-month period Tim and his wife participated in an awareness-enhancing program that first provided them with information about their situation and then gradually helped them apply it to their own lives. They were helped to experience Tim's residual symptoms and preserved strengths, and to use this information to set therapy goals. They were also encouraged to look at the long-term implications of what they were learning for their vocational situation. The client moved from complete unwillingness to consider compensation strategies to consistent use of a system. He learned to use a daily written list to guide his schedule and to organize his day. He also became more proficient at reading as he learned a reading comprehension strategy. He reported that he was able to read the newspaper on a daily basis, which had not previously been possible. However, he continued to perseverate about his belief that he had not initially received adequate care, as well as his feelings of anger toward the driver who had caused his accident. He also continued to exhibit decreased self-awareness about his behavior, as he did not alter his discussion of these themes in a group setting, even if others indicated that they were uncomfortable. Thus Tim was more productive during his day and became more proficient at several skills that were important to him. He did, however, continue to suffer significant cognitive and self-awareness problems.

REFERENCES

Allen, C., & Ruff, R. M. (1990). Self rating versus neuropsychological performance of moderate versus severe head injured patients. *Brain Injury, 4*, 7–17.

Beardmore, S., Tate, R., & Liddle, B. (1999). Does information and feedback improve children's knowledge and awareness of deficits after traumatic brain injury? *Neuorpsychological Rehabilitation, 9*(1), 45–62.

Bergquist, T. F., & Jacket, M. P. (1993). Awareness and goal setting with the traumatically brain injured. *Brain Injury, 7*(3), 275–282.

Berti, A., Ladavas, E., & Della Corte, M. (1996). Anosognosia for hemiplegia, neglect dyslexia, and drawing neglect: Clinical findings and theoretical considerations. *Journal of the International Neuropsychological Society, 2*, 426–440.

Biach, E., Vallar, G., Perani, D., Papagano, C., & Berti, A. (1986). Unawareness of disease following lesions of the right hemisphere: Anosognosia for hemiplegia and anosognosia for hemianopia. *Neuropsychologia, 24*, 471–482.

Burgess, P. W., Alderman, N., Wilson, B. A., Evans, J. J., & Emslie, H. C. (1996). The Dysexecutive Questionnaire (DEX). In B. A. Wilson, N. Alderman, P. W. Burgess, H. C. Emslie, & J. J. Evans (Eds.), *Behavioural assessment of the*

Dysexecutive Syndrome. Burry, St. Edmunds, England: Thames Valley Test Company.

Cavello, M. M., Kay, T., & Ezrachi, O. (1992). Problems and changes after traumatic brain injury: Differing perceptions within and between families. *Brain Injury, 6,* 327–335.

Chittum, W. R., Johnson, K., Chittum, J. M., Guercio, J. M., & McMorrow, M. J. (1996). Road to Awareness: An individualized training package for increasing knowledge and comprehension of personal deficits in persons with acquired brain injury. *Brain Injury, 10*(10), 763–776.

Cicerone, K. D., & Giacino, J. T. (1992). Remediation of executive function deficits after traumatic brain injury. *Neuropsychological Rehabilitation, 2*(3), 12–22.

Crosson, B., Barco, P. P., Velozo, C. A., Bolesta, M., Cooper, P. V., Werts, D., & Brobeck, T. C. (1989). Awareness and compensation in postacute head injury rehabilitation. *Journal of Head Trauma Rehabilitation, 4,* 46–54.

Damasio, A. R. (1994). *Descartes' error: Emotion, reason, and the human brain.* New York: Putnam.

Deluca, J. (1992). Rehabilitation of confabulation: The issue of unawareness of deficit. *Neuropsychological Rehabilitation, 2,* 23–30.

Dywan, J., & Segalowitz, S. J. (1996). Self and family ratings of adaptive behavior after traumatic brain injury: Psychometric scores and frontally generated ERPs. *Journal of head Trauma Rehabilitation, 11*(2), 79–95.

Fleming, J. M., Strong, J., & Ashton, R. (1996). Self-awareness of deficits in adults with traumatic brain injury: How best to measure? *Brain Injury, 10,* 1–15.

Fordyce, D. J., & Roueche, J. R. (1986). Changes in perspectives of disability among patients, staff and relatives during rehabilitation of brain injury. *Rehabilitation Psychology, 31,* 217–229.

Giacino, J. T., & Cicerone, K. D. (1998). Varieties of deficit unawareness after brain injury. *Journal of Head Trauma Rehabilitation, 13*(5), 1–15.

Godfrey, H. P. D., Partridge, F. M., Knight, R. G., & Bishara, S. N. (1993). Course of insight disorder and emotional dysfunction following closed head injury: A controlled cross-sectional follow-up study. *Journal of Clinical and Experimental Neuropsychology, 15,* 503–515.

Hart, T., Giovannetti, M. S., Montgomery, M. W., & Schwartz, M. F. (1998). Awareness of errors in naturalistic action after traumatic brain injury. *Journal of Head Trauma Rehabilitation, 13*(5), 16–28.

Langer, K. G., & Padrone, F. J. (1992). Psychotherapeutic treatment of awareness in acute rehabilitation of traumatic brain injury. *Neuropsychological Rehabilitation, 2,* 59–70.

Lebrun, Y. (1987). Anosognosia in aphasics. *Cortex, 23,* 251–263.

McGlynn, S. M., & Schacter, D. L. (1989). Unawareness of deficits in neuropsychological syndromes. *Journal of Clinical and Experimental Neuropsychology, 11*(2), 143–205.

Prigatano, G. P. (1991). Disturbances of self-awareness of deficits after traumatic brain injury. In G. Prigatano & D. Schacter (Eds.), *Awareness of deficit after brain injury: Theoretical and clinical implications* (pp. 115–135). New York: Oxford University Press.

Prigatano, G. P., & Altman, I. M. (1990). Impaired awareness of behavioral limitations after traumatic brain injury. *Archives of Physical Medicine and Rehabilitation, 71,* 1058–1064.

Prigatano, G. P., & Klonoff, P. S. (1998). A clinician's rating scale for evaluating impaired self-awareness and denial of disability after brain injury. *Clinical Neuropsychologist, 12,* 56–67.

Rebmann, M. J., & Hannon, R. (1995). Treatment of unawareness of memory deficits in adults with brain injury: Three case studies. *Rehabilitation Psychology, 40*(4), 279–287.

Roueche, F. R., & Fordyce, D. J. (1987). Perceptions of deficits following brain injury and their impact on psychosocial adjustment. *Cognitive Rehabilitation, 1,* 4–7.

Schacter, D. L., Glisky, E. L., & McGlynn, S. M. (1990). Impact of memory disorder on everyday life: Awareness of deficits and return to work. In D. E. Tupper & K. D. Cicerone (Eds.), *The neuropsychology of everyday life: Assessment and basic competencies (*pp. 231–257). Boston: Kluwer Academic.

Schlund, M.W. (1999). Self awarenesss: Effects of feedback and review on verbal self reports and remembering following brain injury. *Brain Injury, 13*(5), 375–380.

Sohlberg, M. M., Glang, A., & Todis, B. (1998a). Improvement during baseline: Three case studies encouraging collaborative research when evaluating caregiver training. *Brain Injury, 12*(4), 333–346.

Sohlberg, M. M., Mateer, C. A., Penkman, L., Glang, A., & Todis, B. (1998b). Awareness intervention: Who needs it? *Journal of Heat Trauma Rehabilitation, 13*(5), 62–78.

Sohlberg, M. M., Todis, B., & Glang, A. (1999). *Changes in self awareness among students with brain injuries.* Wake Forest, NC: Lash & Associates.

Stuss, D. (1991). Disturbances of self-awareness after frontal system damage. In G. P. Prigatano & D. L. Schacter (Eds.), *Awareness of deficit after brain injury: Clinical and theoretical issues* (pp. 63–83). New York: Oxford University Press.

Stuss, D. T., & Benson, D. F. (1986). *The frontal lobes.* New York: Raven Press.

Sunderland, A. (1990). Clinical memory assessment: Matching the method to the aim. In D. E. Tupper & K. D. Cicerone (Eds.), *The neuropsychology of everyday life: Assessment and basic competencies* (pp. 169–183). Boston: Kluwer Academic.

Tepper, S., Beatty, P., & Dejong, G. (1996). Outcomes in traumatic brain injury: Self-report versus report of significant others. *Brain Injury, 10*(8), 575–581.

Weinstein, E. A., & Friedland, R. P. (1977). Behavioral disorders associated with hemi-inattention. In E. A. Weinstein & R. P. Friedland (Eds.), *Advances in neurology* (Vol. 18, pp. 51–62). New York: Raven Press.

Weinstein, E. A., & Kahn, R. I. (1955). *Denial of illness: Symbolic and physiological aspects.* Springfield, IL: Charles C. Thomas.

Wilson, B.A., Alderman N., Burgess, P., Emslie, H., & Evans, J. (1996). *Behavioral Assessment of Dysexecutive Syndrome.* Burry, St. Edmunds, England: Thames Valley Test Company.

Zhou, J., Chittum, W. R., Johnson-Tomkins, K., Poppen, R., Guercio, J., & McMorrow, M. J. (1996). The utilization of a game format to increase knowledge of residuals among people with acquired brain injury. *Journal of Head Trauma Rehabilitation, 11*(1), 51–61.

APPENDIX 9.1

SELF-AWARENESS OF DEFICITS INTERVIEW

1. Self-awareness of deficits.

Are you any different now compared to what you were like before your accident? In what way? Do you feel that anything about you, or your abilities, has changed?

Do people who know you well notice that anything is different about you since the accident? What might they notice?

What do you see as your problems, if any, resulting from your injury? What is the main thing you need to work on/would like to get better?

Prompts

Physical abilities (e.g., movement of arms and legs, balance, vision, endurance)?

Memory/confusion?

Concentration?

Problem solving, decision making, organizing and planning things?

Controlling behavior?

Communication?

Getting along with other people?

Has your personality changed?

Are there any other problems that I haven't mentioned?

2. Self-awareness of functional implications of deficits.

Does your head injury have any effect on your everyday life? In what way?

Prompts

Ability to live independently?

Managing finances?

Look after family/manage home?

Driving?

Work/study?

Leisure/social life?

Are there any other areas of life that you feel have changed/may change?

3. Ability to set realistic goals.

What do you hope to achieve in the next 6 months? Do you have any goals? What are they?

In 6 months' time, what do you think you will be doing? Where do you think you will be?

Do you think your head injury will still be having an effect on your life in 6 months' time?

If yes, how?

If no, are you sure?

Scoring

1. Self-awareness of deficits.

0 Cognitive/psychological problems (where relevant) reported by the patient/client in response to general questioning, or readily acknowledged in response to specific questioning.

1 Some cognitive/psychological problems, but others denied or minimized. Patient/client may have a tendency to focus on relatively minor physical changes (e.g., scars) and acknowledge cognitive/psychological problems only on specific questioning about deficits.

2 Physical deficits only acknowledged; denies, minimizes, or is unsure of cognitive/psychological changes. Patient/client may recognize problems that occurred at an earlier stage but denies existence of persisting deficits, or may state that other people think there are deficits, but he/she does not think so.

3 No acknowledgment of deficits (other than obvious physical deficits) can be obtained, or patient/client will only acknowledge problems that have been imposed on him/her, e.g., not allowed to drive or drink alcohol.

2. Self-awareness of functional implications of deficits.

0 Patient/client accurately describes current functional status (in independent living, work/study, leisure, home management, driving), and specifies how his/her head injury problems limit function where relevant, and/or any compensatory measures adopted to overcome problems.

1 Some functional implications reported following questions or examples of problems in independent living, work, driving, leisure, etc. Patient/client may not be sure of other likely functional problems, e.g., is unable to say because he/she has not tried an activity yet.

2 Patient/client may acknowledge some functional implications of deficits but minimizes the importance of identified problems. Other likely functional implications may be actively denied by the patient/client.

3 Little acknowledgment of functional consequences can be obtained; the patient/client will not acknowledge problems: except that he/she is not allowed to perform certain tasks. He/she may actively ignore medical advice and may engage in risk-taking behaviors, e.g., driving, drinking.

3. Ability to set realistic goals.

0 Patient/client sets reasonably realistic goals, and (where relevant) identifies that the head injury will probably continue to have an impact on some areas of functioning, i.e., goals for the future have been modified in some way since the injury.

1 Patient/client sets goals that are somewhat unrealistic, or is unable to specify a goal, but recognizes that he/she may still have problems in some areas of function in the future, i.e., sees that goals for the future may need some modification, even if he/she has not yet done so.

2 Patient/client sets unrealistic, or is unable to specify a goal, and does not know how he/she will be functioning in 6 months' time, but hopes he/she will return to pretrauma, i.e., no modification of goals has occurred.

3 Patient/client expects without uncertainty that in 6 months' time, he/she will be functioning at pretrauma level (or at a higher level).

Note. From Fleming, Strong, and Ashton (1996). Copyright 1996 by Taylor & Francis, Inc./Routledge, Inc., http://www.routledge-ny.com. Reprinted by permission.

APPENDIX 9.2

MEDICAL RECORDS REVIEW

Name _____ Date: _____

Sources of Information _____

Mechanism of Injury: (Explain how your brain was injured.) _____

_____

Types of Cognitive Problems: (Explain what kinds of thinking problems are
the most obvious and bothersome to you; you can use the list or write in your
own responses. Examples: Concentrating; dealing with distractions;
remembering what I am supposed to do in the future; remembering people I
used to know; trying to learn new information or procedures; getting started
on projects; organizing myself; figuring out what I am supposed to be doing;
figuring out how to fix my mistakes; other.)

1. _____

2. _____

3. _____

4. _____

5. _____

Cause of Cognitive Problems: (You can choose from list or write in other
response. Examples: Parts of the brain that are involved in these abilities
were injured; my heart stopped and not enough oxygen got to my brain,
resulting in brain damage; bleeding in my brain damaged places that are
important for thinking; chemicals affected thinking centers in the brain; tumor
caused damage by pressing on parts of the brain involved in thinking; other.)

_____

_____

Cognitive Strengths: (List types of thinking that are not as much of a
problem for you; you can use the previous list or make up your own.)

1. _____

2. _____

3. _____

4. _____

5. _____

Ways to Deal with Cognitive Problems: (List types of strategies that might be helpful for dealing with the thinking problems that you identified; you can use the list or make up your own. Examples: Turning off the TV or shutting the door when I am trying to concentrate; making checklists with the steps I need to do to get something done; organizing my home or hospital room by posting reminders on bulletin board, refrigerator, mirrors, etc.; using a notebook, date book, or appointment book with things-to-do lists and calendars; using reminder devices like a watch alarm, egg timer, or pill box with an alarm; learning specific memory tricks like making up rhymes to remember names of my medications; working on therapy exercises; other.)

1. _____

2. _____

3. _____

4. _____

5. _____

My Therapy Plan: (Explain therapy goals and what you will be working on.)

_____

_____

_____

_____

_____

_____

APPENDIX 9.3

SELF–OTHER COMPARISON RATING

We want to learn which things are challenging for you (him or her) due to having had a brain injury. I'm going to describe different abilities and then ask you whether each one represents (5) a major problem, (4) a medium problem, (3) a small problem, (2) no problem or no change, or (1) an area in which you perform (he or she performs) above average.

The first area is cognition or thinking skills.

___ 1. How would you describe your (his/her) **attention/concentration?** This is the ability to keep focusing on a task not to get too distracted, or to hold on to information long enough to get it into your (his or her) memory.

___ 2. How about **visual/perceptual abilities?** This is *not* how well your eyes work with or without glasses. It is being able to judge distances or put a puzzle together, to see a whole piece of paper or TV screen, or to coordinate your (his or her) eyes and hands.

___ 3. What about **memory and learning new things?** How would you describe your (his or her) ability to remember events, to remember what people have told you, or to learn new procedures?

___ 4. The next area is **reasoning and problem solving.** How would you describe your (his or her) ability to figure things out if you are confused?

___ 5. The next area is **planning and organization.** How would you describe your (his or her) ability to organize time, to get errands done, or to get to appointments?

___ 6. How would you describe your **language or communication?** Can you (he or she) express what you want (he or she wants) to say? Do you seem (does he or she seem) to understand what other people say?

___ 7. How would you describe your (his or her) **math** abilities?

___ 8. How would you describe your (his or her) **reading** abilities?

Self Subtotal I ___

Other Subtotal I ___

The second group of questions pertains to social and emotional issues.

___ 9. How would you describe your (his or her) **interpersonal skills** or your people skills—that is, your (his or her) ability to get along with others?

___ 10. How about your (his or her) **self-control** or ability to monitor emotions or behaviors? This area covers how you control (he or she controls) your (his or her) anger, anxiety/worry, or impulses.

__ 11. The next question is about your (his or her) **adjustment or acceptance** to having had a brain injury.

__ 12. I'm interested in whether **depression** is an issue for you (him or her).

__ 13. How would you describe your (his or her) **social support network?**

Self Subtotal II ____

Other Subtotal II ____

The next group of questions has to do with daily living skills.

__ 14. How about **personal care** such as grooming and dressing?

__ 15. How about **household management**—that is, taking care of your (his or her) living quarters, doing chores such as dishes and cleaning, and so on?

__ 16. How about **accessing the community** or getting around in town? How would you describe your (his or her) ability to get to places like the store, post office, or other places outside the house or apartment?

__ 17. Tell me about your (his or her) ability to **manage money**. How do you (does he or she) do with budgeting, keeping track of money, doing banking, and so on?

Self Subtotal III ____

Other Subtotal III ____

The next few questions have to do with physical abilities.

__ 18. How would you describe your (his or her) **endurance** or stamina?

__ 19. How would you describe your (his or her) **balance and coordination**?

__ 20. How would you describe your (his or her) **hands** for activities such as writing or doing the dishes?

__ 21. How would you describe your (his or her) ability to **manage physical limitations** and only do what is safe and within your (his or her) capabilities?

Self Subtotal IV ____

Other Subtotal IV ____

The last group of questions pertains to leisure or free time.

__ 22. Do you (does he or she) have enough **ideas and interests** for things to do during your (his or her) free time?

__ 23. How would you describe your (his or her) **leisure planning,** or ability to plan things to do during free time?

__ 24. How about your (his or her) **involvement in the community?** Do you (does he or she) do things out in the community with other people?

Self Subtotal V ____

Other Subtotal V ____

Self Total ____

Other Total ____

10

Communication Issues

TYPES OF COMMUNICATION CHALLENGES

Acquired brain injury can affect multiple aspects of communicative functioning. Although relatively rare, aphasic disturbances following brain injury do occur. More common, however, are difficulties with communication due to cognitive impairments. Cognitively based verbal impairments encompass a wide variety of symptoms. Examples include language that is confabulatory, tangential, fragmented, and/or devoid of content. Cognitive and psychosocial issues may also give rise to *pragmatics* deficits, or decreased ability to use language effectively in a social or verbal exchange. Frequent pragmatics symptoms include poor regulation of turn taking, poor topic maintenance, and reduced sensitivity to one's communication partner. Pragmatics deficits are perhaps the most socially punishing and chronic communication problems associated with acquired brain injury.

Aphasia and Brain Injury

Aphasia is the reduced capacity to interpret and formulate language symbols. It is most commonly a symptom of cerebrovascular accidents that affect the language centers or circuitry in the brain. These are usually housed within the left hemisphere, which for most people is dominant for language. The reported incidence of aphasia following closed head injury varies. Differences in subject selection criteria and in measures of aphasia make it difficult to compare studies. One study evaluated 750 patients with head injury who were admitted to a city hospital over a 10-month period, and found that only 13 of them (1.7%) exhibited aphasia (Heilman, Safran, & Geschwind, 1971). A similar study identified aphasia in only 34 cases out of 1,544 (2.2%) (Constantinovici, Arseni, Iliescu, Debrota, & Gorgia, 1970). Other reports, however, suggest much higher incidences (nearly 50%) (Levin, Grossman, & Kelly, 1976; Thompson, 1975).

More interesting and relevant than the frequency of aphasia are the types of aphasic disturbances observed following brain injury. The most common aphasic disturbance is *anomia,* characterized by impairments in visual naming and word association processes (Sohlberg & Mateer, 1989). Patients may present with more frank aphasic disturbances early following a brain injury, which eventually resolve into a mild residual anomia (Groher, 1977; Penn & Clary, 1988; Weinstein & Keller, 1963).

Cognitively Based Linguistic Deficits Following Brain Injury

Early research attempted to differentiate linguistic deficits of an aphasic nature from those that might be manifestations of other cognitive problems. Sarno (1980) identified a subgroup of patients with closed head injury, whom she labeled as having "subclinical aphasia." Aphasic symptoms were not observed in conversational speech; however, linguistic deficits were identified upon evaluation. Other researchers distinguished "confused language" from aphasia by describing the memory and orientation impairments resulting in language problems (Groher, 1977; Halpern, Darley, & Brown, 1973). Similar to aphasia, confused language often resolves over the initial weeks following a brain injury.

More recently, research revealing the nature of information-processing deficits following brain injury has been used to explain changes in communicative functioning. This research shifted from examining subjects' comprehension of single-sentence utterances to their comprehension of multiple-sentence utterances, or *discourse* (Nicholas & Brookshire, 1995). One study compared the comprehension of spoken narrative discourse in four groups: adults with left-hemisphere brain damage, with right-hemisphere brain damage, with traumatic brain injury, and without brain injury (Nicholas & Brookshire, 1995). Results suggested that a resource allocation model of discourse comprehension was useful in explaining the performance of all four groups. All groups displayed more difficulty as comprehension tasks became more complex. They were more accurate on comprehension questions testing main ideas than on questions testing details, and on questions testing stated information than on questions testing implied information. This is consistent with the resource allocation model, which suggests that human cognitive activities rely on a restricted supply of processing resources. When the demand for resources exceeds the available resources, cognitive processing suffers and performance declines.

Discourse processing, which involves a complex interplay of linguistic and cognitive abilities (e.g., attention and memory), is impaired in many persons who sustain a severe brain injury (Chapman, 1997). Such impairments involve failure to retain the important information conveyed in conversation and an inability to maintain organization of the information.

Consequently, oral and written language tends to unfold as incoherent fragments of information (Chapman, 1997; Chapman et al., 1997). The relative contributions of linguistic and cognitive deficits to communication breakdown are not well understood. However, the evidence supports cognitive mechanisms as primary sources of impairments. The fact that the formal aspects of language are usually well preserved sometimes masks existing communication impairments. Discourse processing is an important part of a cognitive–communicative evaluation for persons with brain injury.

Reduced verbal memory is another common cognitive impairment following acquired brain injury that has direct implications for communication abilities (Turkstra, McDonald, & Kaufmann, 1995). For example, verbal expression will necessarily be affected by an inability to recall the initial portion of a proposition.

Cognitive impairments such as decreased memory and attention are frequent explanations for communication impairments. However, linguistic deficits may also account for changes in ability. A comparison of adolescents with head injury and matched noninjured peers suggested that the former were significantly less competent in the interpretation and comprehension of linguistic humor (Docking, Murdoch, & Jordan, 2000). The subjects with head injury had difficulty completing a humor test that required them to say why different linguistically based items were funny (e.g., double meanings for words). This subject group also performed significantly below the comparison group on expressive and receptive measures of language, although many scores were still within normal limits. The authors noted the presence of subtle linguistic deficits affecting important language abilities such as the comprehension of humor.

In summary, consideration of how changes in both cognitive and linguistic processing affect communication constitutes an important part of an evaluation for persons with brain injuries.

Pragmatics Deficits and Brain Injury

Pragmatics constitute a comprehensive set of skills required for competence in naturalistic, functional use of language. The term can be broadly defined as the use of language for communication in specific contexts (Friedland & Miller, 1998). Pragmatics behaviors transcend isolated word and grammatical structures; they make up the system of rules clarifying the use of language in terms of situational or social contexts. People with brain injury often demonstrate normal basic linguistic skills, but have difficulty adapting their communication to specific contexts; for example, they may exhibit tangential speech, poor verbal organization, or inadequate turn taking (McDonald, 1993).

The recognition of pragmatics as a key consideration in brain injury rehabilitation is not new. Milton, Prutting, and Binder (1984) evaluated pragmatic skills in five persons with and five persons without brain injury; they concluded that following brain injury, "people talk better than they communicate." This is different from an aphasic syndrome, in which patients often "communicate better than they talk" (Holland, 1982). Although heterogeneity in the types of pragmatics deficits observed following brain injury is one of the hallmarks of the population, the pervasiveness of these disorders and the social isolation they cause are almost universal.

The sources of pragmatics deficits following brain injury often involve an interaction between cognitive and affective factors. Decreased self-awareness also contributes to reduced pragmatics. Damage to frontal brain structures, which house executive functions (see Chapter 8), frequently results in impaired social communication. For example, a person with deficits in self-regulation due to trauma involving frontal brain circuits may exhibit inappropriate topic selection, excessive interruption, and poor perspective taking in conversation. Because such individuals demonstrate normal linguistic functions (i.e., no difficulties with word finding, speech, or verbal fluency), their communication partners may not understand that the underlying cause of observed communication difficulties is brain damage. These people may quickly become socially ostracized for poor pragmatics.

Research suggests that pragmatics deficits do not spontaneously improve over time. Snow, Douglas, and Ponsford (1998) followed the conversational discourse abilities of 24 subjects with severe brain injuries for a minimum of 2 years after injury. The results of their assessment provided evidence that conversational skills remain compromised over time. Of particular concern was the finding that the discourse skills of one-third of their sample actually deteriorated over the follow-up period. Snow and colleagues (1998) suggest that both changes in executive functions and a diminished social circle account for reduced pragmatics.

The importance of pragmatics to successful community integration following neurological damage has encouraged clinicians to prioritize the assessment and treatment of pragmatics deficits. Although the shift to assessing and treating language use within naturalistic contexts is not new, it has been difficult. The complexity of naturalistic settings makes it difficult to develop and evaluate assessment and treatment procedures. To address pragmatics skills, a clinician or researcher must look beyond the linguistic functioning of an individual and, together with the client, take a broad view of the social communication context relevant to that individual.

Due to the predominance of pragmatics deficits in the population with brain injury, and the close association of such deficits with impaired cognitive functioning, the remainder of this chapter is devoted to the assessment and treatment of pragmatics functioning. For remediation of specific linguistic deficits that occur following brain injury, the reader is referred to other existing texts covering aphasia rehabilitation. Aphasia treatments, similar to cognitive interventions, exist along a recovery–compensation continuum. One end of the continuum is linguistic recovery, which targets impairments in semantic, syntactic, and phonologic processes, usually through direct treatment or stimulation approaches. The other end of the continuum hosts treatments that help individuals compensate for communication deficits, such as gesturing or using alternative communication modes. Remediation of pragmatics is often provided in conjunction with language remediation. Information specific to the remediation of underlying cognitive impairments responsible for pragmatics deficits (e.g., therapies to increase attention, memory, awareness, etc.) is discussed in other chapters within the present text.

ASSESSMENT OF PRAGMATICS

The Challenge of Assessing Pragmatics

There is widespread agreement that pragmatics assessment is a critical component of a cognitive evaluation following brain injury. Poor communication skills, which are common following brain injury, present a serious handicap and a major barrier to community reintegration; they are the probable cause of social isolation and decrease in vocational ability (Galski, Tompkins, & Johnston, 1998; Newton & Johnson, 1985). However, tools and information for assessing pragmatics are scarce. Turkstra and colleagues (1995) delineate a number of reasons for this shortcoming in the clinical research literature. They note that it is difficult to systematically quantify pragmatics deficits that emerge in real-world communication exchanges. Structured language evaluations do not capture pragmatics skills. Abilities in pragmatics functioning are best revealed by evaluation of functional communication, which can be time-consuming and subjective.

Another research limitation responsible for our lack of understanding of pragmatics deficits is the field's reliance on group data. As discussed below, there is a great variation in the characteristics of pragmatics deficits in persons with brain injury, which makes it imperative to evaluate individual performance data. A related problem is the lack of knowledge about "normative" pragmatic functioning. It is difficult to study and develop assessment tools in the absence of comparative data. The context-specific and value-laden nature of pragmatics renders it difficult to operationalize functioning "within normal limits."

Heterogeneity of Pragmatics Deficits

The heterogeneity of and difficulty in defining pragmatics deficits have been obstacles to the development of assessment tools. Some studies have documented clear differences in communication between persons with and without brain injury, while others have failed to identify such distinctions (Galski et al., 1998). For example, Mentis and Prutting's (1987) analysis of topic introduction and topic maintenance found that a subject with closed head injury produced fewer units containing novel information not specifically requested, more units containing information, specifically requested, fewer clarification and confirmation requests, and more agreement and acknowledgment units. In contrast, an analysis by Wozniak, Coelho, Duffy, and Liles (1999) of conversation in subjects with and without brain injury did not reveal different patterns of interaction between the two groups. Subjects in a study by Coelho, Liles, and Duffy (1991) highlighted the heterogeneity of communication disorders in persons with brain injury. In one subject, the content of discourse was appropriate, although it was poorly organized. In the second subject, the authors reported the reverse pattern: This subject demonstrated sufficient verbal organization, but impoverished content.

The identification of pragmatics behaviors commonly disrupted following brain injury is dependent upon the type of discourse analysis performed. One study compared the productions of 2 subjects with closed head injury to those of 12 subjects without brain injury (McDonald, 1993). The productions were generated by having the subjects explain a novel procedure to a blindfolded person. A "cohesion analysis" (i.e., an analysis of the degree to which strings of sentences operated together to make a unified whole, as opposed to a confused, fragmented production) suggested that the explanations generated by the subjects with brain injury were similar in cohesion to those of the control subjects. However, an "informational analysis" revealed differences between the subjects with and without brain injury, as well as differences between the two subjects with brain injury. Unlike the control subjects, the two subjects with brain injury both demonstrated substantial difficulty meeting the informational needs of the listener. Both of their productions were disorganized; the sequencing of propositions in their text was different from that of the controls. They differed from each other, however, in that one subject produced a text that was rated as overly repetitive, whereas the other subject produced too little detail. The author discusses how each of the subjects' production problems were characteristic of their particular "frontal deficits" (McDonald, 1993). These findings support the notion that pragmatics deficits following brain injury are heterogeneous. Clinicians need to include assessment of pragmatics or adaptive language functioning in their evaluations.

Methods for Assessing Pragmatics

Currently the most common methods used to assess the wide variety of possible pragmatics deficits are (1) informal observation of a client in conversation, and (2) the solicitation during interviews of the client's and others' reports of pragmatics functioning. Obviously such methods present grave limitations, because of their subjectivity and their inadequacy in elucidating environmental determiners of pragmatics skills. It is difficult to identify specific contextual factors in short observations or standardized checklists, and even harder to document change or responsiveness to an intervention. There is a critical need for ongoing research to develop practical methods to assess pragmatics. In the meantime, three existing assessment techniques that may be employed to evaluate pragmatics more fully are (1) systematic observation, (2) conversational analysis (CA), and (3) the use of elicitation tasks to illuminate specific pragmatics behaviors of interest.

Systematic Observation of Conversation

Researchers agree that in order to understand the nature of pragmatics deficits, it is critical to observe naturally occurring conversation. Systematic observations are facilitated by the use of checklists or indices that list the communication parameters one is interested in assessing.

The Pragmatic Protocol. Several existing protocols list a variety of pragmatics behaviors and may facilitate the observation process. As noted, however, use of such measures may be time-consuming and may require special expertise in scoring and analysis. Again, because of the pervasiveness of pragmatics deficits and their widespread effect on the lives of those with brain injury, prioritizing such an assessment is a worthy clinical investment.

The Pragmatic Protocol (Prutting & Kirchner, 1983, 1987) remains the "gold standard" for observational checklists. It presents a taxonomy of 32 pragmatics behaviors in four categories, extrapolated from a breadth of developmental and adult theories of communication discussed across a broad range of literature. These categories are as follows:

1. The *utterance act,* which includes verbal, nonverbal, and paralinguistic behaviors related to how the message is presented.
2. The *propositional act,* which refers to the linguistic meaning of the sentence.
3. The *perlocutionary act,* which relates to the effects of the speaker on the listener.
4. The *illocutionary act,* which refers to the speaker's intention.

The last two areas regulate the discourse between the speaker and listener and contain a number of pragmatics items. Each of the items refers to one unique dimension of communicative competence and is mutually exclusive

(Prutting & Kirchner, 1983). Appendix 10.1 provides a complete listing of the components of the Pragmatic Protocol.

The authors suggest that the Pragmatic Protocol should be completed after observing an individual engaged in spontaneous, unstructured conversation with a partner. It is recommended that a clinician observe at least 15 minutes of a conversation sample and then complete the protocol. Each item on the protocol is judged as "appropriate," "inappropriate," or "not observed." The guideline for judging an item's appropriateness is whether it is judged to facilitate the communication exchange or is neutral (appropriate) or whether it detracts from the exchange and/or socially penalizes the individual (inappropriate).

In the aforementioned study of five adults with brain injury and five without brain injury who were matched for age, sex, and education, Milton and colleagues (1984) found that the group with brain injury differed from the control group primarily in illocutionary and perlocutionary behaviors. The authors suggested that communication breakdown occurred most frequently in the ability to regulate discourse. The types of behaviors observed to be the most problematic for individuals with brain injury included prosody (e.g., intonation, stress, timing); topic selection (e.g., restricted range of topics); topic maintenance (e.g., topic change occurred following minimal speaking turns); turn-taking initiation, pause time, and contingency (e.g., awkward phrasing of new information added to the ongoing exchange); and quantity/conciseness (e.g., redundant information or excess detail). These authors concluded that the Pragmatic Protocol was useful in identifying strengths and weaknesses in conversational competence in persons with brain injury, and that it helped direct treatment efforts.

The Communication Profiling System. Facilitating unstructured observation essentially requires the clinician to structure an unstructured communication sample. In recent years, researchers have begun to appreciate the sensitivity of communication performance to different contextual factors, such as partner, topic, setting, and factors internal to the client (Friedland & Miller, 1998). It may not be possible to evaluate pragmatics deficits in a 15-minute contrived communication sample.

An ecologically valid communication assessment procedure called the Communicative Profiling System (Simmons-Mackie & Damico, 1996), developed for evaluating communication skills in persons with aphasia, offers an alternative (albeit more intensive) methodology for assessing naturalistic communication. Simmons-Mackie and Damico suggest: "To develop a socially broader, more ecologically valid perspective, aphasiologists must view the behaviors of individuals with aphasia from a socially sensitive perspective—looking for explanations of behaviors rather than judging behavior based on preconceived notions of appropriateness" (p. 549).

Such a view also applies to the assessment of pragmatics deficits following brain injury. Rather than using structured tests, questionnaires, or checklists, the Communication Profiling System requires gathering information from real-life communication partners and situations. It involves a cyclical collection and analysis of naturalistic communication data, divided up into the following four phases:

- *Phase 1: Glean a broad-based perspective.* Interviews are conducted with at least two different people familiar with the targeted individual, to gather their perspectives on relevant communication factors (e.g., which persons the individual typically talks to, what activities he or she participates in, what communicative behaviors or difficulties have been noted, etc.). A Communication Profile is generated from these interviews.
- *Phase 2: Systematic observation and analysis.* Actual data are gathered in authentic contexts. The clinician engages in direct observation of actual communication exchanges as determined from the interview. The clinician also facilitates several communication partners, keeping anecdotal notes on communication activities for a specified period of time. Based on this data, the clinician refines the Communication Profile.
- *Phase 3: Videotaping and analysis.* The clinician observes videotapes of a variety of communicative events, and compares and contrasts performance to identify any relevant patterns.
- *Phase 4: Introspection.* The clinician considers the data and tries to take the perspective of the various communication partners. The impact of different social contexts on specific behaviors is noted, and ideas for compensatory strategies or target skills that would be useful are generated.

Functional Assessment. The Communication Profiling System shares many features with functional assessment. In the past, clinicians were quick to select the target communication skill and begin the training process. For example, in a manual describing exercises to improve pragmatics skills in persons with brain injury, Sohlberg and colleagues (1992) detail the training steps for a variety of communication exercises and assume that the clinician will choose the appropriate communication target from among these five pragmatics categories: initiation, topic management, turn taking, verbal organization, and listening skills. More recently, we have come to understand the importance of identifying classes of functionally equivalent behaviors (Carr, 1988) before beginning a communication skills training process (Ducharme, 1999).

Ducharme (1999) describes *functional equivalence* as a behavioral phenomenon in which two distinctly different responses meet the same communication goal. In terms of assessment, the clinician identifies the functions or reinforcement accessed by the maladaptive communication or social behavior (e.g., "getting attention," "avoidance," "limiting load on memory"). The target communication or social skill that is selected for training should serve the same or an equivalent adaptive function. Although the assessment requires more time initially, it helps ensure that the skill that is trained will be adopted. For example, consider the communication problem of interrupting behavior. Frequent interrupting is an example of lack of response inhibition seen following frontal lobe injury. A clinician might reflexively use skills-based training to teach turn-taking skills after observing frequent interrupting. However, if part of the reason (reinforcement) for the interrupting behavior is that the client is fearful of forgetting his or her point, training turn-taking skills will not be effective in reducing the frequency of interruptions. Identifying a functionally equivalent communication skill that serves the same purpose as the problem behavior—in this case, compensating for a memory impairment—may be the most successful tactic. Instead of focusing on number of turns (a goal of training appropriate turn taking), the clinician may teach the client to interrupt "politely" in important circumstances, using such prefaces as "Excuse me for interrupting, but . . . "

Conducting a functional assessment requires that the clinician determine the functions or classes of reinforcement maintaining or stimulating the problem behavior by careful observation and measurement (O'Neill, Horner, & Albin, 1990). The clinician will want to observe the client in natural communication settings, in order to form hypotheses about existing pragmatics deficits. These hypotheses can be evaluated by further observation, measurement, and discussion with natural communication partners. These examples of hypotheses about communication deficits that we have addressed in our clinical work are shown in Table 10.1.

The following questions can aid the clinician in identifying functionally equivalent communication behaviors:

1. What is the communication behavior that is of concern?
2. Who is troubled by the communication problem?
3. In which context(s) does the communication problem occur most frequently? Note the conversation partners, topics, response of partner(s) before and after communication problem, time of day, and purpose of communication exchange.
4. Are there any communication contexts when the communication problem does *not* occur?

In order to respond to these questions, it will be critical for the clinician to observe "typical" communication exchanges and sample common conversational situations, or at least to train a family member or significant other to make the observations (Sohlberg, Glang, & Todis, 1998). In the past several years, the literature has clarified the difficulty of attempting to draw conclusions about communication behavior when the partner

TABLE 10.1. Examples of How Identifying Functionally Equivalent Behaviors May Lead to Appropriate Interventions for Pragmatics Deficits

Communication problem	Underlying dysexecutive symptoms	Sample hypotheses for what is maintaining and reinforcing problem behavior	Functionally equivalent adaptive communication behaviors	Intervention approach
Constant arguing; inability to listen to another perspective; very disruptive in group therapy.	Disinhibition; rigid thinking	Client engages in loud arguing when conversation turns to topics that are morally charged, such as religion and sex. Unable to inhibit aggressive responding during groups where participants frequently make jokes or discuss such topics.	Conversation on topics that are not emotionally charged for client	Environmental management: Set up group to avoid problem trigger topics. Skills-based training: Train client to state position on common trigger topics, using practiced, pat phrases that will also help desensitize client.
Looks bored and uninterested in conversation; sits without initiating conversation or responding to others' conversation.	Lack of initiation	Lack of initiation is most prominent when there is some pressure or expectation to talk, and partner begins to ask client direct questions.	Talking when there is little pressure about high-interest, very familiar topics	Environmental management: Have "props" that stimulate talk about high-interest, familiar topics, such as photo albums, books, personal mementos. Skills-based training: Give client lots of practice talking using "props"; work with client and relevant communication partners in using appropriate "communication starters" that do not pressure client.
Can't get to the main point; takes a long time to take a turn in conversation.	Reduced verbal organization; difficulty with generative thinking	Occurs most frequently when client is trying to tell a story about an event or occurrence in response to a question from spouse.	Structured storytelling	Skills-based training: Work with client and spouse together, and teach client to use sequence markers at the beginning of each sentence (e.g., start sentence with "First I . . . Next . . . Finally . . . ").

is a designated examiner or clinician and/or the communication event is artificial (Wozniak et al., 1999). The Pragmatic Protocol (Appendix 10.1) may be useful for the initial identification of possible communication deficits. Subsequent analysis can then be conducted to generate and evaluate hypotheses about the factors reinforcing and maintaining problematic communication behaviors.

Conversational Analysis

CA is a relatively recent method for analyzing pragmatics deficits following brain injury. Natural conversations are tape-recorded, transcribed, and analyzed (see, e.g., Snow et al., 1998). The analysis involves detailing the sequential interaction between two speakers. CA is a data-driven approach to examining communication; every aspect of an exchange is considered important, from global behaviors (such as repair of communication breakdowns) to small pauses in a conversation (Friedland & Miller, 1998).

One study attempted to determine whether CA could capture the types of communication breakdowns observed after brain injury, and to look at the relationship between CA and formal test results (Friedland & Miller, 1998). The authors interpreted the results of their single-case study as support for the benefit of using CA in identifying pragmatic impairments in conversation. They further suggested that use of CA in conjunction with formal test results can appropriately direct treatment. For example, the CA revealed difficulty with topic maintenance and topic shift. Formal testing showed impairment in divergent thinking, including idea generation. Friedland and Miller (1998) suggested that the subject's limited topic choice may have been linked to the impairment in divergent thinking.

The time commitment required to complete CA may prevent its clinical use in current service delivery models. However, it could be argued that spending more time on assessment may result in less time needed for therapy, because the determinants of communication impairments are accurately identified (Friedland & Miller, 1998). In any case, CA remains a useful research tool to elucidate the nature of pragmatics deficits in the population with brain injury.

The Use of Elicitation Tasks

Currently there are no widely used standardized tests of pragmatics. For the reasons discussed in the previous sections, it is difficult to structure naturalistic communication. However, progress has been made in using semistructured tasks to elicit information regarding pragmatics.

In a line of research conducted by Turkstra and colleagues, various tasks have been developed and evaluated to assess receptive and expressive pragmatics skills in adolescents with brain injury. Turkstra and colleagues

(1995) describe four such tasks, which tap distinct pragmatics abilities and differentiate adolescents with brain injury from those without brain injury:

• *Negotiating requests.* Subjects are given verbal descriptions of common everyday situations, and are asked what they would say in each situation in order to be as polite and convincing as possible. (For example, "If you want to go camping with your friend but your parents do not like him or her, what would you say?")

• *Hints.* Examinees are required to ask for something indirectly by hinting. (For example, they are asked to hint that they would like a ride to some place.)

• *Semistructured discourse elicitation task.* Examinees are asked to explain a simple board game that they have learned to someone who does not know how to play the game.

• *Sarcasm.* Subjects read statements uttered by different pairs of speakers, one of whom is being sarcastic. They then answer questions based on their interpretation of the message.

Reliable scoring for these pragmatics tasks is described by the authors. Turkstra and colleagues (1995) administered this pragmatics assessment battery to 3 adolescent subjects with brain injury and 36 of their uninjured peers. The pragmatics test scores were able to differentiate between distinct pragmatics abilities in the two groups. However, there was a lack of correlation between performance on these pragmatics tests and a vocabulary measure closely associated with overall intelligence; this lack of correlation suggests that performance on these pragmatics tasks is a unique aspect of communication behavior. The authors suggest that linguistic skills contribute less to social communication than do the abilities to perceive incongruity, abstract, infer, and solve problems.

The use of elicitation tasks that are sensitive to specific pragmatics skills has the advantage of being time-efficient and semiobjective. Using elicitation tasks, the study by Turkstra and colleagues (1995) showed unique profiles of pragmatic functioning in both groups. However, much more research is needed to identify tasks that are able to measure the broad range of pragmatics functioning critical for social communication. Future studies also need to evaluate more fully possible changes in pragmatics occurring after brain injury. For example, there was relatively good performance by the subjects with brain injury on the sarcasm task, which only looked at interpretation of sarcasm. Turkstra and colleagues suggest that although poor problem-solving skills and reduced self-regulation may affect the *production* of sarcasm, such deficits do not necessarily impair the capacity to *comprehend* social nuances. A complete assessment would need to evaluate the production and comprehension of sarcasm. Future inquiry using standardized pragmatics tasks may shed light on this and related clinical theories about pragmatics functioning.

MANAGEMENT OF PRAGMATICS DEFICITS

The evolution of different approaches to manage communication deficits following brain injury has been heavily influenced by paradigm shifts in aphasia therapy. Early treatments for aphasia focused on remediating the underlying cause of aphasia by stimulating the damaged language functions of the brain (see, e.g., Schuell, 1974). Later, functional treatments emerged that emphasized the development of compensatory tools and skills (Aten, 1994; Holland, 1982). Most recently, aphasia treatment has evolved toward socially based interventions that promote a person's autonomy and control within naturalistic communication contexts (see, e.g., Fox & Fried-Oken, 1996; Lyon et al., 1997).

There has been an analogous shift toward emphasizing the naturalistic context in the management of pragmatics deficits following brain injury. Initially, research and clinical efforts focused on remediating specific communication impairments by training the deficient skills (see, e.g., Sohlberg et al., 1992). The cognitive rehabilitation field gradually moved from approaching pragmatics impairments as a uniform pathology toward a focus on individual patterns of deficit and the need to train people to utilize tailored compensatory strategies and/or to adopt specific environmental modifications (Sohlberg & Mateer, 1989; Wozniak et al., 1999). More recently, there have been efforts to develop collaborative, client-centered treatment models that focus on real-life contexts (see, e.g., Glang, Todis, Cooley, Wells, & Voss, 1997).

Examination of a subgroup of subjects with brain injury whose conversational skills were monitored for several years following their injury suggested that the small number of speakers whose conversational abilities improved over time had received significantly more months of formal speech–language pathology services (Snow et al., 1998). This study calls for more intensive services to identify and remediate changes in communication abilities in the early period following brain injury. In the remainder of this chapter, three different approaches to managing pragmatics deficits—approaches that reflect the movement toward treatment in naturalistic contexts—are reviewed. These include individualized communication skills training, group intervention, and building social networks.

Individualized Communication Skills Training

There is high agreement that dysexecutive syndromes commonly associated with brain injury (see Chapter 8) are devastating to communication abilities. As discussed there, the nature of the impairments is extremely variable. The need for individually tailored intervention makes skills-based training a useful methodology for addressing communication deficits (Helfenstein & Wechsler, 1981). This approach to intervention identifies specific deficiencies in communication skills through either the implementation of functional assessment or the use of the Communication Profiling System. Examples of the broad range of communication skills that might be deficient are found on the Pragmatic Protocol. After specific skills or sets of skills are identified, exercises are selected to target those functions. Clients are then provided sufficient practice with the target skills. Often, as clients improve, more challenging aspects of naturalistic communication contexts are introduced to the practice sessions (e.g., introduction of different communication partners). The same effective instructional and behavioral principles reviewed in Chapter 7 with respect to teaching the use of external memory aids, and in Chapter 11 with respect to managing problem behavior, can be employed in teaching communication skills. The steps involved in communications skills training, and examples of pragmatics behaviors that may be addressed in such training, are summarized in Box 10.1.

Group Intervention

There are many advantages to using a group therapy context to address pragmatics deficits. Two obvious benefits are the opportunities provided for modeling target skills and the promotion of generalization (Sohlberg & Mateer, 1989). Therapists can demonstrate and reinforce (both directly and vicariously) the pragmatics skills they wish to encourage in group participants. Groups also offer a controlled microcosm of a larger community, which allows clinicians to systematically introduce interactional challenges in order to facilitate generalization of skills to more naturalistic contexts.

Within a group therapy context, pragmatics may be addressed in several different formats. Commonly, exercises or activities are utilized in which clients practice effective social communication behaviors. In addition, groups may focus on introspection or reflection about how to improve communication behavior. Such an emphasis may involve increasing people's awareness of strengths and weaknesses, and heightening their appreciation of the effects certain behaviors have on other individuals. Similarly, groups may target learning communication principles that can be applied across situations. Examples of group practice exercises, awareness activities, and the teaching of communication principles are described below.

Practice Exercises

Numerous workbooks and therapy manuals provide examples of activities that give clients practice with specific pragmatics behaviors (e.g., Sohlberg et al., 1992). The same steps described in Box 10.1 for training individual communication skills can be implemented within the group context. An example of a group activity that enables an individual to practice a specific

BOX 10.1. Skill Instruction with Appropriate Communication Partner(s) in Naturalistic Contexts

Steps Involved in Training

- Identify the target communication skill(s) and the context(s) that can be addressed to reduce the communication problem. (The Communication Profiling System or functional assessment methods may be useful in this identification process.)
- Demonstrate or model the target skill for both partner and client, using errorless instruction.
- Make sure instructions are clear and concise.
- Record data on client and partner performance and on clinician prompting.
- Provide sufficient practice until client and partner can independently demonstrate communication behaviors. Make sure they are giving each other feedback. Use of videotaping and modeling is very helpful.
- As client and partner master the skills, introduce elements from other contexts in which they will be functioning (e.g., different people, topics, etc.).
- Provide lots of practice with all of the different types of situations/contexts.
- Make sure to incorporate client's and partner's ideas and opinions in the training.
- Establish a plan for ongoing monitoring of communication skills, including identification of what to assess and a method for collecting and acting upon performance or outcome data (e.g., sample videotaping, asking partners to give feedback, etc.).

Examples of Pragmatics Behaviors Addressed in Training

- Initiating appropriate social greetings
- Decreasing interrupting
- Checking for understanding (e.g., paraphrasing instructions)
- Avoiding troublesome topics
- Asking questions of a listener, in order to reduce monologue behavior
- Increasing eye contact
- Reducing the tendency to invade a communication partner's "personal space"

---

pragmatics skill is to *increase initiation of conversation* through the use of a token system. The group member is given a target number of tokens at the start of a group session, and each time the person initiates a comment, a token is relinquished. The goal is for the person to end the group session with no tokens. Depending upon the skill level of the client, conversation prompts may be provided. Role plays or communication scenarios that provide opportunities to apply the skills being practiced are perhaps the most common methods for practicing communication behaviors within a group. Scenarios that resonate with real-life challenges are most helpful; they frequently involve conflict resolution, problem solving, and perspective taking, which are often affected by brain injury and represent areas of pragmatics difficulty. The success of exercises that provide practice in target pragmatics skills depends greatly upon the selection of skills that are functional for each individual and can be reinforced within naturalistic contexts.

Awareness Activities

It is difficult for people to effortfully modify their communication style, if they do not believe there is a need to change it. Either concurrently or prior to practicing skills, clients may benefit from feedback within a group on the strengths and weaknesses of their communication behavior. A group format provides opportunities for participants to gain a realistic perception of their functioning by listening to peer appraisal, which can be more powerful than that of a clinician. Viewing oneself on videotape can be very helpful for an individual. Structuring viewing opportunities to facilitate observation of key behaviors (e.g., having a person who tends to monopolize conversations track the number of questions directed toward the partner, and comparing that to the number of questions directed toward the client) can be effective. It is important to balance any discussion or observation of areas that might benefit from attention with observing and measuring areas of strength. It is also important to stress positive performance, as viewing a videotape can be a negative experience for clients. (See Chapter 9 on increasing awareness.)

Teaching Communication Principles

In their workbook, McGann and Werven (1999) focus on teaching students with pragmatics problems the social framework within which communication occurs, rather than focusing only on specific communication skills. They offer a curriculum for students between the ages of 8 and 11 years, which teaches seven communication principles by providing concrete examples and role play:

1. Communication involves sending and receiving messages (e.g., "Amy and Karla talk about the movie they saw together").
2. Communication involves people (e.g., "Ms. Thompson introduces the new student to the class").
3. Everyone communicates differently (e.g., "Louie and Chi-fa say hello in different ways").

4. Communication is stating what we think, feel, and believe (e.g., "Carrie and Mark have different opinions on a subject").
5. Places and people change the way we communicate (e.g., "Wendy starts whispering when she enters the library").
6. The way we communicate affects those around us (e.g., "Karn's joke made Ben feel sad").
7. Communication is always changing (e.g., "When Adam's dad was a boy, he used to say, 'Groovy' ").

McGann and Werven suggest that these communication principles are constant and exist independently of personal skills and abilities. If they are internalized by students with communication issues, this can help them apply specific skills they may be practicing in therapy more effectively.

An Application of Group Intervention Approaches

All three of the above-described approaches to improving pragmatics within a group context were incorporated in a pilot group for adolescent girls with pragmatics deficits that interfered with school integration. A description of this group will serve to illustrate the application of these clinical practices. An interview with the speech–language pathologist who was the group facilitator, and a parent of a student in the group (which met at one of our clinics), suggested that the following activities were useful in improving pragmatics behavior:

1. *Perspective-taking activities.* An example of such an activity was painting each other's fingernails. The girls worked on satisfying the requests of their partners, even when they did not like the color or request. Another activity involved decorating cookies for others in the group and thinking about what they might like.

2. *Role play.* The group acted out scenarios highlighting specific pragmatics skills that the students had identified as ones they wanted to improve (e.g., eye contact, monitoring voice volume, asking questions about the other person).

3. *Commercially available communication games.* There are many games (Guesstures, Taboo, Pictionary, etc.) that promote interaction or help people work in teams. The group played such games and focused on one or two specific skills at a time.

4. *Field trips.* Going out into the community to practice target skills as a group was an important activity. An example was going to a nearby bookstore to buy a card for someone as part of a perspective-taking unit.

5. *Building self-esteem.* At each weekly session, each of the stu-

dents brought an example of something she was proud to share from the last week and something nice she had done for someone else.

General principles for conducting the pragmatics group included the following:

1. *Focusing the treatment goals.* The group worked on only one or maybe two skills at a time.

2. *Homogeneous groupings.* It helped that the group was fairly homogeneous—not necessarily in the actual skills, but in general levels of cognitive and social ability.

3. *Clear demonstration and ample opportunity to practice.* It was important to demonstrate every target skill. Initially, the group spent too much time *talking* and not enough time *doing*. Although it was important to achieve closure and talk briefly about activities when they were completed, progress was not achieved without lots of practice.

4. *Use of compensation lists.* The students responded well to developing and using lists of functional rules they could use in communication situations at school. For example, they developed "a list of what to do when I meet someone":

a. Use eye contact.

b. Shake the person's hand.

c. Tell my name.

d. Ask two things about the person.

5. *Client-centered goals.* It was important to make sure that the goals that were generated were chosen by the students and their families.

6. *Specific homework.* Specific homework assignments with feedback sheets seemed to promote generalization. It helped if the homework was a step or so below the level of what was being addressed in the group.

7. *Repetition.* Repeated practice of the target skills proved beneficial.

8. *Allowing time to brainstorm solutions.* It was helpful to review problems that might have occurred since the last session.

The effectiveness of different therapeutic strategies for managing pragmatics deficits is woefully underresearched. Most reports, like the one just presented, are anecdotal case reports. There is a need for more studies such as one by Helfenstein and Wechsler (1981), which examined the effectiveness of interpersonal skills training. They compared changes in communication skills in a group of persons with brain injury who received communication skills training with a control group who received "nontherapeutic attention." The training consisted of clients reviewing and processing videotaped interactions of themselves and a therapist and rehearsing deficient skills. The results of the study showed that the experimental group benefited from the training and improved in their communication skills as assessed by professional staff members who were not aware of group placement. Given the profound consequences pragmatics deficits can have on affected individuals, the field of cognitive rehabilitation needs to make evaluation of pragmatics interventions a higher clinical priority.

Building Social Networks

A different approach to managing pragmatics deficits is to focus on altering the environment or context in which a person functions. Table 10.1 gives several examples of environmental modification to address a specific communication issue. A broad-based form of environmental modification is to facilitate the building of social networks.

Zencius and Wesolowski (1999) note that the following people may be included in a social network: family, relatives, work colleagues, friends, church or club members, acquaintances from a frequently visited store (e.g., grocery or hair salon), or any other member of the community with whom an individual has frequent contact or whom the individual can ask to provide assistance on an emergency basis. Their work suggests that individuals with brain injury have significantly smaller social networks than nonclients, and that a diminished or limited social network can be a serious obstacle to successful community integration. Their investigation of 70 individuals with brain injury revealed that they had significantly fewer members in their social networks than members of a control group did, and that the makeup of the social networks was different. Family members were the primary constituents in the social networks of the persons with brain injury, whereas the networks of the noninjured subjects consisted of friends, acquaintances, coworkers, and family members, in that order.

The Building Friendships Process (Glang, Todis, Cooley, Wells, & Voss, 1997), designed to decrease the social isolation of three students with brain injury, is one of the only interventions dedicated to increasing social networks that has been validated with research for the population with brain injury (Glang et al., 1997). It was a collaborative group intervention that brought together students and support people in the school environment to identify goals and strategies for increasing the students' social opportunities. The students' teams met frequently to review progress toward identified social goals. Examples of goals might be to join a school organization, to designate a specific person as a peer, or to establish a lunch buddy program. Team members (including each student) took responsibility for implementing strategies to meet the goals. See

Table 10.2 for an outline of the four phases involved in the Building Friendships Process.

The primary outcome measures used to evaluate the Building Friendships Process (Glang et al., 1997) were the frequency of students' social contacts with nondisabled peers, parent and educator social validation ratings, and observation data. The number of social contacts for each of the three subjects increased over baseline levels and was maintained over the course of the study. Parents, teachers, and students were generally satisfied with the process and with the concomitant increases in the students' degree of social integration. However, these improvements were not maintained over time when the primary facilitators were no longer involved. This study suggests the importance of ongoing active facilitation.

Results from this study are consistent with other work (Ylvisaker & Feeney, 1998) suggesting that intervention for social or pragmatics issues should have the following characteristics:

1. It should be delivered in the natural, "everyday" setting.
2. Individuals and their relevant support persons should be engaged in planning their own intervention and making choices whenever possible.
3. The intervention should be delivered in the context of, and designed to effect change in, daily routines.

The Building Friendships Process can be easily adapted to adult clients. Spouses, employers, neighbors, peers, children, and friends may all be selected to participate in the group planning and review meetings. Once

---

TABLE 10.2. Four Phases of the Building Friendships Process

Phase 1: Information gathering. Interviews with key people (e.g., the student, parents, school staff, and peers) are conducted by the facilitator, in order to identify opportunities and contexts within the school and community settings to increase social contact and to enhance current friendships.

Phase 2: Recruit team members. The facilitator works with the student and family members to recruit team members. Participation is flexible, as team members may participate over a long period of time or just once.

Phase 3: Conduct initial team meeting. Information is shared to create social goals. The student has veto power over any goals or strategies that are selected.

Phase 4: Regular review meetings. Every 2–3 weeks, team members meet to review progress, to revise goals and strategies, and to reevaluate team membership and responsibilities.

Note. From Glang, Todis, Cooley, Wells, and Voss (1997). Copyright 1997 by Aspen Publishers, Inc. Adapted by permission.

again, we call for continued research on effective methods for addressing the pragmatics deficits that are common following brain injury.

SUMMARY

The greatest communication concern for individuals with cognitive impairments is compromised pragmatics. Although the types of observed pragmatics deficits vary among persons with neurogenic damage, the devastating effects on social integration are universal. Effective assessment is dependent upon observations and/or analysis of conversations and social interactions occurring in naturalistic contexts with typical communication partners. There are several options for assessing pragmatics, including structured observation using pragmatics ratings scales or profiling communication behaviors. CA of transcripts of naturalistic communication samples is another assessment options; it provides a detailed, quantitative measurement of conversational abilities. Assessment of pragmatics has also been attempted using elicitation tasks that are sensitive to the types of pragmatics disorders seen in patients.

Treatment of pragmatics deficits may be approached from a variety of perspectives, including individualized communication skills training, group interventions, and building social networks. Specific communication behaviors may be targeted and trained in individual therapy sessions. This therapy is most effective when therapists identify functionally equivalent communication behaviors and consider the real-world situational factors. Skills as well as knowledge about effective principles of communication may also be targeted within group therapy and utilize peer interactions as part of the treatment regimen. Finally, pragmatics issues may be addressed by building or enhancing social networks and helping the environment become more receptive to accommodating the individual who presents with pragmatics deficits. Much research remains to be done in the domain of pragmatics assessment and intervention; this represents a rehabilitation issue with high clinical priority.

REFERENCES

Aten, J. L. (1994). Functional communication treatment. In R. Chapey (Ed.), *Language intervention strategies in adult aphasia* (pp. 266–276). Baltimore: Williams & Wilkins.

Carr, E. G. (1988). Functional equivalence as a mechanism of response generalization. In R. Horner, G. Dunlap, & R. L. Koegel (Eds.), *Generalization and maintenance: Life-style changes in applied settings* (pp. 221–241). Baltimore: Paul H. Brookes.

Chapman, S. B. (1997). Cognitive–communication abilities in children with closed head injury. *American Journal of Speech–Language Pathology, 6*(2), 50–58.

Chapman, S. B., Watkins, R., Gustafson, C., Moore, S., Levin, H. S., & Kufera, J. A. (1997). Narrative discourse in children with closed head injury, children with language impairment and typically developing children. *American Journal of Speech–Language Pathology, 6*(2), 66–75.

Coelho, C. A., Liles, B. Z., & Duffy, R. J. (1991). Discourse analysis with closed head injured adults: Evidence for differing patterns of deficits. *Archives of Physical Medicine and Rehabilitation, 72,* 465–468.

Constantinovici, A., Arseni, C., Iliescu, A., Debrota, L., & Gorgia, A. (1970). Considerations on post traumatic aphasia in peacetime. *Psychiatric Neurolo-Neurochirugy, 73,* 105–115.

Docking, K., Murdoch, B. E., & Jordan, F. M. (2000). Interpretation and comprehension of linguistic humour by adolescents with head injury: A group analysis. *Brain Injury, 14*(1), 89–108.

Ducharme, J. M. (1999). A conceptual model for treatment of externalizing behaviour in acquired brain injury. *Brain Injury, 13*(9), 645–668.

Fox, L., & Fried-Oken, M. (1996). Interactive group treatment for aphasia: An AAC alternative [Abstract]. *ISAAC 1996 Proceedings: The 7th Biennial Conference of the International Society for Augmentative and Alternative Communication,* 390–391.

Friedland, D., & Miller, N. (1998). Conversation analysis of communication breakdown after closed head injury. *Brain Injury, 12*(1), 1–14.

Galski, T., Tompkins, C., & Johnston, M. V. (1998). Competence in discourse as a measure of social integration and quality of life in persons with traumatic brain injury. *Brain Injury, 12*(9), 769–782.

Glang, A., Todis, B., Cooley, E., Wells, J., & Voss, J. (1997). Building social networks for children and adolescents with traumatic brain injury: A school-based intervention. *Journal of Head Trauma Rehabilitation, 12*(2), 32–47.

Groher, M. (1977). Language and memory disorders following closed head trauma. *Journal of Speech and Hearing Research, 20,* 212–223.

Halpern, H., Darley, F., & Brown, J. R. (1973). Differential language and neurologic characteristics in cerebral involvement. *Journal of Speech and Hearing Disorders, 38,* 162–173.

Heilman, K., Safran, A., & Geschwind, N. (1971). Closed head trauma and aphasia. *Journal of Neurology, Neurosurgery and Psychiatry, 34,* 265–269.

Helfenstein, D. A., & Wechsler, F. S. (1981). The use of interpersonal process recall (IPR) in the remediation of interpersonal and communication skill deficits in the newly brain-injured. *Clinical Neuropsychology, 4*(3), 139–143.

Holland, A. L. (1982). Observing functional communication of aphasic adults. *Journal of Speech and Hearing Disorders, 47,* 50–56.

Levin, H., Grossman, R., & Kelly, P. (1976). Aphasia disorder in patients with closed head injury. *Journal of Neurology, Neurosurgery and Psychiatry, 39,* 1062–1070.

Lyon, J. G., Cariski, D., Keisler, L., Rosenbek, J., Levine, R., Kumpula, J., Ryff, C., Coyne, S., & Blanc, M. (1997). Communication partners: Enhancing participation in life and communication for adults with aphasia in natural settings. *Aphasiology, 11,* 693–708.

McDonald, S. (1993). Pragmatic language skills after closed head injury: Ability to meet the informational needs of the listener. *Brain and Language, 44,* 28–46.

McGann, W., & Werven, G. (1999). *Social communication skills for children: A workbook for principle-centered communication.* Austin, TX: Pro-Ed.

Mentis, M., & Prutting, C. A. (1987). Cohesion in the discourse of normal and head-injured adults. *Journal of Speech and Hearing Research, 30,* 88–98.

Milton, S. B., Prutting, C. A., & Binder, G. (1984). Appraisal of communicative competence in head injured adults. In R. H. Brookshire (Ed.), *Proceedings of the Clinical Aphasiology Conference* (pp. 114–123). Minneapolis, MN: BRK.

Newton, A., & Johnson, J. A., (1985). Social adjustment and interaction after severe head injury. *British Journal of Clinical Psychology, 24,* 225–234.

Nicholas, L. E., & Brookshire, R. H. (1995). Comprehension of spoken narrative discourse by adults with aphasia, right-hemisphere brain damage, or traumatic brain injury. *American Journal of Speech–Language Pathology, 4,* 69–81.

O'Neill, R. E., Horner, R. H., & Albin, R. W. (1990). *Functional analysis of problem behavior: A practical assessment guide.* Sycamore, IL: Sycamore Press.

Penn, C., & Cleary, J. (1988). Compensatory strategies in the language of closed head injured patients. *Brain Injury, 2*(1), 3–17.

Prutting, C., & Kirchner, D. (1983). Applied pragmatics. In T. M. Gallagher & C. A. Prutting (Eds.), *Pragmatic assessment and intervention issues in language* (pp. 29–68). San Diego, CA: College-Hill Press.

Prutting, C., & Kirchner, D. (1987). A clinical appraisal of the pragmatic aspects of language. *Journal of Speech and Hearing Disorders, 52,* 105–119.

Sarno, M. T. (1980). The nature of verbal impairment after closed head injury. *Journal of Nervous and Mental Disease, 168,* 685–692.

Schuell, H. (1974). *The Minnesota Test for the Differential Diagnosis of Aphasia.* Minneapolis: University of Minnesota Press.

Simmons-Mackie, N., & Damico, J. S. (1996). Accounting for handicaps in aphasia: Communicative assessment from an authentic social perspective. *Disability and Rehabilitation, 18*(11), 540–549.

Snow, P., Douglas, J., & Ponsford, J. (1998). Conversational discourse abilities following severe traumatic brain injury: A follow-up study. *Brain Injury, 12*(11), 911–935.

Sohlberg, M. M., Glang, A., & Todis, B. (1998). Improvement during baseline: Three case studies encouraging collaborative research when evaluating caregiver training. *Brain Injury, 12*(4), 333–346.

Sohlberg, M. M., & Mateer, C. A. (1989). *Introduction to cognitive rehabilitation: Theory and practice.* New York: Guilford Press.

Sohlberg, M. M., Perlewitz, P. G., Johansen, A., Schultz, J., Johnson, L., & Hartry, A. (1992). *Improving pragmatic skills in persons with head injury.* Tucson, AZ: Communication Skill Builders.

Thompson, I. V. (1975). Evaluation and outcomes of aphasia in patients with severe closed head trauma. *Journal of Neurology, Neurosurgery and Psychiatry, 38,* 713–718.

Turkstra, L. S., McDonald, S., & Kaufmann, P. M. (1995). Assessment of pragmatic communication skills in adolescents after traumatic brain injury. *Brain Injury,* *10*(5), 329–345.

Weinstein, D., & Keller, W. (1963). Linguistic patterns of misnaming in brain injury. *Neuropsychologia, 1,* 79–90.

Wozniak, R. J., Coelho, C. A., Duffy, R. J., & Liles, B. Z. (1999). Intonation unit analysis of conversational discourse in closed head injury. *Brain Injury, 13*(3), 191–203.

Ylvisaker, M., & Feeney, T. J. (1998). *Collaborative brain injury interventions: Positive everyday routines.* San Diego, CA: Singular Press.

Zenicus, A. H., & Wesolowski, M. D. (1999). Is the social network analysis necessary in the rehabilitation of individuals with head injury? *Brain Injury, 13*(9), 723–727.

PRAGMATIC PROTOCOL

Taxonomy	Modality	Description and Coding
Utterance act	Verbal/ paralinguistic	The trappings by which the act is accomplished
1. Intelligibility		The extent to which the message is understood
2. Vocal intensity		The loudness or softness of the message
3. Voice quality		The resonance and/or laryngeal characteristics of the vocal tract
4. Prosody		The intonation and stress patterns of the message; variations of loudness, pitch, and duration
5. Fluency		The smoothness, consistency, and rate of the message
6. Physical proximity	Nonverbal	The distance from which speaker and listener sit or stand from one another
7. Physical contacts		The number of times and placement of contacts between speaker and listener
8. Body posture		Forward lean is when the speaker or listener moves away from a 90° angle toward other person; recline is when one party slouches down from waist to head and moves away from the partner; side to side is when a person moves to the right or left
9. Foot/leg movements		Any movement of foot/leg
10. Hand/arm movements		Any movement with hand/arm (touching or moving an object or touching part of the body or clothing)
11. Gestures		Any movements that support, complement, or replace verbal behavior
12. Facial expression		A positive expression is when the corners of the mouth are turned upward; negative is a downward turn; neutral expression is when face is in a resting position
13. Eye gaze		When one looks directly at the other's facial region; mutual gaze is when both members of the dyad look at each other

Propositional act	Verbal	Linguistic dimensions of the meaning of the sentence
1. Lexical selection/ use		
A. Specificity/ accuracy		Lexical items of best fit considering the context
2. Specifying relationships between words		
A. Word order		Grammatical word order for conveying message
B. Given and new information		Given information is that information already known to the listener; new information is information not already known to the listener
a. Pronominalization		Pronouns permit the listener to identify the referent and form one of the devices used to mark givenness
b. Ellipses		Given information may be deleted
c. Emphatic stress		New information may be marked by stressing various items
d. Indefinite/ definite article		If new information is signaled, the indefinite article is used; if old information, then the definite article is used
e. Initialization		Given information is stated prior to new information
3. Stylistic variations		
A. The varying of communicative style	Verbal, paralinguistic, nonverbal	Adaptations used by the speaker under various dyadic conditions, e.g., polite forms, different syntax, vocal quality changes
Illocutionary and perlocutionary acts	Verbal	Illocutionary (intentions of the speaker) and perlocutionary (effects on the listener)
1. Speech act pair analysis		The ability to take both speaker and listener role appropriate to the context
		Directive/compliance: personal need, imperatives, embedded imperatives, permissions, directives, questions, directives, hints

	Query/response: requests for confirmation, neutral requests for repetition, requests for specific constituent repetition
	Request/response: direct requests, indirect requests, inferred requests, request for clarification, acknowledgment of the request, perform the desired action
	Comment/acknowledgment: descriptions of ongoing activities in immediate subsequent activity, of state or condition of objects, persons, naming, acknowledgments that are positive, negative, expletive, indicative
2. Variety of speech acts	The variety of speech acts or what one can do with language, such as comment, assert, request, promise, etc.
A. Topic	
a. Selection	The selection of a topic appropriate to the context
b. Introduction	Introduction of a new topic in the discourse
c. Maintenance	Maintenance of topic across the discourse
B. Turn taking	Smooth interchanges between speaker and listener
a. Initiation	Initiation of speech acts
b. Response	The responding as a listener to speech acts
c. Repair/revision	The ability to repair a conversation when a breakdown occurs and the ability to ask for a repair when misunderstanding, ambiguity, etc., has occurred
d. Pause time	When pause time is excessive or too short between words or in response to a question or between sentences
e. Interruption/ overlap	Interruptions between speaker and listener; overlap is when two people talk at the same time

f. Feedback to speaker   Verbal behavior to give the speaker feedback such as "yeah," "really"; nonverbal behavior such as head nods up and down can be positive; side to side can express negative effect or disbelief

g. Adjacency   Utterances that occur immediately after the partner's utterance

h. Contingency   Utterances that share the same topic with the preceding and that add information to the prior communicative act

i. Quantity/conciseness   The contribution should be as informative as required but not too informative

Note. From Prutting and Kircher (1983). Copyright 1983 by College-Hill Press. Reprinted by permission.

INTERVENTIONS FOR BEHAVIORAL, EMOTIONAL, AND PSYCHOSOCIAL CONCERNS

Managing
Challenging Behaviors

Changes in behavior and behavioral control are extremely common following acquired brain injury. Although behavioral problems are often
among the most troubling consequences of brain injury for family, friends,
and professional staff, the biggest impact of disruptive and difficult-to-
manage behavior is on the client. Behavioral problems can limit the injured
person's participation in, and ability to benefit from, valuable treatment
activities. They typically result in a dramatic decrease in the number and
quality of social interactions. Behavioral difficulties, particularly aggressive
or impulsive behaviors, can be frightening and dangerous. They are often
an important factor in short- and long-term placement decisions that may
ensure the safety of the injured person and others. However, many of these
safety measures also severely limit the individual's independence and
choice. Moderate to severe behavior disorders can present significant long-
term obstacles to community integration and contribute to instability of relationships, difficulty with maintenance of work, and problems with the
law (Lezak, 1978).

MODELS OF BEHAVIOR CHANGE
FOLLOWING ACQUIRED BRAIN INJURY

Several models have been put forward to describe various influences on the
behavioral and psychosocial difficulties observed following acquired brain
injury. Prigatano (1992; Prigatano et al., 1986) has identified three important factors in the evolution of behavioral problems following brain injury.
The first involves organic factors related to the site, source, and severity of
injury, and includes such consequences as impulsivity, distractibility, and

337

cognitive difficulties. The second involves reactive factors, primarily behavioral changes associated with feelings of loss and frustration. The third involves characterological factors related to the person's premorbid level of behavioral control, social interaction style, self-esteem, personality style, and history of motivation and achievement. Sbordone (1990) has articulated the P-I-E-O model, which includes similar constructs. *P* stands for *person* and reflects important aspects of the person's history and personality style. *I* stands for *injury* and involves the specific physical, cognitive, and behavioral impairments resulting from the injury. *E* stands for *environment* and emphasizes the importance of the environment in which the person is functioning, including the supports available to the person and the expectations or demands made of him or her. *O* stands for *outcome* and involves the history of successes and failures the person has experienced since the injury. All of these factors are proposed to contribute to the profile of the injured person's behavior, personal and social adjustment, and functional adaptation.

COMMON BEHAVIORAL PROBLEMS
ASSOCIATED WITH ACQUIRED BRAIN INJURY

The most commonly reported behavioral problems in individuals with acquired brain injury are disinhibition, impulsivity, socially inappropriate behavior, and lack of initiation. Such individuals appear to act quickly on partial information or with little provocation. It is as if the normal checks on behavior are no longer operative. A person may, for example, use language that is not appropriate to the social situation, exhibit sexually explicit behavior, act out in an aggressive manner when angry or frustrated, or seek attention in unusual or self-injurious ways. Such individuals also often do not seem to be aware of the impact of their behavior on others and act in ways that appear selfish, rude, or otherwise unmindful of others. Although perhaps not as disruptive to others, problems with initiation and persistence on tasks can contribute substantially to long-term disability.

Different behavioral profiles are typically seen at different stages after injury. As the individual with a brain injury regains consciousness and begins to progress, a variety of challenging behaviors may emerge. Early behavioral consequences often include restlessness and agitation associated with confusion and disorientation. During this period, crying, moaning, flailing, kicking, and hitting are common. In the earliest stages these behaviors may seem unrelated to external provocation, but in later stages the agitation is more clearly seen in response to environmental events. Tolerance for medical, nursing, or physical management procedures and/or for therapeutic activities is often markedly reduced, and dressing, washing, or range-of-motion exercises may trigger perseverative and disruptive behaviors. Current beliefs hold that these behaviors are in part by-products of confusion, fear, pain, and dyscontrol. The primary goals of behavior management at this stage are to reduce the frequency and intensity of the behaviors, so as to reduce the likelihood of further injury to the self or others; to support basic care and treatment goals; and to prevent the person from developing learned patterns of inappropriate behavior through inadvertent reinforcement. It is important, for example, not to reinforce withdrawal responses or noncompliance. Inconsistent reactions from family and professional staff may contribute unintentionally to the evolution of behavioral problems.

At this stage following a severe injury, the caregivers must assume most, if not all, of the responsibility for the behavior of an injured person. The person may have little capacity for self-regulation, and indeed may have limited awareness of his or her behavior or circumstances. The behaviors are often triggered by environmental stimuli that seem to have gained control of behavior. The strategies that are most effective at this stage focus on factors external to the individual. They involve structuring the environment, conducting behavioral analyses to clarify the antecedents and consequences of the behavior, and implementing behavioral interventions. At the same time, therapists gradually try to increase the person's awareness of his or her circumstances.

As individuals go through the stages of recovery, they typically regain orientation, and the behaviors associated with generalized confusion and agitation decrease. They also begin to demonstrate better self-control for familiar or routine activities. However, changes in routine, changes in the environment, higher levels of stimulation, and/or expectations for more complex or demanding cognitive activities are frequently associated with increased confusion and deterioration of behavioral control. Problems with impulse control, cooperation with treatment activities, and appropriate social interaction may increase at this stage. Some of these behavioral difficulties are probably associated with cognitive impairments. Distractibility, perceptual problems, poor decision making, impaired judgment, poor comprehension of language or other cues for social monitoring, and difficulty shifting from one activity to another can all contribute substantially to behavioral difficulties. Such difficulties are frequently compounded by lack of insight and awareness.

Behavioral problems may be worsened by fear and profound depression as the individual confronts problems and gradually begins to recognize and experience the frustration of losses and limitations. Fear, frustration, and anxiety may be manifested as avoidance, refusal to participate, acting out, and aggression, while depression and hopelessness are often evident in withdrawal and occasionally even suicidal gestures or other forms of self-harm. As the individual gains insight and awareness, and begins to develop better inhibitory control, the form of treatment needs to change gradually. Effective interventions in this later stage focus on facilitating successful behavioral routines and training compensatory and self-regulatory strategies. Assistance with developing insight and awareness, and with coming to grips with permanent losses or changes in ability, is also more likely to be effective at this stage.

This shift in emphasis from a focus on environmental management and behavioral intervention to self-regulatory strategies is illustrated in Figure 11.1. Essentially, when an individual is minimally aware of difficulties and has little capacity for inhibiting responses to environmental triggers, interventions focused on changing the environment are likely to be most effective. As the individual recovers some insight and capacity for self-regulation, the focus turns to facilitating awareness and providing training in the use of compensatory strategies and self-regulation. Interventions must be dynamic, such that they allow progression from external control to internal self-control of behaviors. More discussion of these issues is found in this text's chapters dealing with unawareness, executive functions, and the development of compensatory strategies (see Chapters 7–9).

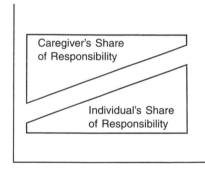

Time since Injury

Intervention approaches

Primarily "external"	Primarily "internal"
Environmental modifications	Cognitive-behavioral interventions
Behavioral strategies	Metacognitive/self-regulatory strategies
Cues, prompts, and checklists	Training in use of compensation strategies
Teaching task-specific routines	Practice in task management
Pharmacological interventions	Awareness training and psychotherapy

FIGURE 11.1. Time-based shifts in responsibility for the safety and behavior of an individual with brain injury, and in the interventions likely to be most successful.

MULTIPLE ORIGINS OF CHALLENGING BEHAVIORS

As suggested earlier, challenging behaviors usually have multiple origins—including factors related to the brain injury, various sources of emotional distress, and personality variables. In terms of the underlying neurobiology of behavioral difficulties, disturbances of various regions of the frontal cortex and their connections are most commonly cited (Levin, Goldstein, Williams, & Eisenberg, 1991; Stuss & Benson, 1986). Individuals with damage to the orbitofrontal cortex are likely to display disinhibited behavior and impulsivity, whereas damage to the dorsolateral region of the prefrontal cortex is more likely to result in cognitive problems with working memory and planning. Damage to the ventromedial area of the frontal lobe has been associated with behavioral inactivity/inertia and apparent uninterest or lack of concern. These same patients may demonstrate perserwative behavior, motor automatisms, and utilization behavior. Many individuals demonstrate a mixed clinical picture; for example, a patient with frontal lobe injury may sit quietly and apparently without interest for long periods, but react quickly and aggressively when stimulated or requested to do something.

Sources of emotional distress that may affect behavior include fear or startle responses, confusion, lack of understanding of what is expected, and fatigue. Such factors may hamper the person's ability to respond appropriately or to cope with even seemingly simple activities or requests. Another source of emotional distress may be others' requests for involvement in activities that are beyond the person's level of competence. These may include requests to undertake difficult activities as part of a cognitive assessment, or involvement in more complex and integrative activities such as shopping. New or unfamiliar social situations with expectations for greeting and talking with people the person does not know well may also cause considerable distress. Lastly, there may be substantial internal sources of distress, such as trying to meet personal expectations that are unrealistic or unachievable at the present time. Any of these sources of emotional distress can contribute to problems with behavior or behavioral regulation.

Finally, some behaviors may reflect a preinjury style of interacting with others or responding to challenges. The person may premorbidly have had a low frustration tolerance for working on what appear to be school-like activities. There may have been problems with impulse control or disinhibition that not only predated the accident, but also contributed to it. The person may have had prior problems with complying with school, parental, or family demands, and may feel anger and resentment at any attempts perceived as controlling or limiting. An understanding of such preinjury dynamics can be useful in evaluating the origins of current behavior.

It is easy to misinterpret behaviors as meaningful or intentional, when in fact they may reflect underlying cognitive difficulties or attempts to reduce an injured person's own stress or fear. There is often an attempt to determine whether behaviors are deliberate or nondeliberate. Whereas the early disorganized and confused behaviors associated with brain injury can be seen as almost entirely out of the person's control, over time, most individuals regain some control over their behavior. Behavior is, however, influenced by a complex set of biological factors, social controls and constraints, and personal drives and motivations, many involving maintenance of equilibrium and a sense of security. Although aggressive behaviors may be deliberate, they likely serve not as a means to hurt others, but as a means to avoid frustration, anxiety-producing activities, or emotionally painful realities. It is useful to consider a range of potential triggers to dyscontrol. It is useful to run through a number of questions such as the following before assuming that a behavior is purposeful or results from an attempt to hurt or manipulate others. Many of these involve organismic influences especially important in the early stages after injury.

- Is the person confused and not understanding what is expected of him or her?
- Is the person easily distracted and/or forgetful (i.e., the person does not recall or is unaware of what he or she is being asked to do)?
- Is the person potentially able to perform an expected behavior, but somehow is inadequately trained or supported in doing so?
- Is the person adequately motivated to participate?
- Is the person able to learn the task without substantial external support?
- Is the person fearful, angry, or depressed, and is this preventing him or her from focusing on or cooperating with the task at hand?
- Is the person avoiding activities that are frustrating, painful, or boring?
- Is the person getting enough sleep? Ample rest periods?

It is also important to recognize that it is people around the injured person who usually identify and define challenging behavior. Caregivers, including family members and professionals, are more likely to see behaviors as disruptive or challenging if they are unable to carry out therapeutic or social activities effectively with the person, or if they feel threatened, vulnerable, or frustrated by the person's behavior. Before the behavior itself is addressed, it is important to determine how the behavior is affecting others around the person. It may be that the impact on the caregivers can be altered or reframed through education or the provision of coping skills and strategies.

In the later stages of recovery from brain injury, direct organismic influences (e.g., fatigue, confusion, limited processing capabilities) are likely to diminish and behaviors become more purposeful. During those stages, the following basic assumptions are helpful in the functional assessment of problem behaviors:

- Problem behaviors do not occur randomly. Problem behaviors are related to events and the circumstances that precede and follow them.
- Problem behavior often serves a function or purpose. In many instances, problem behaviors are instrumental in changing the situation or have communicative intent.
- One problem behavior can serve multiple purposes. The function of behavior is more important than the form of behavior.
- For lasting change to occur, the intent, purpose, or function of the behavior needs to be understood and acknowledged.

APPROACHES TO WORKING
WITH CHALLENGING BEHAVIORS

There are various approaches to working with individuals who demonstrate difficult, disruptive, or maladaptive behaviors. As indicated earlier, approaches that focus on altering the environment in which the behaviors are observed are often the most effective in the early stages after injury. Another important approach is managing what can be called the *social–communicative environment*. This involves attending to (and, if necessary, modifying) the expectations, communication style, and knowledge of caregivers with regard to ways in which behavior is likely to be altered. These approaches are sometimes combined with more structured behavioral interventions. In the later stages of recovery and/or with individuals who are more self-aware, treatment can more productively focus on self-regulatory strategies (Mateer, 1997). A brief description of each of these approaches is provided below.

- *Environmental management therapies.* The goal of these interventions is to establish external, situational, and contextual influences on behavior. Someone regulates these influences other than the client—typically a therapist, another staff member, or a family member. They can include physical changes in lighting, seating, regulation of visitors, noise level, and the like. Use of a Craig bed, for example, provides safety and reduces the potential for overstimulation.
- *Caregiver communication strategies.* Management strategies in this domain include facilitating changes in expectations and modifying communication patterns on the part of caregivers (family members, staff members, and others). These techniques can be used in almost any situation and require little formal structure. Although they can be quite effective, it may take considerable effort and tact to educate caregivers about their use, and

to provide practice. Such techniques also require consistency, and family members in particular may need considerable support in persisting with them.

• *Behavioral therapies.* Behavioral therapies tend to be more structured, and are usually employed when one or more behaviors are particularly persistent or disruptive. These treatments rely on identifying relevant stimulus cues, systematically charting behaviors, and developing specific reinforcement contingencies in order to reestablish appropriate behavioral functions. The goal is to establish adequate behavioral responses in specific situations, with the hope that external cues and contingencies can eventually be reduced or withdrawn with maintenance of the desired behavior. It is usually more productive to increase adaptive behaviors than simply to focus on decreasing negative, disruptive, or maladaptive behaviors. Antecedent control is often more effective than consequent control.

• *Metacognitive self-regulatory therapies.* Therapeutic approaches in this domain attempt to reestablish the conscious and volitional links between social/environmental demands and the deliberate responses of the individual. The goal is to change behaviors via self-control strategies. Training stages typically involve providing information/knowledge about the behaviors in question, training self-observation and analysis, training strategy use in controlled and natural conditions, and training self-monitoring for verification of strategy use and error recognition.

These various strategies are elaborated on below, but before we proceed, it may be important to reframe the terms *behavior management* and *behavior modification.* Historically, these terms have sometimes had negative connotations, related to the impressions that such therapies are methods of controlling someone else, taking away free will, or deciding for another what is considered proper or acceptable behavior. Traditional behavioral interventions were often seen as depersonalized, coercive, and even degrading. In response to these concerns on the part of individuals with disabilities and their families, and to a much greater appreciation of behavioral complexity, there has been a shift in the basic values inherent in what might be called *behavioral programming.* Whereas the traditional behavioral modification literature tended to emphasize decreasing problem behaviors, the emphasis is now on increasing skills and adaptive behaviors. In addition, there tended to be more emphasis in the past on manipulating consequences, whereas the emphasis in most current behavioral interventions now is on modifying antecedent events and circumstances. Perhaps more importantly, whereas it used to be that the *form* of the behavior was most important, there is now greater appreciation of the importance of the *function* of behavior. Most behaviors are now believed to be instrumental in some fashion—that is, to have a function or effect some change in the circumstances. Understanding how behavior is instrumental can help in finding ways to meet the same need or achieve the same outcome, and thus to reduce or eliminate the problem behavior. Today, there is also much more integration of functional, instructional, cognitive, psychoemotional, and behavioral interventions. Finally, there is a much stronger emphasis on collaborative involvement in the design and implementation of behavioral interventions among clients, family members, and professionals. In working with clients who have behavioral difficulties and their families, operating with these contemporary principles in mind can help to reduce the fear and apprehension that may interfere with effective planning and strategy selection.

Environmental Management

A number of basic techniques within the domain of environmental management are relatively easy to employ and may go a long way toward reducing disruptive behaviors. A careful analysis of events and conditions associated with both positive and negative behaviors can suggest ways to modify those events and conditions. It is important to undertake any plan to respond to an individual's behavior with respect, and in ways that are appropriate to the person's age. Among the most effective aspects of the environment that can be manipulated are the level and nature of sensory stimulation. Preventing overstimulation is a key factor here. Reducing visual or auditory distraction through placement of the client in the room, the use of blinds or drapes, and modulation of noise levels is an easy first step. Another is the introduction of calming stimuli in the form of familiar, previously enjoyed music; familiar objects; pictures of family or friends; or pets, if pets are allowed. Providing comfortable, well-fitting, and familiar clothing that allows a maximum of movement is important.

In some cases, various forms of restraint (e.g., wrist, belt, bed, or personnel) may be necessary to ensure safety. However, these should be used only as a last resort for safety of patient and caregivers. Their implementation should be decided upon and monitored carefully, with inputs from staff and family. If restraint is a potential intervention, it should be explained to the family in advance if at all possible. Even when they realize it is necessary, many family members and some staff experience a strong visceral reaction to mechanical restraint. Other options should always be explored. For example, having a family member stay in the room to provide some supervision and familiar support may minimize or eliminate the need for restraint. Engaging in shorter but frequent therapeutic interactions is usually more effective than trying to engage the individual for longer sessions. Some times of day will also be more conducive than others to interaction and therapeutic involvement.

Caregiver Communication Strategies

The following caregiver communication strategies can be helpful in reducing disruptive behavior. Although some of these may sound simple, caregivers often benefit from modeling, practicing, and being supported in implementing such communication strategies.

- *Selectively ignoring behaviors.* Any response to a behavior may inadvertently increase the likelihood of its reoccurrence by providing attention, social reinforcement, a sense of social control, or escape from an undesirable activity. Caregivers' simply proceeding with what they are doing and failing to react to the behavior may extinguish it. Many behaviors (e.g., swearing or lewd language, physically aggressive or sexualized behaviors) are particularly difficult for family and staff to ignore. Such actions are often personally offensive and trigger emotions that are hard to control. In addition, extinction of a behavior is very hard to achieve, and partial reinforcement (responding only some of the time) has consistently been demonstrated to make the behavior more resistant to extinction. There is also the potential for one unreinforced behavior (e.g., screaming) to be replaced with another (e.g., throwing things) if that particular behavior has succeeded in drawing attention.
- *Redirecting the person's attention.* Disruptive behaviors sometimes reflect perseveration. They may also reflect anger or frustration in response to something that has happened, or something that has been requested but has not been provided. Ignoring such a behavior may have minimal if any effect, as the behavior is not attention-seeking or instrumental. Redirecting the person's attention to another activity in a neutral manner is often effective. Engagement in a new activity often breaks the cycle of perseveration or frustration and allows the person to move on. In some circumstances, a sudden and unexpected response can be effective (e.g., singing can sometimes stop an emergent tantrum). Although it may not be useful on a regular basis or in many situations, production of an unexpected behavior on the part of the therapist can have its place.
- *Providing choices.* A hallmark of adult behavior is that there is a certain amount of personal choice in activities. Following a brain injury, choices may be drastically reduced, and the injured person may feel controlled, coerced, and manipulated. Giving options for what activity or activities to do, and for when, where, and how they will be done, can often go a long way toward fostering feelings of personal independence and self-esteem. The choices must be real and not only for appearance, and these choices must be honored.
- *Reducing expectations.* There is much to work on following a brain injury—new skills to learn and old ones to regain. Family and treatment staff are committed to helping the client move forward, and they work

hard to provide assistance to the injured person. However, they may under-estimate the level of effort required on the part of the patient, the toll of emotional response to injury, or the degree of confusion and fragility of cognitive systems. Signs of withdrawal or agitation often indicate that the person is feeling overwhelmed and backing off. Making something simpler, or providing additional cues and supports, may be necessary to avoid fur-ther behavioral deterioration or disruption.

• *Backing off and trying again.* Behaviors are in part related to the en-vironment and to immediate antecedents. The fact that a behavior was produced before in response to a request does not mean that it will be con-sistently produced again. Given a minute or two to calm down, refocus, and perhaps to integrate the consequences of the last action, the person may respond quite differently to the same request. Sometimes simply changing the staff or family member who is making the request (e.g., changing from a male to a female staff member) can help to improve the chance of success by changing some aspect of the stimulus set. Indeed, bringing in a third party to diffuse conflict is a classic, often effective tech-nique.

• *Speaking quietly and maintaining a neutral stance.* Behavioral prob-lems often trigger strong emotions in caregivers. Fear, anger, and frustra-tion are common and understandable responses to behavior that seems dangerous, self-defeating, and purposeless. It is important, however, to maintain a neutral stance and not to display or get caught up in the emo-tion. To do so will probably result in further escalation of the behavior, and further breakdown of the intervention and the relationship. Caregivers may need assistance in learning to control their own emotions and to re-main calm when dealing with such circumstances. A first step in this pro-cess is learning to identify one's own signs of distress and choosing the best techniques to reduce one's own stressful feelings and emotions. For staff members working with behaviorally disordered clients, formal training in crisis intervention is extremely valuable.

• *Identifying signs of the patient's escalating distress.* Although a pa-tient's disruptive behaviors can sometimes feel as if they came out of no-where, in most instances there are subtle signs of increasing distress. An in-crease in muscle tension, perhaps evident in a swinging leg, a tightened jaw, or a furrowed brow; an increase in the pitch, intensity, or level of strain in the voice; or an increase in breathing or heart rate can signal an escalation of distress and an increased likelihood of a behavioral outburst. Caregivers need to learn to identify such signs and respond by backing off, redirecting, or otherwise modifying the situation. Individuals with acquired brain in-jury typically have less emotional resilience when they are fatigued, hungry, or in pain. Identifying times during the day when energy levels are high, and scheduling more demanding activities during such times, may be bene-ficial.

• *Avoiding confrontation and power struggles.* Negative behaviors often spark confrontations and power struggles in which there will be no winners. Indeed, power struggles can have rewarding or reinforcing properties in and of themselves. Confrontation may only further entrench or reinforce the challenging behaviors, and should thus be avoided.

Behavioral Therapies

Applied Behavior Analysis

Effective prevention and management of behavioral problems require an appreciation for the multiple contributions to behavioral difficulties. In some situations, it is important to carry out a detailed analysis of behavior to identify the specific factors that influence the client. *Applied behavior analysis* is a technique designed to evaluate these contributions and provide a springboard for development of behavior management planning. In such an analysis the clinician observes and records targeted aspects of behavior, and makes careful note of the situation, conditions, and/or setting in which the behaviors occur. Careful observation is also made of any and all responses to the behaviors on the part of others. The underlying premise is that situational variables trigger or influence the frequency or intensity of certain behaviors, and that consequent events either increase or decrease the probability of the behavior's occurring again in that setting or circumstance. A detailed applied behavior analysis can provide substantial information about the behaviors and suggest effective interventions. The acronym A-B-C refers to the systematic identification and quantification of *antecedent events*, *target behaviors*, and *consequent events*.

• *Identifying and quantifying target behaviors.* The first step in undertaking an A-B-C analysis is to identify in specific terms the most important targets of intervention. These are typically specific behaviors that are blocking successful participation in rehabilitation, school, or work activities; causing danger or potential harm to the person; and/or contributing to problems in interacting with medical/therapy staff, family, and/or peers. It is important to define the problem behaviors clearly, so that they can be accurately identified. Target behaviors must be overt and recognizable, and it is important to avoid language that labels or attributes an intent or emotion to the behavior. For example, it is more effective to chart instances of "spitting" or "hitting" than instances of "aggressive" or "angry" behavior. The purpose is to establish a baseline for the frequency and/or intensity of certain behaviors. Also, in the focus on and concern about maladaptive or disruptive behavior, many positive behaviors may go unnoticed and unrewarded. It is important to identify specific behaviors that would be helpful if increased (e.g., behaviors that are adaptive, appropriate, and/or prosocial). A substantial literature provides useful examples of target behaviors and behavioral interventions for individuals with brain injury (Burgess & Alderman, 1990; Davis, Turner, Rolder, & Cartwright, 1994; Wood, 1987). There are now also software programs that facilitate recording, reporting, and graphing behavioral data (e.g., ABBY for Windows, available through http://www.compusmart.ab.ca/jhealth).

• *Identifying antecedents.* Antecedents are factors that appear to elicit or trigger both the problem behaviors and more adaptive behaviors. Antecedents actually include a wide variety of factors. They can include environmental factors, such as noise or other forms of stimulation that may contribute to confusion or distractibility. They might also include particular activities, such as physical manipulation for changing dressings or nursing care, or activities with a high cognitive demand in one or more domains. Still other antecedent variables may relate to physiological variables, such as fatigue (perhaps related to time of day the behaviors are most often observed) or medication. Antecedents are also called *occasion setters* or *setting events*, because they set the "occasion" for the occurrence of a particular behavior.

• *Quantifying consequences.* Consequences are the events that follow the behavior and are related to the likelihood of its recurrence. Consequences can either increase or decrease the likelihood that the behavior occurs again. The most typical consequences of interest are the behaviors of the individuals around the person at the time the behaviors are observed. Consequences take the form of verbal responses, facial expressions, and actions in response to the behavior. The intent of a response is not important; rather, the effect of the response is critical. Though caregivers/therapists may believe that their responses will reduce the behavior, their consequent actions may actually serve to reinforce and increase the behavior.

Some further steps need to be added to the A-B-C analysis in work with an individual who has sustained a brain injury. First, it is important to identify cognitive factors that may affect behavioral interventions or suggest additional treatment objectives (e.g., severe memory problems, inability to read social cues, a high degree of distractibility). Second, it is important to evaluate the resources available in the individual's environment for implementing a behavior management plan. This involves an assessment of the structure of the setting, as well as identification of a person or persons (e.g., family member, aide, job coach, or therapist) who are interested, willing, and able to be involved in the behavioral plan. Third, it is important to target functional activities and behaviors that are necessary for adaptive functioning. When reinforcement is used, it must also be meaningful to the individual.

Once the information has been gathered, a plan for managing the difficult or disruptive behaviors can be developed. A decrease or increase in the frequency of particular behaviors is achieved through antecedent control (e.g., making changes in the environment, altering task demands) and/ or through consistent changes in the consequent events (e.g., social reinforcement). The following case example illustrates the use of an applied behavioral analysis, and the treatment plan based on that analysis.

Case Example of Using Applied Behavior Analysis to Develop Interventions

Background

Tom was a 27-year-old man who was struck on the head with a large tree branch while felling timber. He sustained a right penetrating frontoparietal skull fracture, and was unconscious for 2 days. He had a high school education, and was divorced; he had two children. Three weeks following his injury, he was transferred to rehabilitation. Admission notes indicated left-sided hemiplegia and variable orientation. Two weeks later, it was recommended by nursing staff that he be discharged to a step-down unit, as "aggressive behaviors" were preventing him from participating in the rehabilitation program and were interfering with the most basic aspects of care.

Problem Analysis

The staff elected to do an A-B-C assessment over 3 days during the morning nursing shift. Two different nurses and three nurses' aides cared for him over the 3 days. Over these days, the behaviors in the left-hand column were observed and counted. (The right-hand column lists various antecedent activities or circumstances that were associated with various behaviors.)

Hitting	8	Incontinence	5
Pinching	1	Bed baths	10
Kicking	8	Transfers	8
Spitting	2	Dressing	5
Scratching	3	Brushing teeth	2
Verbal abuse	11	Giving medications	4
Refusing medications	4		

The consequences for these behaviors were inconsistent. It appeared that 13 of the 37 problem behaviors were actually reinforced through cajoling, soft talking, and withdrawal from the room, while only 8 of 56 cooperative, prosocial behaviors were reinforced. No clear or consistent differences were seen among the different staff members. Review of the cognitive testing revealed some left-sided neglect, slow speed of information processing, poor attention, poor visuospatial memory, and poor spatial analysis and problem solving.

Conclusions from A-B-C Analysis

"Aggressive behaviors" most commonly occurred during physical manipulations, particularly those that involved discomfort or what would normally be considered the most "personal" of physical care. Cooperative behaviors were minimally reinforced, and there was actually more reinforcement for uncooperative behaviors. Tom's cognitive impairments might be contributing to his startle and fear responses and to processing difficulties during the course of physical care.

Management Program

The following management instructions were developed for Tom's various caregivers:

- Because he shows some left-sided neglect, approach Tom from the right side so that he will not have the experience of someone "suddenly" appearing in front of him. Move slowly to his left side to increase attention to his left visual space.
- Because Tom has difficulties with visual analysis and memory, he may not recognize individuals who are taking care of him. Tell Tom who you are, and remind him that you have worked with him before.
- Before touching Tom, inform him of what you are about to do in short, clear sentences (e.g., "I am going to put your shirt on now; you could help by raising your arm").
- Speak and move slowly, allowing each message to sink in before proceeding. Break down procedures into small steps, and provide reinforcement for cooperative or helpful behaviors. Inform Tom before proceeding to each new step.
- Because Tom has poor attention and is distractible, avoid rapid movement or excessive talking around him. For example, make sure to close curtains and drapes if the environment is distracting, and do not talk with others while you are working with him.
- Increased muscle tension, tremors, and grunting sounds signal Tom's agitation. Upon noticing such signs or encountering resistance, use distraction to focus his attention toward something else. It this is unsuccessful, back off immediately, and try again in a few minutes.
- Use extinction. Remember that any reaction on the part of caregivers, including cajoling, scolding, arguing, or explaining, is potentially reinforcing, as it may provide social reinforcement and delay or deter fearful, anxiety-provoking, or undesired manipulations.
- To the extent possible, be respectful of Tom's need for privacy and distress at having others provide such a personal level of care. Acknowledge his feelings, and facilitate ways in which he might begin to participate in his own care (e.g., giving him the washcloth during bathing). Make sure to put items in his right visual space. Leave sufficient time for care routines so that he will not be rushed in his attempts to care for himself.
- Use extinction in response to verbal abuse or refusal of medications. Ignore any instances of verbal abuse, without arguing, reasoning, or discussing. Do not

show that you are upset or respond emotionally in any way. Remain neutral, as any reaction on the part of caregivers is likely to increase the behavior. When medications are refused, make no response (ignore) and try again in 1 minute without commenting on the refusal. Reinforce all instances when medications are not refused.

This management program was explained and practiced with the nurses, nurses' aides, and attendants. (Positive practice and role playing are often useful when a behavior management plan is implemented with new or inexperienced staff members or with family members.) The program was explained to all treatment staff so that the general principles could be applied in other settings. Data were collected for 2 weeks (see Figure 11.2). The intervention immediately resulted in fewer negative behaviors, though there was an initial increase in negative behaviors specifically associated with bathing. These declined after an initial increase, and there were no further recommendations from the nursing staff to discontinue Tom in active rehabilitation.

Eliciting Desired Behaviors: Basic Techniques

Decreasing the frequency of challenging behaviors is just one side of the coin. The other consists of eliciting, shaping, stabilizing, and reinforcing desired behaviors. The basic techniques used are prompting, shaping, and chaining.

- *Prompts* are verbal requests or other signs or signals to do something. It is important to remember to require only one response unit per cue, and not to ask for more.
- *Shaping* is used when a client's response is not similar enough to the target response to be considered correct. It involves reinforcing variations or forms of the behaviors that increasingly resemble the target response. Guidelines for the trainer include the following:
  1. Keep the terminal goal in mind.
  2. Begin with behaviors in the client's repertoire.
  3. Begin with behaviors that most closely resemble the goal.
  4. Select a step size that can easily, but not too easily, be achieved.
  5. Remain at a step just long enough to stabilize it.
  6. If behaviors appear to begin to disintegrate, drop back a step or two.
  7. Use effective reinforcement procedures throughout.

- *Chaining*, which involves teaching a complete sequence in a particular order, is used when responses require a combination of several different behaviors. In forward chaining, the trainer begins with and stabilizes the first behavior in the sequence, cueing the rest, and repeats until the entire sequence can be repeated. In backward chaining, the trainer starts with

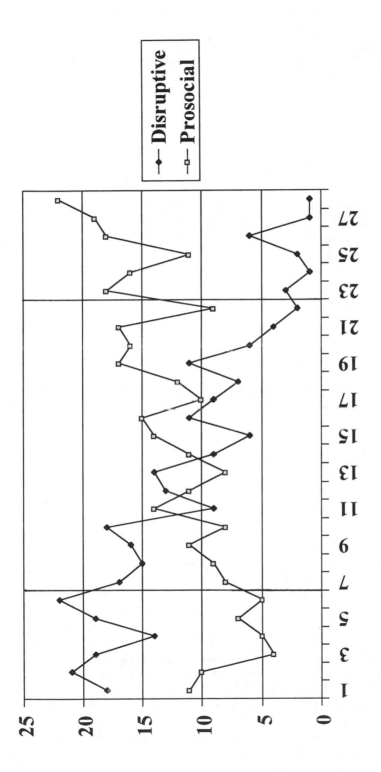
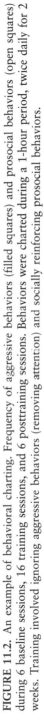

FIGURE 11.2. An example of behavioral charting. Frequency of aggressive behaviors (filled squares) and prosocial behaviors (open squares) during 6 baseline sessions, 16 training sessions, and 6 posttraining sessions. Behaviors were charted during a 1-hour period, twice daily for 2 weeks. Training involved ignoring aggressive behaviors (removing attention) and socially reinforcing prosocial behaviors.

having the client do the last step and works backward to the first. For example, to teach the client to make juice using backward chaining, the trainer starts with drinking it, then stabilizes pouring it, stirring the juice and water, filling the pitcher with water, pouring the juice concentrate in the pitcher, and finally opening the juice concentrate can. This often has the reward of always achieving the end goal right away.

Behavioral interventions have a rich history, and many different principles and approaches have been articulated (Hersen & Bellack, 1988). Many published case studies describe using different forms of behavioral interventions in individuals with brain injury (Jacobs, 1993; McGlynn, 1990; Wood, 1987). The most straightforward approaches are described and illustrated in the case example above. That is, the trainer or trainers provide environmental manipulations based on the person's cognitive and behavioral profile, and then shape and reinforce positive behaviors and extinguish/ignore negative behaviors. However, many more individualized and sophisticated approaches can be adopted. A few examples are provided below.

Discrimination Training

In some situations, a behavior in and of itself is neither inappropriate nor disruptive; the goal is not to extinguish it, but rather to decrease it in particular situations. Blake, Bogod, and Newbigging (1995) described a young man with a brain injury who resided in a care facility, and was very talkative. He appeared to seek out attention and social interaction at every opportunity. However, he was very poor at determining social cues for when someone was otherwise engaged or did not have the time to talk with him. His constant talking with the staff became a problem, in that it was taking up staff time and resources to the detriment of other clients on the unit. Simply telling him that one did not have time to speak or had other obligations had no impact. The staff implemented a behavioral plan involving discrimination training. The client was encouraged to speak with any individuals who had green squares attached to their clothing; these included other program participants who enjoyed talking with him, as well as staff members who were either assigned to him or had responsibilities for general supervision. He was not to speak with any individuals who were wearing red squares. These included other participants who became agitated when he spoke to them, staff members who were assigned to other participants, or staff members who needed to be engaged in other activities. He was reinforced for talking to people with the green squares; however, if he approached people with the red squares, he was told they could not speak to him then and they pointed to the red squares, with no further discussion or explanation. The client learned the discrimination quite easily and with little apparent frustration or agitation. The overt visual cues were gradually made smaller and finally faded, with reliance on the simple verbal cue. The client thus learned to change his behavior in response to a discriminant stimulus.

Reciprocal Inhibition

Reciprocal inhibition is an intervention based on the behavioral principle that engaging in one behavior may preclude engaging in another. Although many behaviors of concern after acquired brain injury fall into the realm of social behavior, other kinds of problematic behavior can be seen, and reciprocal inhibition is often helpful in dealing with these. Hanlon, Clontz, and Thomas (1993) described use of reciprocal inhibition in a 53-year-old woman who had sustained a right subarachnoid hemorrhage involving the right temporal and frontal lobes. Two months following the bleed, she developed involuntary, uncontrollable oral–facial gestures in the form of repetitive involuntary exhalations, involuntary vocalizations, tongue protrusion, lip smacking, and involuntary eye closure. Traditional rehabilitation treatments and pharmacological interventions did not help to reduce these behaviors. The behavioral treatment consisted of introducing and cueing an incompatible behavior, which was to place a plastic drinking straw in her mouth and bite down when she felt the onset of an involuntary movement. She was able to learn to make the reciprocal gesture, despite some residual cognitive difficulty including perseveration and echolalia. With this intervention, there was a decrease in involuntary exhalations and vocalizations, though when the treatment (straw) was withdrawn there was an increase in the movements. She continued to use the device, and 1 month after her discharge she demonstrated good carryover, eventually substituting a lollipop and even an unlit cigarette as more socially acceptable things to have in the mouth.

Response Cost Techniques

Most clinical accounts of behavioral intervention involve incentive-based interventions for prosocial or adaptive behaviors (reward) and the use of extinction (usually ignoring or time-out procedures) to decrease the frequency or duration of difficult or disruptive behaviors. Ignoring typically involves choosing not to respond to a behavior, but the client remains in the setting and is not excluded from the situation. A time-out procedure is exclusionary in that it usually involves removal of social contact—either by having the client sit or stand away from others, or by having the client go into another area altogether (e.g., a special time-out room). There has been a gradual shift away from exclusionary interventions, for several reasons: They are awkward to implement; the meaning behind the behavior is generally not considered; behavior change may not generalize to other settings; and engaging in the time out can itself become rewarding. Time out can also be perceived by the person and others as demeaning or punishing. In addition, disinhibition, impulsiveness, perseveration, and lack of awareness may make it difficult if not impossible for the individual to utilize or learn from this form of feedback.

In a *response cost* technique, the client has something taken from him or her in response to behaviors that are targeted for reduction. In a so-called *token economy*, wherein tokens can be used to gain desired objects, activities, or privileges, response cost approaches involve taking tokens the person has away from him or her in response to specific behaviors. Alderman, Fry, and Youngson (1995; see also Alderman & Ward, 1991) described the use of a response cost technique followed by training in self-monitoring in a 21-year-old woman who was seen for treatment 13 months after contracting herpes simplex encephalitis. She was described as restless, sexually disinhibited, and verbally aggressive. Both her Verbal and Performance IQ were less than 65, and she demonstrated grossly impaired memory, orientation, and attention. The target behavior was fast, loud, repetitive, and stereotyped speech, which was disruptive to group activities and a source of irritation and provocation to other patients. Baseline assessment indicated approximately nine disruptive utterances per minute. In the first stage of intervention, time outs were used, but the utterances actually increased quite dramatically under those conditions. The staff then implemented a response cost program for her within the context of a simple ongoing token economy program. Sixty pennies were placed on the table, and the patient was given cues and instructions with regard to what was an inappropriate response. If she had an outburst, she was prompted to give back a penny and to provide a reason why she was giving it back (with prompting as needed). After 15 minutes, the coins were counted, and she was given praise, an edible, and a token if she had 10 or more remaining coins. Explanations were provided, and tokens could be exchanged later for larger reinforcements. The introduction of the response cost program had an immediate, beneficial impact on the behavior and led to the client's demonstrating much greater inhibitory control. Even during intermittent sessions without the response cost, there was an improvement, though when the treatment was withdrawn completely, speech outbursts increased. Time sampling after treatment indicated an overall increase in inhibitory control 15 months after treatment. Improvements generalized to other situations on the unit, but not to community outings. Because of the difficulty of implementing a token system in the community, the researchers implemented another program that involved the client's learning to self-monitor and eventually to control (decrease) inappropriate verbalizations. Although this latter program is less intrusive, the authors argued that the initial intensive behavioral analysis was necessary to break the cycle of disruptive behavior initially observed.

Supported Behavior Routines

At later stages of recovery, when an individual has returned to home, school, and/or work, new and unforeseen difficulties may be encountered. Early after injury, a great deal of support, direction, and assistance may be provided by family members, teachers, friends, or coworkers. With support and reduced demands for productivity and speed, the person may function relatively well in familiar and routine activities. As time since injury increases, however, the person is often expected to do more and more with less and less assistance, and is faced with new tasks to learn and new challenges to meet. The person may appear to be doing well, and for others in the school or work environment, memory of the injury fades (or there may be no knowledge whatsoever that the injury occurred). It is often during this stage that there is an escalation of behavioral problems, as frustration, feelings of failure, low self-esteem and self-confidence, and a sense of loss begin to mount.

Feeney and Ylvisaker (1995) described this scenario in a research report focusing on three male high school students who had sustained severe traumatic brain injuries. Each of them had been progressing well and had returned to school, but began to develop an escalating pattern of challenging behaviors (including physical aggression) in response to increasing academic demands and expectations. Dependent variables in the study included the frequency of challenging behavior, scores on the Aberrant Behavior Checklist, and the percentage of work completed on specific assignments.

- During a 1-week baseline condition, the young men received just the normal orientation to school tasks and routines. They received verbal reminders about their schedules at the beginning of the day and at several other points during the day.

- Over the next 3 weeks, the research staff implemented four new strategies. First, each student and a staff member reviewed the student's daily routine in detail. Second, the staff member and student engaged in a negotiation with regard to the amount and order of work to be done. Particular emphasis was placed on providing the student with the opportunity to make choices and provide input as to which assignments would be completed and how they would be completed. Third, the student was provided with and oriented to an "advanced organizer." This was a set of photographs that depicted the various activities the student would be involved in over the course of the day. Fourth, the staff member and student engaged in verbal rehearsal and review of the routine for the day. During these 3 weeks, there was a gradual decrease in the frequency and intensity of disruptive behaviors.

- For the next 2 weeks, written cues were substituted for photographic cues. Students and staff members continued to engage in rehearsal and review, and, again, choices were provided. There was an initial increase in disruptive behaviors and then a decrease.

• Students were then returned to the initial baseline condition; that is, they received periodic nonspecific reminders of what was to happen, but were given no photographic or written cues and were not provided with any rehearsal or review. At this point, with removal of positive supports, behavior deteriorated and returned to baseline levels.

The researchers argued that providing structure, choice, and routine were instrumental in reducing the disruptive behaviors, but they also recognized that the young men would continue to need supports for positive behavior and cues for behavioral routines. The supports as described were reinstated.

Follow-up 1 to 2 years later with regard to school and vocational activities suggested positive long-term effects and outcomes. Feeney and Ylvisaker (1995) proposed that the intervention was successful because it was provided in the environment where the students were receiving education and services, and where the behaviors were evident. Staff members already working with the students on a day-to-day basis also carried it out. The investigators pointed out the importance of positive routines and momentum, and the utility of actively involving the students in goal setting, planning, and monitoring. The effect of the advanced support system was to help the students to understand what was required of them, to give them a sense of control and involvement in the process, and to help them remain on task.

This study well illustrates a program weighted toward *antecedent* control, a concept less easily understood than operant control. Ylvisaker and Feeney (1998) stress the need for collaborative interventions using individuals in an adolescent's natural environment, and provide many case examples of facilitating positive everyday routines. These authors stress the importance of helping individuals with brain injury know what they are good at and what is difficult for them, and know that there are things that can help them when tasks are difficult. They highlight the effectiveness of making plans for completing tasks at home, school, or work, and having the individuals pay attention to how well they are doing. They also stress the need to have individuals be able to identify when they are not successful, and to try a new approach to task completion. Their approach stresses the need for consistent modeling and coaching within the context of everyday routines and conversational interactions, not just during instruction or therapy sessions. Although such interventions can be very helpful for social and behavioral difficulties, they do not necessarily address the cognitive problems with attention or memory. The use of learning techniques such as *direct instruction* (an academic teaching approach that emphasizes minimization of incorrect responses), scaffolding of educational material, and the implementation of external aids for memory and organization are important adjuncts to such behaviorally oriented interventions.

Positive Programming

LaVigna and colleagues (Donnelan, LaVigna, Negri-Shoulz, & Fassbender, 1988) emphasize yet another approach to working with challenging behavior. Their work builds on behavioral traditions, yet represents a real shift in terms of how such behavior is viewed and in terms of the focus of intervention. They term their approach *positive programming*, and describe it as a gradual educational process for behavioral change that is based on a functional analysis of the presenting problems and involves systematic instruction in more effective ways of behaving. Whereas traditional procedures for behavioral change have focused on discrete manipulations of specified undesirable behaviors, positive programming stresses long-term skill building rather than specified behavior reduction. It does not have the "on–off" quality of other behavioral interventions, which are either "in effect" or "not in effect." Positive programming can be used to teach new behavior; to teach alternative communication strategies as substitutes for unconventional behaviors that serve a communicative function for an individual; to teach more appropriate alternative behaviors; and to assign meaning to the individual's behavior even when its intentionality is unclear. Examples of these four approaches within a positive programming framework, drawn from Donnelan and colleagues' (1988) training materials, are provided below.

- *Teaching a new behavior.* An 11-year-old boy returned to school after surgery for a benign brain tumor. However, he was failing to attend school several days a week; he either played truant or claimed that he was not feeling well. After a functional analysis, it was suspected that he did not attend school because of problems with the other children in the schoolyard. A social skills training program taught him to be more assertive and less frightened of his peers.
- *Facilitating communication strategies.* A woman with intellectual disabilities who was also deaf and blind (though she had been able to develop a fairly extensive sign vocabulary) demonstrated frequent aggressive and self-abusive behavior. It was hypothesized that she could not predict when using signs would "work" for her because she could not hear or see if anyone was nearby, and that she used these more disruptive behaviors to get attention, ask for help, or get a break. She was given a desk bell and taught to ring it to draw attention before she signed. The bell as a communication device, paired with the signs, eliminated her aggressive and self-injurious behavior.

• *Teaching more appropriate alternative behaviors.* Following a severe head injury, a 21-year-old woman was able to return to her parents' home. However, she would repeatedly pull all of her clothes out of her dresser and then fold them and put them back in. Her job coach got her a position in a local thrift store. She pulled clothes out of bags and folded them or sorted them into bins; she also learned to empty or stock clothing racks. She worked with fabric and clothing all day, which she liked, and received a wage for doing it as part of her supported work plan.

• *Assigning meaning to apparently unintentional behaviors.* A young boy with autism was nonverbal and rarely initiated social interaction. Periodically, he would place himself close to instructors. Staff members decided to respond to this behavior as if it were intentional and communicative. They would treat his approach as an invitation of social interaction and begin to converse with him, or would treat it as a request for an object and give him something he liked. Over time, his movements appeared to become increasingly intentional, and the staff was able to shape additional gestures.

The advantages of positive programming begin with its affirmative and constructive nature. New behaviors are taught, minimizing the risk of the development of new problem behaviors. It has long-term and lasting effects, as new behavioral repertoires are built and maintained by natural contingencies in the environment. This increases the likelihood of generalizing such gains over time. The approach is also efficient, in that it relies on whatever limited resources are available in a given setting. It stresses social validity, in that the concerns and feelings of both the learner and the others in his or her environment are addressed. Finally, it contributes to dignity, in that it enables learners to participate actively in managing their own behavior and in making their own decisions.

Metacognitive/Self-Regulatory Strategies

Behavioral interventions of the types described above can be extremely valuable and important components of a treatment plan. In the long run, however, it is often difficult to maintain a high level of support for an individual with brain injury, and reinforcement in home, school, and work environments (even with the best of intentions and training on the part of caregivers) is likely to be somewhat inconsistent and intermittent. Indeed, fading procedures are necessary and important if generalization of behavioral changes in the natural environment is to be promoted and stabilized. In addition, maximum independence and self-management are well-recognized goals of rehabilitation. Correspondingly, the ultimate goal of interventions in the area of behavioral management is internalized self-regulation of behavior. This includes self-monitoring, self-inhibiting, self-evaluating, problem solving, and other skills necessary for deliberate self-control of behavior. Teaching self-regulation can make behavior changes more robust and resilient in relation to changes in the environment, and can provide for substantially more flexibility and adaptive capability. However, such abilities typically require a higher level of cognitive ability, insight, self-awareness, and motivation than the other approaches to behavior management that have been discussed thus far. The goals of metacognitive/self-regulatory strategy training include not only reducing maladaptive or undesirable behaviors, but also developing the behavioral skills and routines necessary for successful living and social interactions.

Effective training of self-regulatory strategies requires breaking down the strategy training to provide sufficient and consistent opportunities for success. Most strategies involve training individuals to be more aware of their own behavior in a particular setting, and then moving through a set of steps or procedures to manage their behavior in the situation. Supportive coaching and positive reinforcement are the most appropriate and ultimately successful means to establish more appropriate behaviors. Examples of self-regulatory strategies include stress and anger management (see Chapter 12); assertiveness training; and a variety of pragmatics interventions designed to address such areas as conversation initiation, turn taking, and topic maintenance (see Chapter 10). Once self-regulatory skills are trained in the clinical setting, high levels of cues, prompts, and reinforcement must be systematically faded, and the responsibility for cueing, monitoring, and self-evaluation should gradually be taken over by the client (though specific practice and training in target environments are crucial). Over the course of metacognitive training, there is a systematic and reciprocal withdrawal of support for increasingly difficult tasks and/or in increasingly difficult environments.

Metacognitive strategy training principles were primarily developed in the context of working with students who have developmental learning problems (Graham & Harris, 1989; Harris, 1990). Many of the traditional techniques included self-regulatory strategies to facilitate adaptive behaviors that would lead to better learning and retention in an academic context. They were later adapted for use with individuals with brain injury. Stuss, Delgado, and Guzman (1987) used a verbal self-regulation strategy (self-reminding) to sustain motor actions in two patients who were unable to persist in a motor activity. Although the strategy helped when it was cued, there was little generalization. Cicerone and Wood (1987) described use of a self-instructional technique that involved initially overt, and then more and more covert, self-cueing on a problem-solving task. Lawson and Rice (1989) have described a self-monitoring paradigm summarized by the acronym WSTC. While doing an activity, a person learns to say to him- or herself, "What am I supposed to be doing?" (W); "Select a strategy" (S); "Try the strategy" (T); and "Check the strategy" (C). (For further discussion of WSTC and other self-regulatory techniques, see Chapter 8 on the management of executive disorders.)

In attempts to train any metacognitive strategy, at least three training components are involved. First, the individual must be provided with information regarding the need for a strategy and knowledge about the basic principles of the strategy. Second, the individual must be taught the skills and techniques necessary to use the strategy through systematic practice. Third, generalization must be implemented to ensure use of the strategy in novel, more complex, and more demanding environments. Metacognitive strategies were initially designed as approaches for cognitive activities, but they have been adapted for use in dealing with difficult behaviors, physical sensations, and emotions. They have been used successfully in dealing with anxiety responses, anger, pain, and specific fears or phobias.

When a self-regulatory strategy is used with individuals who have sustained a brain injury, several modifications may need to be made in implementing the strategy. The instructions may need to be more explicit, and it will help if they are written down and available for cueing and for review. Additional training may be necessary to recognize problem behaviors secondary to limited awareness. Additional frustration may be present and need to be dealt with, as the individuals may recall having had better abilities and skills prior to their injury. The following case example illustrates the use of metacognitive/self-regulatory strategies to deal with outbursts of anger.

Case Example of Using Self-Regulatory Strategies for Anger Management

Jerry was a 24-year-old man who sustained a moderate traumatic brain injury in a motor vehicle accident. He had a high school education and had worked before the accident in auto body repair. There was some history of substance abuse, but he had maintained steady work in two jobs and a steady relationship for 3 years. He and his partner had two young children. Following the injury, he was in and out of consciousness for 2 days, but then made a relatively rapid recovery of orientation, motor functions, and speech–language abilities. Residual difficulties involved some impulsivity, irritability, and low frustration tolerance; cognitive testing revealed problems with mental rigidity, complex attention, and problem solving. He was discharged from inpatient rehabilitation after just 3 weeks. He attempted to return to work twice over the next 6 months. Although his ability to do the work seemed relatively intact, he lost both jobs due to anger outbursts (with his boss, coworkers, and customers). He expressed anger verbally, and also threw and hit things. His partner was still with him, but she felt she couldn't cope with Jerry's anger much longer, and she feared for the children. He had never hit her or the children, but she felt uncomfortable and threatened. He had recently punched a hole in the wall of their apartment.

Treatment involved several components. First, Jerry was provided with information in the form of films, readings, and discussions about the common effects of traumatic brain injury and frontal lobe damage. A particular focus was on problems with irritability and anger. Jerry was aware that things were not going well, but tended either to blame others for his outbursts or to feel that his anger came on so suddenly he had no way to control it. Second, Jerry was trained to identify signs of escalating distress and anger, of which he was apparently unaware. Discussions were held on mildly provocative topics, and the examiner signaled him about any signs of growing irritation (e.g., clenching of his fists or jaw, more rapid breathing, increased rate of speech, a loud voice, forward-leaning posture). A list was made of these behaviors, and Jerry "imitated" them when he was not irritated, in order to become more aware of them. He then watched videotapes of himself and the examiner and was asked to identify the salient behaviors on the tape. Exercises were set up in which he matched his judgments against those of the therapist. Third, Jerry practiced identifying his own behaviors as he was talking with the examiner about increasingly sensitive or anger-provoking topics. Fourth, after he was able to identify signs of growing irritability and anger, he was asked to keep an anger log outside the treatment sessions. He was asked to record the date and time, what happened, his level of anger (according to the Anger Management Scale provided in Appendix 11.1), what he did, and what he felt. During this phase, Jerry observed that although he loved his children, he found the noises associated with their playing almost unbearable. Fifth, Jerry was trained to take a time out, basically removing himself from the situation for a few minutes (or, if this was not possible, counting to 100 while breathing deeply). He practiced these techniques in therapy sessions, during which one of the exercises involved doing a task while listening to recordings of his children playing. He learned to rate his level of irritation and to initiate appropriate strategies. He then began using the technique at home. He recorded any angry feelings/behaviors, along with his response in the situation, in his record book ("What happened? What did I do? Did I take a time out? How did it work?"). The therapist also worked with him to develop a list of activities he could do to relax following an escalation of anger (e.g., walk or exercise, listen to music, play with the dog, meditate). He was also coached in how to know when he could go back into the situation and how to decide what he needed to do. A list of anger signs and techniques to try was printed on an "anger cue card" that he carried in his wallet (Figure 11.3).

At the same time, Jerry's partner was seen and provided with information about acquired brain injury and the associated problems with anger. She asked for and was given help in learning to ignore Jerry's outbursts, avoid confrontations, and recognize signs of his escalating distress. The couple was helped to identify jointly a set of signals she could give him when they were at home or in public, to help him notice anger signs. After 3 months of biweekly treatment sessions, Jerry felt that he had relatively good control of his anger. He returned to work again, and although he continued to feel more easily frustrated and irritated than before his injury, he was able to control those feelings and maintained both his employment and his relationship. He continued to carry and use his anger cue card.

Step 1:   *Identify my anger signs.*
          Pacing
          Loud voice
          Fast breathing
          Tight jaw
          Thoughts getting blocked

Step 2:   *Block the anger cycle.*
          Stop and say, "I'm starting to feel angry. I need to take a time out."
          Go outside or to the bedroom.
          Walk.
          Take long, deep breaths.

Step 3:   *Return to the situation.*
          When I can smile, I am ready to go back.
          Decide what I need to do, if anything:
              Apologize?
              Explain?
              Set time to talk?

Step 4:   *Evaluate.*
          How did I do?
          What did I do well?
          What might I have done better?

Step 5:   *Complete anger journal.*
          Date and time
          What was happening?
          What was my anger level (1–10)?
          What did I do?
          What did I feel?

FIGURE 11.3. Jerry's anger management cue card.

FAMILY AND STAFF EDUCATION AND TRAINING

The first step in working with family members, professional staff, and other caregivers around behavioral problems often involves education with regard to the origin of the behaviors. In the early stages of recovery, when the injured person is confused and agitated, professionals will be familiar with the common behavioral signs and symptoms displayed. But family members are often shocked, confused, and/or filled with fear. Education about the normal stages of recovery, and about the behaviors they may observe or expect, is critical. In the later stages of recovery, however, it is not uncommon for professionals as well as family members to misinterpret problem behaviors. Repetitive question asking can be seen as something done to annoy or gain attention, whereas the injured person may genuinely not remember asking the question or no longer has the appropriate skills to get attention. An injured person whose memory seems to fluctuate from day to day may be seen as not trying or as displaying "sick behavior," whereas such fluctuation is actually normal during recovery; memory may be affected by environmental distractions, attention, or the importance or relevance of a specific memory to the injured person. When caregivers can develop more accurate perceptions about the reasons for behavioral difficulties, they are often able to respond more consistently and appropriately, and with less negative emotion.

Behaviors will be best managed if all of the significant individuals—including family members, professionals (including nurses, therapists, aides, and teachers), and other caregivers—are provided with education and training with regard to the behavior management plan, and indeed are involved in the design and implementation of the plan. All of these individuals should be involved in structuring the environment as effectively as possible to avoid behavioral difficulties, in learning to identify antecedents of behavioral outbursts, and in providing consistent and appropriate consequences or feedback to the individual when the behaviors occur. All caregivers need to learn how to reduce the likelihood of difficult behaviors by making sure that performance demands are reasonable and consistent. They also need to be taught the skills to work through difficult behaviors and deal with behavioral crises. This will be particularly critical when the injured individual displays aggressive or self-injurious behaviors.

Describing the behavioral intervention is a useful first step, but it is often important (and indeed critical) actually to observe family members, staff members, or other caregivers as they engage in the interaction. They may be unknowingly providing cues or responses that are reinforcing difficult behaviors, or they may be failing to recognize opportunities for reinforcing positive behaviors. In addition, it is important to acknowledge that dealing with challenging behaviors is often frustrating, stressful, and even fear-provoking. Interacting with someone who may be verbally abusive and/or who may physically assault others, either knowingly or unknowingly, can be extremely anxiety-provoking. A caregiver may develop a great deal of anticipatory anxiety and fear prior to engaging in the interaction. Family members often speak of feeling as if they are "walking on eggshells," not knowing when or at what seemingly insignificant provocation their injured relative may have an outburst of anger or aggression. It is often helpful for caregivers to prepare for a potentially stressful interaction (e.g., changing the person's bed or clothing) by reminding themselves of what they are going to do and how they are going to respond to difficult behaviors if these occur. Repeated self-reminding that the behaviors are secondary to brain injury, are not fully under the person's control, and should not be taken personally can be helpful during a potentially difficult interaction. Adjunct education for stress reduction and management, and other forms of therapeutic support, can be a valuable addition to the behavior management plan. Feedback regarding a caregiver's performance, constructive suggestions for other ways to deal with a difficult behavior, and praise for handling a situation well can also be invaluable (Meichenbaum, 1985).

Caregivers should be familiar with all stages of the intervention plan. This includes the use of preventative strategies, a plan for moving through challenging behaviors, and training and practice in crisis management techniques. Caregivers need to know that target behaviors may actually increase immediately after implementation of a behavior management plan. Many solid behavioral plans have been abandoned too early when the target behaviors increased after intervention, although this pattern is common, and persistence with a well-conceived plan usually results in successful reduction in the behavior. Isolated episodes of undesirable behavior or behavioral outbursts do not represent failures in the management plan, but opportunities to learn more about how the plan is working and how it might be altered or refined.

Sohlberg, Glang, and Todis (1998) designed a study to look at the effectiveness of training caregivers to provide appropriate cognitive support to persons with brain injury within their own natural living and working environments. The goal of the original research project included evaluating a collaborative mode of interaction with the subjects and their support persons; the caregivers and subjects were instrumental in designing the intervention and collecting performance data. Support persons were given information about the need for careful measurements before intervention was attempted. The data presented on three subject–caregiver groups all demonstrated improvement in the target behaviors during the baseline period. In one case, teachers were asked to measure a student's homework performance. Homework assignments were rated as being turned in at a very high level, whereas prior to the study this had been a major concern. Upon interview, it was concluded that teachers modified their behavior in response to being interviewed by the experimenters, and were clearer and more deliberate in making sure the student understood the assignments. In another case, measurements were taken of workplace performance. Performance improved dramatically after the subject's coworkers were contacted to participate in the project. They described feeling that they hadn't known what to do with their injured colleague, but, with the promise of assistance from the experimenters, they provided more support to the injured worker and became more aware of his needs. Sohlberg and colleagues (1998) proposed that the very act of measuring client performance changed the behaviors of the support persons and resulted in positive changes in baseline levels. These authors stressed the need to examine the implementation of support by the individuals most closely involved in a client's daily functioning, and the potential power of consistent behavioral observations and charting in actually effecting behavioral change. Also critical in their analysis of the results of the study was the notion of a bidirectional approach, in which professionals are not seen as primary in the intervention. Caregivers are seen as experts in their own right, and what is encouraged is collaborative work involving clients, family members or other caregivers, and professionals.

SUMMARY

Changes in behavior and problems with self-regulation of behavior are the most common and potentially disruptive consequences of acquired brain injury. Neurological, social, emotional, and other factors all contribute to behavioral difficulties. Different approaches to management of behavioral difficulties are appropriate at different stages after injury and with individuals with different cognitive, emotional, behavioral, and personality profiles. Altering the environment and/or environmental demands, implementing a variety of caregiver communication strategies, employing behavioral interventions (including positive programming), and training and implementing self-regulatory strategies have been highlighted. Education, training, and involvement of family members, professionals, and other caregivers are critical to the success of any intervention for behavioral difficulties.

REFERENCES

Alderman, N., Fry, R. K., & Youngson, H. A. (1995). Improvement of self-monitoring skills, reduction of behavior disturbance and the dysexecutive syndrome: Comparison of response cost and a new programme of self-monitoring training. *Neuropsychological Rehabilitation, 5*(3), 193–221.

Alderman, N., & Ward, A. (1991). Behavioral treatment of the dysexecutive syndrome: Reduction of repetitive speech using response cost and cognitive overlearning. *Neuropsychological Rehabilitation, 1*, 65–80.

Blake, G., Bogod, N., & Newbigging, T. (1995). *Establishing stimulus control over the attention seeking behaviors of a memory impaired, brain injured adult.* Paper presented at the meeting of the International Applied Behavior Analysis Conference, Washington, DC.

Burgess, P. W., & Alderman, N. (1990). Rehabilitation of discontrol syndromes following frontal lobe damage: A cognitive neuropsychological approach. In R. L. Wood & I. Fussey (Eds.), *Cognitive rehabilitation in perspective* (pp. 183–203). London: Taylor & Francis.

Cicerone, K. D., & Wood, J. C. (1987). Planning disorder after closed head injury: A case study. *Archives of Physical Medicine and Rehabilitation, 68*, 111–115.

Donnelan, A. M., LaVigna, G. W., Negri-Shoulz, N., & Fassbender, L. L. (1988). *Progress without punishment: Effective approaches for learners with behavior problems.* New York: Teachers College Press.

Davis, J. R., Turner, W., Rolder, A., & Cartwright, T. (1994). Natural and structured baselines in the treatment of aggression following brain injury. *Brain Injury, 8*(7), 589–597.

Feeney, T. J., & Ylvisaker, M. (1995). Choice and routine: Antecedent behavioral interventions for adolescents with severe traumatic brain injury. *Journal of Head Trauma Rehabilitation, 10*(3), 67–86.

Graham, S., & Harris, K. R. (1989). A component analysis of cognitive strategy instruction: Effects on learning disabled students' compositions and self-efficacy. *Journal of Educational Psychology, 81*, 353–361.

Hanlon, R., Clontz, B., & Thomas, M. (1993). Management of severe behavioural dyscontrol following subarachnoid haemorrhage. *Neuropsychological Rehabilitation, 3*(1), 63–76.

Harris, K. R. (1990). Developing self-regulated learners: The role of private speech and self-instructions. *Educational Psychologist, 25*, 35–50.

Hersen, M., & Bellack, A. S. (Eds.). (1988). *Dictionary of behavioral assessment techniques*. New York: Pergamon Press.

Jacobs, H. E. (1993). *Behavior analysis guidelines and brain injury rehabilitation: People, principles, and programs*. Gaithersburg, MD: Aspen.

Lawson, M. J., & Rice, D. N. (1989). Effects of training in use of executive strategies on a verbal memory problem resulting from closed head injury. *Journal of Clinical and Experimental Neuropsychology, 11*, 942–954.

Levin, H. S., Goldstein, F. C., Williams, D. H., & Eisenberg, H. M. (1991). The contribution of frontal lobe lesions to the neurobehavioral outcome of closed head injury. In H. S. Levin, H. M. Eisenberg, & A. L. Benton (Eds.), *Frontal lobe function and dysfunction* (pp. 318–338). New York: Oxford University Press.

Lezak, M. (1978). Living with the characterologically altered brain damaged patient. *Journal of Clinical Psychology, 39*, 592–598.

Mateer, C. A. (1997). Rehabilitation of individuals with frontal lobe impairment. In J. Leon-Carrion (Ed.), *Neuropsychological rehabilitation: Fundamentals, innovations and directions* (pp. 285–300). Delray Beach, FL: GR Press/St. Lucie Press.

McGlynn, S. M. (1990). Behavioral approaches to neuropsychological rehabilitation. *Psychological Bulletin, 108*, 420–441.

Meichenbaum, D. (1985). *Stress inoculation training*. New York: Pergamon Press.

Prigatano, G. (1992). Personality disturbances associated with traumatic brain injury. *Journal of Consulting and Clinical Psychology, 60*, 360–368.

Prigatano, G., Fordyce, D. J., Zeiner, H. K., Roueche, J. R., Pepping, M., & Wood, B. C. (1986). *Neuropsychological rehabilitation after brain injury*. Baltimore: Johns Hopkins University Press.

Sbordone, R. (1990). Psychotherapeutic treatment of the client with traumatic brain injury: A conceptual model. In J. S. Kreutzer & P. Wehman (Eds.), *Community integration following traumatic brain injury* (pp. 125–138). Baltimore: Paul H. Brookes.

Sohlberg, M. M., Glang, A., & Todis, B. (1998). Improvement during baseline: Three case studies encouraging collaborative research when evaluating caregiver training. *Brain Injury, 12*, 333–346.

Stuss, D. T., & Benson, F. D. (1986). *The frontal lobes*. New York: Raven Press.

Stuss, D. T., Delgado, M., & Guzman, D. A. (1987). Verbal regulation in the control of motor impersistence. *Journal of Neurological Rehabilitation, 1*, 19–24.

Wood, R. (1987). *Brain injury rehabilitation: A neurobehavioral approach*. London: Croom Helm.

Ylvisaker, M., & Feeney, T. (1998). Everyday people as supports: Developing competencies through collaboration. In M. Ylvisaker (Ed.), *Traumatic brain injury: Children and adolescents* (pp. 429–464). Newton, MA: Butterworth-Heinemann.

APPENDIX 11.1

SAMPLE ANGER MANAGEMENT SCALE

Behaviors and actions—related to how angry or frustrated you are	Scale	Acceptable limit of behavior
No anger or frustration; relaxed; no muscle tension; no increase in voice; easy breathing	0	Acceptable in all situations
Some frustration; slight increase in breathing; increased voice; increased speed of talking; changes in posture	1	Acceptable in all situations
Getting more frustrated; getting a little warm; further increase in breathing; raising voice; slight increase in heart rate	2	Maximum acceptable level for work
Increased frustration; loud voice; tapping foot; pointing finger; moving around; agitated; starting to clinch fist	3	Maximum level at home or social situations
Increased frustration/anger; face gets red; loud voice; angry face; leaning toward person; making fist; wide-eyed; aggressive	4	Requires time out and relaxation
Increased frustration/anger; swearing; short quick breaths; use of swearing in one out of three sentences; hitting fist on knee/table	5	Maximum level for therapy situations
Breaking pencils; rapid speech in loud voice; gritting teeth; tight jaw; fast heartbeat	6	Unacceptable in all situations
Hitting desks or objects; throwing objects; heart starts to pound; very agitated; angry	7	Unacceptable in all situations
Yelling; short, rapid breaths; very agitated and threatening; can't think clearly; very hot/warm	8	Unacceptable in all situations
Noticeable swearing; sweating; highly agitated	9	Unacceptable in all situations
Hitting walls, objects, persons; mouth dry; screaming; driving recklessly, out of control	10	Unacceptable in all situations

12

Management of Depression and Anxiety

As the field of brain injury rehabilitation has evolved, attention has increasingly focused on identifying and minimizing the most important roadblocks to successful community reintegration. It is widely acknowledged that the emotional, behavioral, and psychological effects of brain injury are often the most enduring and problematic barriers to community reentry (see, e.g., Ben-Yishay & Daniels-Zide, 2000; Lezak, 1987; Rosenthal & Bond, 1990). Despite their importance, there are still few theories or techniques for assessing changes in mood and anxiety levels following brain injury. The complex interaction among the biological, psychological, and environmental variables poses a significant challenge to understanding, evaluating, and managing changes in these domains.

This chapter focuses on treatment strategies to manage some of the more common psychoemotional issues that emerge following acquired brain injury. Many individuals who have suffered a brain injury experience reactive depression (e.g., Adjustment Reaction with Depressed Mood) and/or anxiety reactions (e.g., Posttraumatic Stress Disorder, Panic Disorder). They may also exhibit difficulties with affect regulation, including emotional lability, irritability, and anger. Emotional changes are noted to occur after head injuries of a range of severity, and with little correlation found between injury severity and degree of emotional disturbance by 12 months after injury (McCleary et al., 1998). An individual with acquired brain injury may also have had premorbid personality traits or disorders that interact with the brain injury to affect the outcome significantly.

BASIC TERMINOLOGY

Mood is usually understood as the frame of mind or emotional state of a person—the internal experience of feeling (Hinsie & Campbell, 1970). Normally it is defined by the internal state of mind, not the external behavioral manifestations, and as such is typically assessed by self-report measures.

Affect, in contrast, connotes behaviors or external manifestations of feeling, mood, or emotion. Affect can include pervasive and enduring characteristics of behavior and temperament, and/or momentary or rapidly changing manifestations of fluctuating emotional states. Characteristics ascribed to affect include facial expressions, tone of voice, and body language; these constitute the outward expression of the inward feeling, and may or may not be associated strongly with ideation or cognition. The fact that observed affect sometimes does not coincide with an individual's mood is well recognized, particularly in the context of a number of neurological disorders. Dissociations of mood and affect are striking symptoms, for example, of psuedobulbar palsy (Lieberman & Benson, 1977), and right-sided cerebrovascular accidents (Bryden & Ley, 1983).

Emotion is far more difficult to define, and the term is often used broadly and vaguely. It is usually considered as an internal affective state in which strong or excited mental or mood states (e.g., joy, sorrow, fear) are experienced. It links affective behavioral responses with underlying thoughts and feelings, and is influenced by arousal.

Personality is usually thought of as the sum of characteristics or qualities that make an individual a unique self. It is manifested in individual, and to some extent predictable, behavior–response patterns that each person evolves both consciously and unconsciously in response to internal and external demands. "The personality functions to maintain a stable, reciprocal relationship between the person and his [sic] environment" (Hinsie & Campbell, 1970).

Psychosocial behavior and *interpersonal skills* are considered to be the behaviors displayed in interactions with other individuals in social situations. They incorporate verbal and nonverbal communication, adherence to social norms, and the individual's general attitude and approach toward others.

ASSESSMENT OF PSYCHOSOCIAL DIFFICULTIES IN THE CONTEXT OF BRAIN INJURY

Acquired brain injury can affect an individual's mood both directly, as a result of damage to those parts of the brain involved in affect regulation, and indirectly, as a result of the consequences and sequelae of the injury itself.

Although much has been written about the assessment and management of anxiety and depression (Beck, 1991), there are additional considerations when the client presenting with these difficulties has a concomitant brain injury. Lewis (1991) has proposed a psychosocial evaluation model consisting of four components:

- *The neurological syndrome.* This consists of the specific neurological and associated cognitive and behavioral difficulties.
- *The psychological impact of the injury.* This includes the meaning and impact of the deficits for an individual. It also includes such potential factors as guilt, fear, loss, shame, and entitlement, to name but a few.
- *Psychological factors independent of the injury.* This includes the premorbid personality style and traits, family dynamics, and relationship issues that influence how the individual responds to the injury. It includes such constructs as premorbid adjustment, self-satisfaction, self-awareness, motivation, goal orientation, stage of life, coping skills, and *locus of control* (the degree to which the person feels a sense of control over his or her life and circumstances).
- *Social context of the injury.* This includes the makeup of the client's family, peer group, and work systems, as well as the ways these groups respond to the client's injury and its consequences (e.g., how empathic, protective, dismissive, etc., members of these groups are).

There are obvious overlaps between this model and the one presented by Sbordone (1990) as discussed in Chapter 11. Both encourage clinicians designing interventions to look at the neurological and neuropsychological factors specific to the injury; preinjury factors; the role of the family; and community issues related to work, leisure, and the social environment. Both taxonomies also anticipate individual variability in response to a neurological event. Consideration of these four components should guide a clinician's assessment and subsequent planning of any psychosocial intervention. The following profile of a client who sustained a brain injury illustrates application of the model.

Case Example of Applying the Lewis Assessment Model

Prior to receiving a moderate brain injury in a motor vehicle accident, Janet was a 31-year-old high-achieving individual who worked in the fast-paced world of emerging Internet technology. Her identity was very much tied to her profession and to her accomplishments at work (significant *psychological factors independent of the injury*). She had always been a strong student, and prior to the injury had spent an average of 50 hours a week at work. This information was gleaned through interview; a review of her academic, vocational, and social history; and administration of a personality inventory. A review of her medical records suggested that relevant *neurological syndrome variables* included the fact that there was a 40-minute loss of consciousness, and that she had been resuscitated at the scene. She had remained somewhat agitated and had demonstrated rather florid confabulations for several days, suggesting some possible executive function impairment. A neuropsychological assessment 15 months after the injury suggested generally very strong recovery, but revealed some persisting difficulties with divided attention, working memory, and executive functions. An interview with Janet further suggested these important *social context variables*: She had felt she needed to get back to work as soon as possible, and thus she had attempted to return to full-time employment (with no change in her work duties or schedule) within 2 months of her discharge from a 5-day hospital stay. Finally, a review of medical records, and phone interviews with her employer and her significant other, indicated that *relevant psychological impact variables* included the fact that she was reporting headaches, decreased concentration, and problems with irritability following the injury. Janet had "blown up" at others several times at work, and she had received the first negative work evaluation in her career. She had sought medical attention and was told that neurologically she appeared to have no residual effects from the accident and was probably experiencing difficulties with stress management. Interview and a depression inventory further substantiated that Janet was feeling depressed and despondent.

Systematically considering each of the four components in Lewis's (1991) model as a framework to organize the assessment results revealed that the client had a vulnerable preinjury personality and lifestyle (she had been a high achiever in a highly competitive employment field). This might have put her at higher risk for a dysfunctional and prolonged response to brain injury (Kay, Newman, Cavallo, Ezrachi, & Resnick, 1992). Second, although there was clear evidence in the medical record of a brain injury, her neurological recovery had been very strong, to the extent that medical doctors were no longer viewing brain injury as a basis for her complaints. Third, she had taken very little time for recovery and returned fully to her work and home responsibilities within a short time of her injury. This increased the likelihood that she would experience difficulties, which would further contribute to the development of negative emotional reactions. Finally, she had experienced significant "failure" since the accident, which (in the absence of supportive education or intervention) resulted in loss of confidence, shaken identity, and depression. Based on these findings, treatment might include a plan to educate and support her with regard to the brain injury and to address the identity issues, while simultaneously recommending strategies to manage real and/or perceived changes in attention/concentration, memory, and organization (e.g., pacing, note taking, etc.).

Although a detailed discussion of diagnostic techniques and tools for the evaluation of mood and other psychiatric disturbances is beyond the scope of this chapter, it is important to stress that care must always be taken in sorting out what may be symptoms of an emotional nature, and

TABLE 12.1. Potentially Confusing "Emotional" Symptoms of Brain Damage

Psychogenic/psychiatric symptoms	Neurogenic syndrome
Denial	Anosognosia (lack of awareness of impairment)
Anger and irritability	Frustration, catastrophic reaction, reduced information processing, lowered anger threshold
Depression	Lack of initiative, impaired emotional expressiveness, lowered crying threshold, fatigue
Rigid compulsive/hypervigilant symptoms	Distractibility, inability to deal with more than one task at a time, dependence on external controls
Emotional lability (rapid fluctuation of the feeling state)	Lability of emotional expressiveness (rapid fluctuation of affect, but not necessarily of the underlying feeling state)
Social withdrawal	Lack of initiative
Sense of futurelessness	Impaired planning
Thought disorder	Aphasia, anomia, confabulation, or confusion
Personality or conduct disorder	Impulsivity, social disinhibition

what may be symptoms characteristic of the neurological effects of brain injury (see Table 12.1). Hence the alert clinician must carefully ascertain the correct differential diagnosis of an individual with an acquired brain injury. Diagnosis of mood and other psychiatric disorders should only be undertaken by individuals with appropriate training and experience.

COMMON EMOTIONAL REACTIONS TO ACQUIRED BRAIN INJURY

Various emotional changes following brain injury may best be considered as normal, understandable reactions to changes in an individual's circumstances and in capabilities. The most common reactions to acquired brain injury, particularly in the postacute state, include depression, anxiety, lowered self-esteem, dependency, and perplexity.

• *Depression.* The clinician evaluating the psychosocial status of a person with acquired brain injury must be very cautious about making a diagnosis of a Major Depressive Episode. Even though this syndrome can be seen in this population, there is a great deal of overlap between the symptoms of depression and other psychosocial and cognitive sequelae of brain injury. Examples of overlapping symptomatology include decreased energy; decreased initiation; irritability; difficulty with decision making; concentration and memory problems; lack of concern regarding physical appearance; decreased libido; sleep disturbance; self-criticism; and flattened affect. Moreover, it has been suggested that when an individual sustains an injury to the frontal convexity (lateral cortical surfaces) the result is a psuedodepression, with decreased initiation and deficiencies in thought formation (Blumer & Benson, 1975). Depressed symptoms most commonly can be seen as a result of Adjustment Reaction with Depressed Mood. This can occur as a consequence of losses resulting from an injury (e.g., losses in independence, ability to engage in normal activities, ability to function effectively at work). Adjustment Reaction with Depressed Mood can occur without any premorbid history of depression, whereas a Major Depressive Episode is more commonly associated with a history of depression. Accurate diagnosis is important, particularly because antidepressant medications may be overused in individuals with reactive depression.

• *Anxiety.* Anxiety is typically manifested as nervousness, insecurity, or fear. Individuals with anxiety often appear outwardly tense, hypervigilant, and tight in their movements. They may also demonstrate tremor in their voice and movement, nervous mannerisms, rapid speech, rapid pulse, and rapid breathing. Anxiety typically reflects an individual's difficulty in coping with stressful situations. Panic attacks and stress-induced "neurological events" are also included in this category, although it should be noted that organic factors may precipitate such events. Symptoms include such subjective feelings as tingling or loss of sensation in the fingers and toes, pseudoseizures, sweating, and skin reactions such as hives. In the individual with brain injury, anxiety may arise as a result of realistic perceptions of reduction in functional ability, an increase in experience of failure, and/or a general fear and concern about what the future may hold.

• *Decreased self-esteem.* In individuals without brain injury who are seeking psychotherapy for problems relating to low self-esteem, the underlying causes are commonly misperceptions about people's reaction to them or their performance, depression, and/or a developmental history that may have led to self-devaluation. In the case of individuals with acquired brain injury, they may have experienced a real decline in function, and their perception of the decline in their capacities may well be accurate. This perception can be very damaging to their self-image. Realistic self-appraisal is typically thought to be of value in the recovery from brain injury, so treatment may include support, encouragement, and a focus on the objective nature of the impairments and on spared or recovered abilities.

• *Dependency.* Feelings of dependency and helplessness are primarily learned. In individuals without brain injury, feelings of helplessness can result when they see themselves as less capable and/or more out of control than they actually are. Psychotherapeutic efforts are designed to increase such individuals' sense of competence. The feelings of helplessness in persons with brain injury may well have emerged from very real decreases in ability to control and manage the environment, particularly in the acute stages of recovery. For many of these individuals, increased feelings of capability and control will decrease subjective feelings of need for help. In other patients, excessive emotional and physical dependency on others may develop and be manifested as exaggerated fear or distress at being alone or separated from a certain person, and/or reliance on others to provide constant or unneeded reassurance and assistance. Again, achieving a realistic perception of skills, abilities, and practical needs is a critical step in assisting someone to achieve a maximally independent, yet safe and supportive, living and work situation.

• *Perplexity.* Many patients with acquired brain injury experience confusion and bewilderment regarding their own reduced or unreliable skills and abilities; this phenomenon is often termed *perplexity.* Such individuals may suddenly find themselves at a loss for even simple words in a conversation, unable to remember an important point in a conversation made just moments before, or unable to add the numbers in a simple game of cards. These problems can be particularly confusing to a patient with a minor head injury who has not been told to expect problems, and who appears to others to be functioning well.

Several large-scale studies have recently addressed the incidence of mood and other psychiatric disturbance following acquired brain injury. Hibbard, Uysal, Kepler, Bogdany, and Silver (1998) looked at the incidence, comorbidity, and patterns of resolution of *Diagnostic and Statistical Manual of Mental Disorders,* fourth edition (DSM-IV; American Psychiatric Association, 1994) disorders and episodes in 100 adults with traumatic brain injury (TBI). The Structured Clinical Interview for DSM-IV (SCID) was used to determine diagnoses prior to the brain injury, during the acute phase of TBI recovery, and in the postacute phase. Prior to TBI, a significant percentage of individuals presented with substance use disorders. After TBI, the most frequent diagnoses were Major Depressive Episode and substance use disorders, followed by select anxiety disorders (i.e., Posttraumatic Stress Disorder, Obsessive–Compulsive Disorder, and Panic Disorder). (See Appendix 12.1 for descriptions of DSM-IV disorders and episodes commonly encountered in persons with brain injury.) Comorbidity was high, with 44% of individuals presenting with two or more DSM-IV diagnoses. Taylor and Jung (1998) also reported that mood disorders and episodes occur after TBI with a higher frequency than in the general population, with estimates approaching 25–50% for Major Depressive Episode, 15–30% for Dysthymic Disorder, and 9% for Manic Episode. These, as well as other recent studies (Bowen, Chamberlain, Tennant, Neumann, & Connor, 1999; McCleary et al., 1998; van Reekum, Bolago, Finlayson, Garner, & Links, 1996), all demonstrate that TBI must be seen as a risk factor for subsequent psychiatric difficulties. Clearly, proactive assessment and timely intervention for these problems in individuals with brain injury are warranted, particularly because of the potential for problems in these areas to have a negative impact on recovery and community reintegration.

An increased incidence of psychiatric and emotional disturbance following TBI-related brain damage is not a surprise, given that such injuries commonly affect regions of the brain that have been recognized as important in the regulation of mood. These include the dorsolateral and orbitofrontal cortex, the basal ganglia, the amygdala, and the temporal lobes. As yet, however, there is insufficient information to postulate a specific neuroanatomical model for post-TBI psychiatric disturbance, given the variable nature of TBI-related injury and the many other pre- and postinjury variables that can affect psychological and psychoemotional functioning.

PRINCIPLES OF PSYCHOTHERAPEUTIC INTERVENTIONS

Laying the Foundations of the Therapeutic Relationship

As in all therapy, it is essential that the clinician build a relationship with a client who has a brain injury, as well as provide the client with all the information needed to make informed choices. The clinician needs to teach the client the necessary skills for eventually managing his or her own emotional difficulties. Several steps are involved in this, including building rapport, validating the client's experience, offering psychoeducation, and teaching relaxation strategies.

Building Rapport

Psychotherapy is a collaborative process that requires much trust on the part of the client. It is crucial that the clinician develop a safe environment where the client feels able to feel and express emotions and thoughts openly. The clinician can maintain good rapport by taking constant care that the client feels respected, and is comfortable and satisfied with the therapy relationship. Working with a psychologist, in particular, often implies to some clients (and families) that something is wrong with them psychiatrically. In building rapport, it may be helpful to steer away from emotionally charged issues initially, focusing on getting to know the person, asking about work, family, and interests. After having "connected" at a more conversational level, clients often volunteer emotional concerns or are less defensive if asked about their reactions.

Some clients may not perceive professionals as having recognized their symptoms, which can heighten vigilance for their own symptoms and can escalate their need for help (Cicerone, 1991). Beginning a therapeutic alliance by conducting an interview that allows a client to describe symptoms, in an atmosphere where he or she does not feel compelled to "convince" the clinician of the validity of the complaints, can be extremely beneficial to addressing psychosocial issues. Such an atmosphere can be fostered when (1) the clinician does not confront the client early on about possible psychoemotional underpinnings for reported physical and cognitive complaints; (2) the clinician offers options for explaining symptoms that include the possibility of an organic basis for symptoms; and (3) the clinician is optimistic about improvement, and indeed anticipates improvement, but in a conservative manner that does not make the client feel he or she will be "cured." If the client is being seen relatively soon after an injury, a number of preventative steps need to be taken, including counseling the client on a gradual return to work/school/home activities and setting realistic time frames for symptom recovery. A more detailed discussion and research support for this approach, with respect to mild TBI in particular, are presented in Chapter 15.

Validating Clients' Experience

Validating clients' experiences or reports of their symptoms is critical both for building a therapeutic alliance and for helping clients with some of the core identity issues that can result in a "shaken sense of self" or loss of confidence (see, e.g., Cicerone, 1992; Kay, 1992, 1993; Sohlberg, 2000). Clinicians need to validate clients' experience in a constructive manner— one that does not further focus them on their deficits, and that feels empathic yet not patronizing.

Use of the Most Troubling Symptom List form (see Appendix 12.2) can assist the interview process by encouraging a client to prioritize those issues that interfere the most with day-to-day functioning, and to reflect on how he or she responds to them. The use of an established protocol may also assist in structuring the client's report to avoid a "stream of consciousness," from which it can be hard to discern needed and salient information. In most cases, obtaining the information via an interview format is preferred to having the client fill out the form independently. An open-ended discussion of concerns and problems is usually preferable to a checklist in identifying the most pressing areas of difficulty.

Psychoeducation

An effective method for helping a client feel validated, while simultaneously increasing his or her knowledge about brain injury and its effects, is to provide structured opportunities to review educational materials. The goal is to demonstrate to the client that "experts" have written about issues with which he or she is personally confronted. The clinician can select either written or visual materials containing helpful information for that client. Examples of such materials may include an article on brain injury written for survivors/families or professionals; videotapes on different aspects of brain injury available from the Brain Injury Association; copies of pages from a book chapter discussing topics germane to that client; or pertinent Internet resources. The clinician can then review the materials with the client, and can structure activities to enhance the validation experience in one or more of the following ways:

• Highlighting in colored pen those sections in written materials relevant to a particular client.
• Giving assignments in which the client (1) summarizes the information, (2) underlines the sections to which he or she relates, (3) writes down questions that the reading evokes, and/or (4) writes more paragraphs to go with the reading that specifically describe his or her situation.
• Having the client "present" the information to other clients in a group therapy situation, or to significant others (see Chapter 9 on how to increase awareness after brain injury).
• Compiling references for families (see Holland & Shagaki, 1998; see also Chapter 13 on collaborating with families).
• Providing, or having the client provide, a list of Internet resources.

The type of exercise that is selected will depend upon the needs of the particular client. The client's psychosocial profile and stage in the treatment process will affect how the educational process is best implemented.

Teaching Relaxation Techniques

It is often beneficial for the clinician to talk with the client about the negative role that tension and anxiety play in physical, mental, and emotional well-being. Excess tension in muscles can exacerbate pain, make it difficult to concentrate, and cause fatigue. The clinician can provide one-on-one training about the sources of tension, how to recognize them, and how to induce relaxation. The techniques should then be practiced. A client will often benefit from listening to relaxation exercises on tape. The client should be encouraged to listen to the tape at least every evening and to practice the techniques throughout the day. Common approaches to relaxing include progressive relaxation exercises (e.g., "Tense your hand and then relax it"), autogenic training (e.g., "Your left arm is heavy and warm"), and visualization exercises (e.g., "Imagine yourself lying on a warm beach"). Different approaches work best with different people, so it may be useful to try a variety of techniques. Individuals who are compromised motorically, for example, may have more trouble relaxing if directed to tense muscles first. Other techniques for physical and mental relaxation may include physical exercise (e.g., stretching, running, walking the dog), taking a warm bath, listening to calming music, or lying down for a short rest. The negative impact of relying on alcohol or other drugs to achieve a sense of reduced tension should be emphasized, as substances can have unpredictable effects in a client with acquired brain injury and may limit recovery. Training in meditation skills may be useful for less compromised clients.

Traditional Forms of Psychotherapy

Historically, there has been a reluctance to recommend traditional forms of psychotherapy for individuals who have suffered brain injury. Proponents of the use of applied behavioral principles, behavioral interventions, and cognitive-behavioral therapy (CBT) in this population cite difficulties in implementing individual psychotherapy with persons who have compromised cognitive functioning. Indeed, some of the common cognitive difficulties following brain injury affect information processing and memory, potentially making traditional "talk-oriented" therapy less effective (Bock, 1987). A further obstacle to the use of traditional psychotherapy arises when clinicians do not have a sufficient background in acquired brain injury to understand changes in behavior and emotion from a neurological perspective (Sbordone, 1990).

There is actually little or no empirical evidence to support the notion that individuals with brain injury do not benefit from psychotherapeutic support. In the emotional realm, psychotherapy can be critical in producing and maintaining arousal for optimum learning; fostering hope, self-confidence, and trust; and combating despair, insecurity, fear, and suspicion. In the cognitive realm, psychotherapy can assist the client in achieving a new and more accurate understanding of his or her problems and ways of dealing with them. Behaviorally, the client is assisted in participating repetitively in activity that leads to behavioral changes outside the clinic situation. Prigatano (1991) views psychotherapy with individuals who have sustained brain injury as a learning experience, which teaches clients how to make honest and fair commitments to work, interpersonal relationships, and the development of individuality. These individuals have suffered a significant loss, and psychotherapy can help them through the grieving process, as well as aid them in accepting a "new self" and the new challenges that they may face.

Increasingly, the skepticism and pessimism regarding the role of psychotherapy with persons who have sustained brain injury have been challenged. Lewis (1991) has suggested that some clinicians' reluctance to treat clients with brain injury is based on their own discomfort rather than factors specific to the client. She proposes that the differences between clients with compromised versus normal neurological functioning have been overemphasized. In their literature reviews, Christensen and Rosenberg (1991) and Ben-Yishay and Daniels-Zide (2000) also make strong cases supporting psychotherapy as a critical part of brain injury rehabilitation. Judd (1999) describes and promotes what he terms *neuropsychotherapy*. It includes forms of intervention that arise out of some more traditional psychotherapeutic traditions, but modifies them so as to adapt to the needs of a person with a brain injury. He emphasizes the importance of providing additional repetition and structure both within and across settings, and the need to support learning and memory by providing written information, notes, frequent review and practice than might be needed for someone without a brain injury.

To some extent, behavioral therapy, CBT, and traditional individual psychotherapy can be viewed on a continuum. In the early stages after injury, when insight and awareness are low and the person is heavily dependent on the environment, environmental modifications and behavioral interventions are likely to be most useful. As the person improves, the training of self-regulation inherent in CBT can be extremely useful. In later stages, when the individual is coming to grips with potentially permanent changes in his or her ability, psychotherapeutic approaches can be helpful in assisting the person to deal with loss, as well as with changes in self-esteem and self-concept. Most clinicians who work with the behavioral, emotional, and psychosocial difficulties of persons who have sustained brain injury use methods drawn from a number of different treatment philosophies and traditions. Indeed, the heterogeneity of brain injury requires that a clinician be comfortable with and have access to tools from behavioral, counseling, neuropsychological, and psychotherapy disciplines.

Determining the source of functional disability after acquired brain injury can be the most challenging part of developing a treatment plan. Psychosocial problems may result from organic changes in brain functioning or from a reaction to real and/or perceived changes in ability across different domains. If, for example, an individual is experiencing anger management problems due to damage to those brain mechanisms involved in impulse control, a clinician may implement behavioral interventions such as those described in Chapter 11, as well as CBT techniques. Alternatively, if the anger problems primarily stem from identity issues or discrepancies between perceptions of one's premorbid and postinjury self, a combination of awareness training, education, and counseling (see Chapter 9) may be most appropriate. In either case, the clinician will need to have grounding in brain–behavior relationships and the nature of brain injury, as well as in traditional counseling methods.

Behavior Therapy

Behavior therapy is based on the notion that changes in behavior will result in changes in mood. Individuals with acquired brain injury often become isolated, and may have difficulty initiating or participating in previously enjoyed activities. The focus of behavior treatment is to facilitate activity, often coupled with diary keeping, to increase awareness of activity levels. This involves having a client identify, plan, and engage in activities that used to be enjoyable or that may be enjoyable now. Examples might include walking, swimming, or other forms of exercise; going to a park, mall, or movie; or going out to breakfast or dinner with friends.

Cognitive-Behavioral Therapy

CBT has been used with increasing frequency in the management of problems after brain injury (Raskin & Mateer, 2000). Indeed, CBT fares extremely well in discussions of evidence-based therapeutic efficacy for a broad range of psychological conditions and disorders in both the general and clinical populations (Task Force on Promotion and Dissemination of Psychological Procedures, 1995). CBT is based on the premise that the beliefs (or *cognitions*) one holds, and the nature of the self-statements one makes, have a large influence on behavior (Dobson, 1990). For example, many people who are depressed express feelings of unworthiness, failure, and incapacity. The content of depressive thinking has been categorized in terms of a *cognitive triad*. This consists of distorted, negative views of (1) the self (e.g., "I'm useless"), (2) current experience (e.g., "Nobody will let me do anything"), and (3) the future (e.g., "I will never get any better"). Such negative and derogatory self-statements and beliefs are usually habitual, automatic, and involuntary, and they actually contribute to and help to maintain depressed mood and can exacerbate a cycle of negativity and withdrawal (see Table 12.2).

Negative beliefs and statements are often quite extreme and unrealistic (e.g., "There is simply no reason to live," "I'll never be able to do anything again"). In part, CBT focuses on identifying and modifying such extreme or unrealistic beliefs—assisting the individual in treatment to see them as extreme, unrealistic, and dysfunctional, and helping him or her to develop more adaptive, coping beliefs and attitudes. Another important aspect of CBT is its emphasis on current behavior in everyday settings. A key component of the treatment is identifying, quantifying, and tracking specific behaviors, as well as the potentially dysfunctional thoughts and self-statements that precede, accompany, or follow specific behaviors. A concrete way to do this is with a Daily Record of Dysfunctional Thoughts form (see Appendix 12.3 for a filled-in example). Another key component of therapy is scheduling and tracking positive events and activities. In its emphasis on behavioral tracking, it is similar to straight behavioral interventions; it is different in that it incorporates and emphasizes the influence of associated thoughts and beliefs about the behaviors. Another similarity to behavior therapy is that it deemphasizes the role of historical factors and/or the ini-

TABLE 12.2. Examples of Common Cognitive Distortions

Overgeneralization: Assuming that outcomes of one event necessarily predict outcomes of future or similar events.
  "I forgot to check the meter. I can't do anything right."

Selective abstraction: Selectively attending to negative aspects of one's experience.
  "I didn't have a moment's pleasure today."

Dichotomous thinking: Thinking in extremes.
  "If I can't do it like I did before, there's no point doing it at all."

Arbitrary inference: Jumping to conclusions on the basis of inadequate evidence.
  "I got angry again last night. This therapy will *never* work for me."

Catastrophizing: Self-statements, thoughts, and images anticipating the worst possible outcome of events and situations.
  "I'll never be able to get another job."

Personalization: Taking responsibility for things that have little or nothing to do with oneself.
  "My speech therapist is moving away. She must hate me."

tial origins of the behaviors or thoughts, instead focusing on the here and now.

Assisting Clients with Accepting their Current Level of Functioning

Many clients with acquired brain injury will face the arduous task of learning to live with the sequelae of their injury. For many, the new self will be rejected in favor of the old sense of who they were. Many clients, for example, talk about the "old me" and the "new me." Two sample therapy activities to work on developing a more realistic and balanced sense of self are described below.

• A clinician can have a client construct a list of positive personal traits that have *not* changed as a result of the accident. Together, the clinician and client can make a list of core traits that have not changed. These traits may include specific abilities such as math or writing skills, or a specific domain of knowledge, as well as personality characteristics such as "being a caring person." The purpose of this task is to encourage the client to build upon existing strengths, instead of focusing on symptoms. Constructing a similar list of "coping skills" can also be valuable. This allows clients to identify useful strategies they can use and see themselves as being able to add new skills if needed.

• For some clients who are very symptom-focused, it can be counterproductive to attempt to "cure," or even to address the "management" of, persistent symptoms. For these clients, it may be most effective to validate their frustration with reported problems and to acknowledge the difficulty the symptoms present. Directing therapy at discussing how to exploit residual talents to achieve future goals (instead of addressing ongoing problems) can be a helpful way in which to approach treatment. Appendix 12.4 is a form that can be used to help such clients reconcile their perceptions of their past, present, and future selves and abilities. Improved self-confidence may result from the focus on strengths. Sometimes, however, there is a somewhat paradoxical response, in that a client actually begins to attempt to convince the clinician that the symptoms are manageable.

Challenging Distorted or Dysfunctional Thoughts

CBT holds that a significant amount of distress and inner turmoil arises from distorted or dysfunctional thoughts. These are often thoughts that emphasize perceived faults or failures, or that focus on the potential negative outcomes of actions or interactions. After any kind of severe loss, it is not uncommon for individuals to begin feeling hopeless and to see their situation in only the darkest fashion. This phenomenon can be further exacerbated in individuals with brain injury, particularly those exhibiting dysexecutive phenomena. These individuals often present as quite rigid and inflexible in their thinking and behaving, seeing things in only one way. They may also tend to "get stuck on" particular thoughts, ideas, and/or themes, which tend to come up again and again (perseveration). Indeed, individuals with brain injury often develop a whole host of negative thoughts and feelings that can limit or prevent their adaptation and recovery.

One approach to dealing with negative beliefs and expectations is to encourage a weekly review of progress, in which the person records aspects of functioning or therapy that week that were successful, as well as ones that are still frustrating or problematic. Another approach, and one that can often be used successfully in a group, is an exercise in taking "balanced perspectives." Examples of extreme or negative statements are selected from the group or from an exercise book, and participants are challenged to come up with (in their minds or on paper) more realistic, rational, or positive statements. We have addressed such dysfunctional thoughts in a number of domains, including avoidance, denial, entitlement, guilt, and feelings of worthlessness. A few examples are provided below.

- Entitlement and victimization

  Examples of extreme or dysfunctional statements

  "I shouldn't have to live this way! It's just not fair!"
  "They owe me! I've suffered, and I'm going to get all I have coming
    to me!"

Examples of rational challenges

"What happened to me wasn't fair, and there is no reason I should like it. But the world isn't fair, and my only options are to make the most of what I have or give up."

"No matter what I get, it will not make what happened go away. My life will be most satisfying and most under my control if I select meaningful and realistic goals and work to achieve them."

- Guilt

Example of extreme or dysfunctional statement

"My injury was punishment (for my wrongdoing)."

Example of rational challenge

"I was not perfect before my injury—just like everyone else—but I was an OK person who didn't deserve bad things. Bad things happen to good people."

- Low self-esteem

Examples of extreme or dysfunctional statements

"I can't do anything right any more. I'm just no good."
"What I'm capable of doing isn't worth doing."

Examples of rational challenges

"I can't do some things as well as before, but I still have some abilities and potential for more improvement."

"I can learn to accept myself as I am by changing some of the ways I measure my self-worth. I am open to new possibilities and goals"

"Progress at any level and of any amount is important. I am gaining mastery and control little by little, day by day."

Once clients have begun to recognize their own dysfunctional thoughts, they can be encouraged to keep a daily record of them. In this context, it is useful to start to tie dysfunctional thoughts to particular situations, mood states, behaviors, and consequences. Appendix 12.3, as noted above, is a filled-in example of a Daily Record of Dysfunctional Thoughts. This form includes spaces for recording the situation, the nature and degree of associated emotions, the automatic (dysfunctional) thoughts, the rational responses, and the outcome. With somewhat higher-level clients, it may be useful to have them provide rating levels for different feelings, or ratings for how much they "believe" a particular statement.

Thought Stopping and Other Self-Regulatory Strategies

It is useful to help clients understand how disruptive their own self-talk and perseverative thinking can be. A client may benefit from the following suggestion: "When you find yourself getting stuck on a particular thought, think or say something aloud to yourself to move past that thought. Pick a few key specific phrases or reminders that work for you." Examples of such phrases could include:

- "Stop! There is nothing I can do about this [some problem] right now. Part of me wants to keep thinking about it, but it's not productive and I can't afford it."
- "Relax. Quiet my thoughts."
- "I'm starting to get stuck in my thinking. I know that now, so I'll *redirect* myself."
- "Time out for *mental control*. I'll think about that after lunch."
- "Easy does it. What am I doing now? What am I supposed to be doing now?"

Some clients find that it is useful to set aside a block of time each day as their designated "worry time." If they find themselves ruminating, then they put off their worry until the designated time. Clients often find that by the time the allotted time has come, the need and desire to worry have passed.

Making Written Plans for Managing Dysfunctional Thoughts and Behaviors

Many clients benefit from constructing a written plan for dealing with emotions and feelings. This is done in the context of a therapy session, and then used by a client as the occasion warrants. In the midst of frustration or confusion, being able to go to a written guide to find out what to do can be very helpful. For example, one young client with a dense amnesia following a brain injury had a section in her memory book called "When I get angry." It listed a number of activities that she could do when she felt angry or frustrated, most of which she generated. They included calling a friend, taking the dog for a walk, listening to music with earphones, tearing up bits of paper, and hitting her pillows. Written plans are only useful if they are easily accessible, so they should be kept in a memory book or organizer, pasted in a conspicuous place in the person's wallet or purse, or (in the case of someone who tends to dwell on things after going to bed) kept on a bedside table. Written plans should not be long or complicated, or they will not be used or read when needed. Rather, they should be simple and have specific key words or phrases that have a clear meaning for the client. It is also useful to incorporate a log or some other way to keep track of how often dysfunctional thoughts, feelings, or emotions occur, and how the person deals with them. Interestingly, simply writing such thoughts down can actually decrease rather than increase recurrent thoughts. These sorts of "action plans" can be added to as needed. They are most functional and likely to be used if the injured person takes a major role in generating the specific words or phrases to be included on the list.

Fostering Personal Empowerment and Self-Sufficiency

Individuals who feel victimized by their injury, or who have lost and are attempting to regain independence, feel powerless and controlled by others. An important component of therapeutic involvement is to increase a sense of self-mastery and self-efficacy. For example, facilitating an understanding of what triggers attentional lapses, and of what steps can be taken to reduce them or their impact, can be enormously empowering. This same approach—that of increasing self-knowledge and increasing self-regulation—can be applied to a broad range of mood states, emotions, and behaviors. Another way to achieve this goal is to increase the client's sense of responsibility both for self and for others. For example, having regular chores, or volunteering even 1 hour a week, can decrease depression and isolation and improve self-esteem. Even having the individual be responsible for selecting and scheduling one "pleasurable event" a week is potentially empowering, and is often a key component of cognitive-behavioral therapy for depression.

The Intervention Sequence

The techniques discussed above can be modified and used to address a wide variety of emotional and psychosocial problems, including difficulties with stress, fear, frustration, irritability, anger, impulsivity, lability, and pain. The most effective approaches combine behavioral charting and monitoring techniques with counseling support. The basic sequence of treatment is listed below.

1. *Identify the target problem behavior or feeling.* This step will necessarily involve interviewing the client and significant others, as well as conducting some monitoring to determine the nature, frequency, and antecedents/consequences associated with the problem.

2. *Generate a list of options for addressing the problem.* During this phase, the clinician describes and enumerates with the client a variety of intervention options that may be helpful for coping with the identified problem. These may include techniques to manage the response to a problem (e.g., stress management techniques for when a client becomes confused),

as well as specific compensatory techniques (e.g., a verbal mediation technique to decrease onset of confusion). This activity, in and of itself, provides a good opportunity to train "brainstorming" skills.

3. *Client selects most appropriate option.* The idea in this step is that the client reviews the list of options and selects the treatment approach seen as most suited to his or her individual situation. The important factor is that the client be given control over the selection to increase personal investment in the options, and to feel personal ownership of the strategy's success. This process may involve modifying some of the treatment options.

4. *Clinician provides training and support for implementing treatment strategy.* The client receives information specific to how, when, and where to implement the selected treatment option. This phase of treatment may involve the client's and/or significant others' completing incident logs and reports. The clinician may also develop some type of structured cueing system to remind the client to implement the strategy (e.g., notes in appointment book, reminder phone calls, Post-It Notes for refrigerator, etc.).

5. *Wean client from clinician support.* The goal of this last step is to ensure maintenance and generalization of the strategy's use beyond the therapy environment. The clinician may gradually decrease the amount and type of cueing as well as the frequency of visits, eventually placing the client on a "follow-up" schedule.

This approach to therapy is grounded in the principles of applied behavior analysis as well as CBT. An important component is the involvement of the client in generating and selecting the specific treatment strategy and in monitoring and describing the problem behavior or feeling. This helps the client take responsibility for the success of the intervention. Incorporating a self-evaluative approach for treatment strategies that the client has endorsed as having potential to fit with his or her lifestyle, personality, and abilities can be very effective for addressing some of the psychoemotional problems that tend to maintain emotional symptoms late after an injury.

Recognizing and Working with Preexisting Personality Features

Premorbid personality characteristics or styles may heighten vulnerability to prolonged dysfunction following brain injury and may interact with treatment efforts. For some individuals, the feelings evoked as a result of the injury and the reactions of others may trigger unresolved emotional issues from the past regarding vulnerability, victimization, fear of abandonment, and loss of control. These feelings and reactions, if not recognized and accommodated within the treatment plan, can result in limited success and feelings of frustration all around. Individuals with characteristics of overachievement and perfectionistic tendencies; grandiosity and narcissistic features; and borderline personality traits and recurrent depression may be at particular risk for prolonged disability and poor response to treatment (Kay et al., 1992). Ruff, Camenzuli, and Mueller (1996) have provided an excellent description of some of the emotional risk factors that influence the outcome of TBI in particular, as well as valuable implications for intervention.

Grandiosity and Narcissistic Features

Individuals who have a premorbid pattern of grandiosity with narcissistic features, by definition, have a strong need to feel and be seen as important. Such clients may report previously "superlative" skills and impress the examiner with prior accomplishments. They may describe their relationships in glowing terms, but further investigation may reveal underlying difficulties and issues of control. They may gather vast amounts of information, juggle newly learned technology, and interact as colleagues with health care professionals. They may tend to see their problems as unique and unable to be understood by the vast majority of people. Such individuals are likely to be very critical of health care professionals and to dismiss them easily. They may be somewhat manipulative of others, frequently missing or wanting to change appointments, and expecting special services. They may verbally embrace the injury and its effects as important, yet reject any suggestion of limitations or restrictions.

With such an individual, it is important to determine the extent to which losses have injured the client's underlying self-image. The clinician must avoid being flattered as a "high-status professional" or the "only one who understands," as this may reflect and feed into the client's need to feel special and unique. Unrealistic expectations must be confronted, since the client may expect special treatment or "magic bullets." Moreover, it is important for the clinician to avoid embracing the client's overly positive outlook, when it is unrealistic. Individuals with narcissistic tendencies tend not to be concerned about the needs of others at the best of times; it may be useful in such a case to work toward the client's understanding that one of the effects of brain injury is often becoming somewhat "selfish," and talking about the need to think about and practice empathy toward others.

Borderline Personality Traits and Recurrent Depression

Individuals who have a premorbid history of borderline personality features tend to have a very unstable sense of self. They may fluctuate rapidly between a sense of emptiness and unworthiness at one extreme and overconfidence at the other. Their sense of self is also very fragile and easily shattered, and they are quick to perceive abandonment. They tend to have intense and unstable personal relationships, with extremes of overideal-ization (where they see primarily positive traits in people) and devaluation (where they see primarily negative traits). They tend to be quite affectively unstable as well, with fluctuating depression, irritability, and anxiety. Anger control may be similarly fragile.

For example, we worked with one young woman who had sustained a brain injury resulting in only mild cognitive impairments, but also in right-sided nerve damage affecting her hand and wrist. She returned to school, where she had been in the top 10% of her first-year medical school class, but saw herself as a total failure after receiving a B on an exam and dropped out. She was quick to blame others for her failure, while at the same time feeling despondent. She felt there was no point in living unless she could go on to her intended career as a cardiac surgeon. Assessment revealed that she had had several emotionally abusive relationships, as well as a history of binge eating and purging.

With such a client, it is important to anticipate distortions and to recognize and avoid adopting the client's all-or-none thinking. The injury and its consequences are likely to further disturb the client's unstable sense of self and to open old feelings of failure. It is also important to monitor impulsivity. Individuals with borderline personality traits are often somewhat impulsive and unpredictable in their behavior. This can be exaggerated by executive dysfunction secondary to injury, putting such individuals at particular risk for self-injury, including suicide. Therapeutic support is essential to deal with reactivity of mood. In addition, when a clinician treating such a patient is working within a rehabilitation team, it is important to be aware of the potential for dividing the staff that the client's characteristics create—especially his or her unpredictable fluctuation between idealization and devaluation of health care professionals. The only person on the team who is seen to "really understand" on one day may be totally dismissed on another. The team will benefit from understanding and working together around such dynamics.

Overachievers with Perfectionistic Tendencies

Individuals with a long-term pattern of high achievement needs, perfectionistic tendencies, and stress may have a complicated recovery from brain injury. This is due to the dysfunctional loops that frequently develop among even minor cognitive failures, perfectionistic tendencies, and heightened levels of stress. They may have had a preexisting focus on work, and may have derived a large part of their sense of identity from their employment. They are also likely to have strong negative reactions to any imperfections they perceive in their work. Such individuals often have a tendency to experience stress in primarily physical symptomatology (e.g., fatigue, headache, dizziness, fluctuating vision). They may also have a somewhat restricted expression of affect and may demonstrate inflexibility and rigidity.

An important implication for working with such an individual, from a rehabilitation perspective, is to evaluate and analyze the stressors the person is experiencing. Next the clinician should determine how the stressors are currently affecting the client, and how stress is being manifested. The next step is to assist the client to understand how perfectionism fuels stress, and how stress and negativity can exacerbate cognitive failures, headaches, and fatigue. Stress management training may need to take into account long-standing difficulty in dealing with stressors. The clinician should also strive to recognize that premorbid daily stressors are now compounded by injury-related stressors. A critical component is to assist the individual in moving from a rigid perspective about perceived demands and needs for flawless performance, and to move to a more multidimensional and relativistic way of thinking.

Premorbid personality features such as the ones described above should not be seen as the cause of symptoms, but as factors that interact with response to and recovery from the common symptoms of brain injury. In addition to the loss of function itself, the meaning the individual assigns to the losses can have a profound impact on recovery (Ruff et al., 1996). The feelings evoked by the injury, as well as the reactions of others, may trigger unresolved emotional issues, reduce the person's strategies for coping, and undermine his or her traditional sources of self-esteem. Understanding these interactions and being able to anticipate some of the potential roadblocks in the recovery process are important components of psychotherapeutic interventions. Similar qualities and behavioral responses can be present in family members and be similarly challenging for the rehabilitation team.

SUMMARY

Effective psychosocial therapy depends on understanding the variety of common emotional and cognitive consequences of brain injury, and the ways they interact with current and premorbid factors. The personality and emotional functioning of a person before and after injury, the injury itself, and the context in which the person must function all affect the outcome and the response to rehabilitation. An eclectic repertoire of skills—including laying the foundations of a therapeutic relationship, and understanding and implementing behavioral interventions, CBT, and other psychotherapeutic techniques—is necessary for providing effective intervention. Personality features and traits have both positive and negative impacts on recovery, and treatment must consider these aspects of individuals to be maximally effective.

REFERENCES

American Psychiatric Association (1994). *Diagnostic and statistical manual of mental disorders* (4th ed.). Washington, DC: Author.

Beck, A. T. (1991). Cognitive therapy. *American Psychologist, 46*, 368–375.

Ben-Yishay, Y., & Daniels-Zide, E. (2000). Examined lives: Outcomes after holistic rehabilitation. *Rehabilitation Psychology, 45*, 112–129.

Blumer, D., & Benson, D. F. (1975). Personality changes with frontal and temporal lobe lesions. In D. F. Benson & D. Blumer (Eds.), *Psychiatric aspects of neurologic disease* (pp. 151–170). New York: Grune & Stratton.

Bock, S. H. (1987). Psychotherapy of the individual with brain injury. *Brain Injury, 2*, 203–206.

Bowen, A., Chamberlain, M. A., Tennant, A., Neumann, V., & Connor, M. (1999). The persistence of mood disorders following traumatic brain injury: A 1 year follow-up. *Brain Injury, 13*(7), 547–553.

Bryden, M. P., & Ley, R. G. (1983). Right-hemisphere involvement in the perception and expression of emotion in normal humans. In K. M. Heilman & P. Satz (Eds.), *Neuropsychology of human emotion* (pp. 6–44). New York: Guilford Press.

Christensen, A., & Rosenberg, N. K. (1991). A critique of the role of psychotherapy in brain injury rehabilitation. *Journal of Head Trauma Rehabilitation, 6*(4), 56–61.

Cicerone, K. D. (1991). Psychotherapy after mild traumatic brain injury: Relation to the nature and severity of subjective complaints. *Journal of Head Trauma Rehabilitation, 6*(4), 30–43.

Cicerone, K. D. (1992). Psychological management of post-concussive disorders. In *Physical medicine and rehabilitation: State of the art reviews* (pp. 129–141). Philadelphia: Hanley & Belfus.

Dobson, K. S. (Ed.). (2000). *Handbook of cognitive-behavioral therapies* (2nd ed.). New York: Guillford Press.

Hibbard, M. R., Uysal, S., Kepler, K., Bogdany, J., & Silver, J. (1998). Axis I psychopathology in individuals with traumatic brain injury. *Journal of Head Trauma Rehabilitation, 13*(4), 24–39.

Hinsie, L. E., & Campbell, R. T. (1970). *Psychiatric dictionary* (4th ed.). New York: Oxford University Press.

Holland, D., & Shagaki, C. L. (1998). Educating families and caretakers of traumatically brain injured patients in the new health care environment: A three phase model and bibliography. *Brain Injury, 12*, 993–1009.

Judd, T. (1999). *Neuropsychotherapy and community integration: Brain illness, emotions, and behavior.* Norwell, MA: Kluwer Academic.

Kay, T. (1992). Neuropsychological diagnosis: Disentangling the multiple determinants of functional disability after mild traumatic brain injury. In *Physical medicine and rehabilitation: State of the art reviews* (pp. 109–127). Philadelphia: Hanley & Belfus.

Kay, T. (1993). Neuropsychological treatment of mild traumatic brain injury. *Journal of Head Trauma Rehabilitation, 8*(3); 74–85.

Kay, T., Newman, B., Cavallo, M., Ezrachi, O., & Resnick, M. (1992). Toward a neuropsychological model of functional disability after mild traumatic brain injury. *Neuropsychology, 6*(4), 371–384.

Lieberman, W. A., & Benson, D. F. (1977). Pseudobulbar palsy. *Archives of Neurology, 34*, 717–719.

Lewis, L. (1991). A framework for developing a psychotherapy treatment plan with brain-injured clients. *Journal of Head Trauma Rehabilitation, 6*(4), 22–29.

Lezak, M. D. (1987). Relationships between personality disorders, social disturbances, and physical disability following traumatic brain injury. *Journal of Head Trauma Rehabilitation, 2*(1), 57–69.

McCleary, C., Satz, P., Forney, D., Light, R., Zaucha, K., Asarnow, R., & Namerow, N. (1998). Depression after traumatic brain injury as a function of Glasgow Outcome Scale score. *Journal of Clinical and Experimental Neuropsychology, 20*, 270–279.

Prigatano, G. P. (1991). Disordered mind, wounded soul: The emerging role of psychotherapy in rehabilitation after brain injury. *Journal of Head Trauma Rehabilitation, 6*(4), 1–10.

Raskin, S. A., & Mateer, C. A. (Eds.). (2000). *Neuropsychological management of mild traumatic brain injury.* New York: Oxford University Press.

Rosenthal, M., & Bond, M. R. (1990). Behavioral and psychiatric sequelae. In M. Rosenthal, E. Griffith, M. R. Bond, & J. D. Miller (Eds.), *Rehabilitation of the adult and child with traumatic brain injury* (2nd ed., pp. 179–192). Philadelphia: F. A. Davis.

Ruff, R. M., Camenzuli, L., & Mueller, J. (1996). Miserable minority: Emotional risk factors that influence the outcome of a mild traumatic brain injury. *Brain Injury, 10*(8), 551–565.

Sbordone, R. J. (1990). Psychotherapeutic treatment of the client with traumatic brain injury: A conceptual model. In J. S. Kreutzer & P. Wehman (Eds.) *Community integration following traumatic brain injury* (pp. 125–138). Baltimore: Paul H. Brookes.

Sohlberg, M. M. (2000). Psychotherapy approaches. In S. A. Raskin & C. A. Mateer (Eds.), *Neuropsychological management of mild traumatic brain injury* (pp. 137–156.) New York: Oxford University Press.

Task Force on Promotion and Dissemination of Psychological Procedures. (1995). Training in and dissemination of empirically validated psychological treatments. *The Clinical Psychologist, 48*, 13–23.

Taylor, C. A., & Jung, H. Y. (1998). Disorders of mood after traumatic brain injury. *Seminars in Clinical Neuropsychiatry, 3*(3), 224–231.

van Reekum, R., Bolago, I., Finlayson, M. A., Garner, S., & Links, P. S. (1996). Psychiatric disorders after traumatic brain injury. *Brain Injury, 10*(5), 319–327.

APPENDIX 12.1

BRIEF DESCRIPTIONS OF COMMON MENTAL DISORDERS AND EPISODES SEEN IN PEOPLE WITH BRAIN INJURY

Disorder/ episode	Features	Duration
Adjustment Disorder	Development of clinically significant emotional or behavioral symptoms in response to an identifiable stressor or stressors. Predominant symptoms may manifest as depression, anxiety, or both	Acute (less than 6 months) or chronic
Major Depressive Episode	Depressed mood; loss of pleasure or interest in all activities; weight loss or gain; insomnia or hypersomnia; psychomotor agitation or retardation; fatigue; feelings of guilt and worthlessness; poor concentration; suicidal ideation.	At least 2 weeks
Dysthymic Disorder	Depressed mood; poor appetite; insomnia or hypersomnia; fatigue; low self-esteem; poor concentration; feelings of hopelessness.	At least 2 years
Manic Episode	Persistently expansive, elevated, or irritable mood; grandiosity; lessened need for sleep; pressured speech; racing thoughts; distractibility; psychomotor agitation; increased risk taking.	At least 1 week
Panic Disorder	Recurring panic attacks; persisting concern about having repeated attacks; worrying about the implications of an attack; avoidance behavior to prevent attacks.	Worry about attacks for at least 1 month
Generalized Anxiety Disorder	Excessive worry and anxiety that are difficult to control; feelings of restlessness; fatigue; poor concentration; irritability; muscle tension; sleep disturbances.	At least 6 months
Obsessive–Compulsive Disorder	Persistent obsessions (intrusive thoughts that lead to distress) or compulsions (repetitive behaviors or mental acts the person must perform in response to obsessions, designed to neutralize the anxiety and distress).	At least 1 hour per day
Posttraumatic Stress Disorder	Exposure to a traumatic event in which the person experienced or witnessed a threat to his or her own physical integrity or that of others, and the person's response was of horror or helplessness. Persisting reexperience of the trauma, avoidance of reminders of the trauma, and persisting symptoms of increased arousal.	At least 1 month
Substance Dependence	Cognitive, behavioral, and physiological symptoms of substance use. Repeated use leads to increased tolerance, withdrawal symptoms, and compulsive substance-taking behavior with or without physiological dependence.	

| Substance Abuse | Recurring substance use that causes failure to carry out major role obligations at work, school, or home; recurring use of substances in situations that may be physically dangerous; recurring substance-related legal problems; continued use of substances despite persisting interpersonal or social problems as a result of the substance use. | Within a 12-month period |

Note. Data from American Psychiatric Association (1994).

APPENDIX 12.2

MOST TROUBLING SYMPTOM LIST

Describe symptom.	When does it occur?	What do I do when it occurs?

APPENDIX 12.3

EXAMPLE OF A FILLED-IN DAILY RECORD
OF DYSFUNCTIONAL THOUGHTS

DATE	SITUATION: What were you doing or thinking about?	EMOTION(S): What did you feel? How bad was it (0–100)?	AUTOMATIC THOUGHTS: What exactly were your thoughts? How far did you believe each of them (0–100%)?	RATIONAL RESPONSE: What are your rational answers to the automatic thoughts? How far do you believe each of them (0–100%)?	OUTCOME: 1. How far do you now believe the thoughts (0–100%)? 2. How do you feel (0–100%)? 3. What can you do now?
Sat 4/11	Watching TV	Sad 70 Empty 90 Lonely 90	No one ever calls me. They're embarrassed to be seen with me. I'll never have friends again. Life is boring. (90%)	There's nothing I can do to alter the fact I had an accident. (100%) I haven't called my friend either. Maybe he is not sure if I can go out now, or if I want to? (80%) At least I can walk now without my cane or braces. I could go to the mall tonight. (70%)	1. 60% 2. Sad 50 Empty 70 Lonely 60 3. Make a plan to call one old friend and plan one outing this weekend.

Note. Drawn from Dobson (2000).

APPENDIX 12.4

RECONCILING PERCEPTIONS OF PAST, PRESENT, AND FUTURE SELF AND ABILITIES

Activity	Current performance	Performance prior to injury	Performance immediately following injury	Anticipated performance in ___ months	Notes/trend

13

Working Collaboratively
with Families

It's not until I'm here and begin to talk with you and I
hear what I'm actually saying that the understanding
comes—I call it the ah-ha feeling. Having a chance to
verbalize my thoughts out loud to someone who listens and
understands helps me figure out solutions to my problems.
                    —MOTHER OF A SON WITH A BRAIN INJURY

WHY INCREASE COLLABORATION WITH FAMILIES?

The following cognitive rehabilitation goals were generated by a clinician
in conjunction with clients and families after careful consideration of cognitive assessment findings. In spite of consultation with families and clients, these program goals designed to generalize cognitive rehabilitation efforts were not successful.

• *Long-term treatment goal: Client will utilize a daily planner to follow a schedule.* But . . . the client's wife does not implement the agreed-
upon program to establish use of the planner at home. She appears more
concerned about embarrassing public behavior displayed by the client due
to his difficulty with impulsivity. She wants to discuss her worry about her
children's social isolation because their father yells at referees, teachers,
and coaches.

• *Long-term treatment goal: Client will prepare simple meals with
children present (increased selective attention).* But . . . the visual prompt
outlining the attention strategy keeps getting misplaced and is not posted.
The husband defends his lack of follow-through by saying that it is just
easier to keep the kids longer at the babysitter's house, in order to avoid

listening to his wife snapping at the children while becoming frustrated during cooking.

- *Long-term treatment goal: Client will independently initiate leisure activities at home.* But . . . the client does not go to the cupboard labeled "Things I can do instead of watching TV" without lots of direct prompting from his mom. Mom says it is just not worth the battle, so she has given up bugging him. She says she's learning to live with constant TV.

As described throughout this text, successful attainment of cognitive rehabilitation goals depends upon well-designed, systematic therapy that accommodates the cognitive impairments and considers relevant environmental variables for each individual client. More recently, we have begun to recognize that rehabilitation success further depends upon a true *collaboration* with the client and family members or other significant support persons in the client's life. The treatment goals described above were not approached in a way that built upon the families' expertise, needs, and concerns. Methods that empower families and create therapeutic partnerships are the focus of this chapter.

Increased family collaboration may be the one silver lining to the dark cloud of restricted rehabilitation services for persons with brain injury. The era of intensive day treatment programs providing months of intervention is medical history (Bontke, 1997). Limited therapy visits deepen the dependence upon the family to maintain, generalize, and facilitate continued cognitive and behavioral recovery. Obviously, families are critical to the treatment process, regardless of the amount of services authorized; however, managed care has encouraged us to identify methods that harness the therapeutic power available in families.

How Collaborative Techniques Have Become More Prominent

The trend toward incorporating families began in the 1970s and focused on using family members as informants to describe changes in the patients. The focus shifted in the 1980s to describing individual family members' responses such as stress and depression, and led to the widespread acknowledgment of the need to adopt a family systems perspective in brain injury rehabilitation (Kay & Cavallo, 1991). In more recent years, the role of families in rehabilitation has expanded to include participation in selecting therapeutic goals (see, e.g., Horwitz, Horwitz, Orsini, Antoine, & Hill, 1998); however, the formation of collaborative partnerships in rehabilitation and educational settings still remains largely an ideal rather than an actual practice.

Techniques to work collaboratively with families are perhaps better established in service fields outside the domain of brain injury rehabilitation and have provided several excellent intervention models. For example, Lucyshyn, Albin, and Nixon (1997) describe a comprehensive, ecological approach to family intervention with a family of a child with severe developmental disabilities. Their study evaluated the benefits of performing a functional assessment of problem behaviors within the context of the family and implementing the support plans developed from that assessment. Results showed the benefits of collaborating with family members and using their expertise on themselves to identify appropriate supports and interventions.

The general field of family therapy is very familiar with techniques to encourage collaboration. Of particular relevance to the field of brain injury rehabilitation are techniques based on the recognition that clients' problems do not *constantly* occur, and if therapists help people focus on problem-absent times, together they can identify solution sequences (de Shazer, 1985, 1988). Solution-focused therapists hold the following basic belief:

> People are competent and, given an atmosphere where they can experience such competency, are able to solve their own problems. . . . Facilitators might consider thinking of themselves not as a leader but as a sort of tour guide, co-discoverer, or co-constructor of solutions. When facilitators take on more prominent roles, clients have less chance of seeing themselves as competent. (Metcalf, 1998, p. 40)

As described in a later section, Sohlberg, Glang, and Todis (1998) have adopted some of these family therapy principles to their work with families coping with the effects of brain injury.

Therapeutic approaches that empower clients with brain injuries and their support persons are beginning to appear in the literature. For example, Horwitz and colleagues (1998) describe a case study of collaboration among family, medical staff, and an insurance case manager in the acute care setting. Following the injury of their daughter, family members became directly involved in caregiving by conducting orientation examinations and calming her during periods of paranoia and agitation. The staff involved the family in decision making for care priorities and methods for achieving goals. The authors concluded that the benefits of collaboration included a shorter than expected hospital stay and significantly reduced anxiety for both the injured daughter and the family. They acknowledged, however, that both parents were in professions that promoted advocacy, which may have increased staff communication and influenced the positive outcome. There is a need to work on collaboration with families unfamiliar with the rehabilitation process.

Lucyshyn, Nixon, Glang, and Cooley (1996) describe elements for creating collaborative partnerships with families affected by brain injury when clinicians are developing plans for behavioral support in everyday settings. They emphasize that true collaboration requires respect for a family's knowledge of the person with brain injury, and recognition of the family's strengths and resources. Their methods involve collaboration with family members throughout the assessment and intervention process. The family participates in intervention and choosing intervention techniques. The family also evaluates progress and intervention acceptability, and determines when interventions are removed or changed.

Ylvisaker and Feeney (1998) offer perhaps the most comprehensive model of collaboration in work with individuals with brain injury. They note that decreased availability of rehabilitation services necessitates involvement of the injured individual's support network (e.g., family, caregivers, paraprofessionals) to create "collaborative alliances." Change occurs through everyday people and contexts, rather than with typical rehabilitation staff and settings. The practitioner serves as an observer and collaborator with injured individuals and their caregivers, and adopts a functional, contextual approach to intervention. The authors emphasize the role of everyday people as coaches and partners for the individual with brain injury; they place the role of interventionists on these individuals.

Collaboration is particularly important in the rehabilitation experiences of adolescents. Ylvisaker and Feeney (1998) emphasize the importance of adolescents' participation and choice, as well as avoidance of power conflicts and the classic negative cycle of control associated with such conflict. For example, they encourage instructional dialogue that highlights a student's goals, choice, decision making, problem solving, and self-evaluation (e.g., "What are you trying to accomplish here?", "Is this useful?", "How do you think this will work?", "It's your decision; do you think this strategy will help?"). Their work further offers a framework to promote collaborative interaction that can be implemented by rehabilitation professionals who are consulting with school teams on the educational needs of students with brain injury. Consultants can help school staff, families, and students frame their issues as hypotheses and then formulate efficient ways to evaluate the competing hypotheses. For example, there may be disagreement on whether a student will profit from a specialized classroom placement. The consultant can help the group form a testable hypothesis, which leads to a 1-month experiment with the student in the specialized placement to evaluate specific possible benefits (Ylvisaker & Feeeney, 1998).

How Collaboration with Families Can Improve Research

Increasing numbers of reports in the literature suggest that family collaboration enhances therapeutic outcome. There are also initial reports suggesting that increased family collaboration will improve our research practices.

Lucyshyn and colleagues (1997) illustrate the benefits of collaborative family intervention research in which families participate in defining the independent and dependent variables of the study and serve as valued partners in the research process.

Sohlberg and colleagues (1998) similarly encourage researchers to partner with families and caregivers of persons with brain injury to define the intervention targets. They present three case studies, which were originally conducted to evaluate a collaborative mode of interaction with the subjects and their support persons. In all three cases, there was improvement in the target behaviors during the baseline period. It appeared that the process of having support persons observe and measure client performance changed caregiver behavior and resulted in positive changes in client performance. The authors suggest that a partnership with families during the baseline period would increase the understanding of important contextual variables, which could then be followed by more controlled experimental analysis with continued involvement of the practitioners and subjects as researchers.

Summary of Reasons for Increasing Collaboration

We have begun this chapter by asking, "Why increase collaboration with families?" The reality is that most clinicians do not have ample time to spend in people's homes, workplaces, or school settings,, and must form partnerships with clients and their relevant support people in order to affect meaningful change. Collaboration (1) facilitates the identification of therapeutic goals that matter to those individuals affected by brain injury; (2) shapes the intervention process so that it will work for real individuals in real-world contexts; (3) acknowledges that family members other than the person with the injury also need support; and (4) can enhance the rehabilitation research process to develop and evaluate effective interventions.

Theoretically, most clinicians agree on the benefits of promoting working partnerships with clients and their support persons. Actually *doing* this, however, is more difficult than one might first suspect. Forming such collaborative relationships requires that clinicians examine their own attitudes, beliefs, and practices, and think creatively about how to facilitate collaboration within the constraints of their own settings.

THE IMPACT OF BRAIN INJURY ON THE FAMILY

Stress and Difficulties

The first step in working collaboratively is to appreciate the effect of brain injury on the family. It is well established that the cognitive, behavioral, and personality changes accompanying acquired brain injury often have a significant negative impact on family members (Kreutzer, Gervasio, &

Camplair, 1994; Prigatano, 1986; Wallace et al., 1998). Over the past two decades, research has documented depression, anxiety, and stress in the relatives of persons with brain injury (Linn, Allen, & Willer, 1994; Mintz, Van Horn, & Levine, 1995). The literature is mixed with regard to the changes in family burden over time. There is some suggestion that the greatest sense of distress is within the first year, and that marriages deteriorate during the initial 12 months (Perlesz, Kinsella, & Crowe, 1999).

A relatively consistent finding in the literature is that family members are more distressed by personality changes and emotional sequelae than they are by physical and some cognitive changes. Emotional and behavioral functioning of the injured family member is a strong factor determining the outcome of family functioning (Kosciulek & Lustig, 1999).

Several studies have attempted to look at the psychosocial outcomes of specific family members, including spouses, parents, and children of individuals with brain injury. In their comprehensive review of the literature, Perlesz and colleagues (1999) found that different relationships (e.g., spousal or parental) are associated with different types of distress. Spouses of persons with brain injury often experience difficulties due to role changes, increased financial stress, reduced sexual intimacy, loss of empathic communication with their partners, and social isolation. Parents, in contrast, report feeling stressed about the future of their injured children and the need to advocate for community supports and manage issues of independence as their children recover.

There is less research examining the effect on children of having a parent with a brain injury, or examining the effect on siblings. There is a suggestion in the literature that rehabilitation professionals, parents, and researchers often ignore the needs of siblings, who tend to be isolated during the hospitalization period and may have restricted access to information at critical times. Perlesz and colleagues' (1999) review again emphasizes the general findings across the literature that *all* family members are affected by brain injury, not just the person with an injury and his or her primary caregiver. Appendix 13.1 is a questionnaire that we use in our own practice for determining what information may be most helpful to provide to older children who have a parent with a brain injury. Similar questionnaires are used for other family members, such as siblings. They help guide the educational process and assist professionals in making recommendations for family support services.

Perlesz and colleagues (1999) critically reviewed 37 studies looking at family outcome following acquired brain injury. Perhaps their most important finding is the lack of research focus on positive, adaptive family outcomes. They encourage further research to determine factors contributing to family resilience and coping strengths following brain injury and to learn from these families' competence. Several research studies are described below that provide preliminary information about positive adaptation.

Positive Adaptation

A study by Kosciulek and Lustig (1999) evaluated 76 families with a member who had a brain injury. Their evaluation differentiated these families into one of three types: "balanced," "midrange," and "extreme." The factors that most clearly differentiated families were the severity of emotional, behavioral, and cognitive difficulties experienced by the person with the brain injury; family adaptation (how each family coped with stress); and age of primary caregiver (extreme families tended to have younger caregivers). Future research on the coping strategies of balanced families may be fruitful.

Karpman, Wolfe, and Vargo (1985) conducted in-depth interviews of 10 adults with brain injury and one of their parents. They identified several themes of positive adaptation: maintaining hope, religious faith, acknowledging internal strengths, increased closeness and cooperation within the family, and accessing outside support.

In his work with Chinese families in Hong Kong, Man (1998) developed an empowerment questionnaire based on a survey of families with a member who had a brain injury. *Empowerment* was defined as the means by which families overcome feelings of powerlessness and attempt to reach personal goals. The survey results suggested four empowerment factors: (1) efficacy (strategies used to solve problems associated with caring for a person with a brain injury), (2) support (attitudes and beliefs that help caregivers cope), (3) knowledge (information and access), and (4) aspiration (anticipation of and planning for future difficulty). According to the responses from 211 families, Hong Kong Chinese family priorities for managing brain injury issues include the need for practical information and the tendency for family members to show support through physical rather than spiritual help. Identification of family needs led to the development of an empowerment program.

Various influences, including culture, severity of injury, and time since injury, will determine how families cope with the burden brought on by brain injury. Karlovits and McColl (1999) described the stresses and coping strategies of 11 adults with severe brain injury during the critical period when they were reintegrating into a new community. Although these investigators did not evaluate the larger family unit, their qualitative study revealed the following three different classes of coping strategies the subjects used to deal with their stresses:

- *Problem-focused strategies* involved behavioral efforts to change a stressful situation. There were four categories of problem-focused strategies: avoiding a problem situation (e.g., taking time out, staying out of people's way); doing things differently (e.g., taking the bus instead of driving); getting involved (e.g., taking a vocational preparation course); and reaching out (e.g., talking to others about a problem, disclosing the need for assistance).

• *Perception-focused strategies* involved cognitive attempts to control the meaning of stressful experiences. There were three categories within this group, including ignoring (deciding not to take notice of the stress), relying on oneself (deciding to follow one's own opinion), and persevering in the face of problems.

• *Emotion-focused strategies* involved attempts to control the emotional response to a stressor. Drug and alcohol use was the only example of this type of strategy.

Karlovits and McColl (1999) concluded that problem-focused coping strategies predicted better outcomes and were most successfully used by persons with brain injury. Integrating this study with the literature on solution-focused therapy suggests that rehabilitation efforts may be enhanced if clinicians work with their clients to identify existing instances of positive coping and then help them expand on using these strategies.

The first step for working collaboratively with families involves acknowledging and developing empathy for the widespread and diverse impact brain injury has on the entire family/community system. The second step is to work with each individual and his or her family in a true partnership.

FORMING TRUE
CLINICIAN–CLIENT–FAMILY PARTNERSHIPS

Any partnership is based on the partners' mutual appreciation of each other's expertise. Because families are the experts on their own situations, capitalizing on this expertise is a critical part of clinicians', clients', and families' becoming rehabilitation partners. Those persons most affected by changes due to brain injury (i.e., the individuals themselves, their families or other significant caregivers, school or residential staff, etc.) often generate and implement effective solutions to their own challenges. Therapy that promotes the opportunity for support persons to systematically observe and take data on issues of concern can promote positive change in the behavior of these persons (Sohlberg et al., 1998). Table 13.1 shows how two different care providers independently responded in a helpful manner to data they were collecting on specific issues of concern.

Sohlberg and her colleagues have continued to investigate the potential therapeutic power when rehabilitation professionals form partnerships with people with brain injuries and their families. Several critical concepts have emerged from their ongoing investigation.* First, clinicians cannot help families uncover the answers to all of their problems simply by being

TABLE 13.1. Two Examples of Data Collection by Care Providers, and Outcomes Based on This Data Collection

Care provider	Issue of concern	Data collected or observations performed by care provider	Outcome
Teachers	Student's not turning in homework	Teachers observed whether student wrote down assignments and/or where student placed homework sheets (e.g., in binder vs. in coat pocket).	Student began turning in homework; student and teachers realized that as they were collecting their data, teachers had become more explicit and clear in making sure student understood the homework.
Paraprofessionals leading support group	Client's interrupting behavior during group process	Number of interruptions during each hour-long group session was noted.	Interruptions decreased; as they collected data, staff members realized they were providing more support to client and avoiding topics that led to interrupting behavior.

Note. Data from Sohlberg, Glang, and Todis (1998).

"good listeners" and validating concerns. Second, the partnerships suggest that interventions may well fail, or at best may have only short-term benefit, if practitioners decide what clients need without considering their individual circumstances and involving family members or other caregivers. When practitioners form *true* partnerships with clients and families, and together prioritize issues and discuss ways to address concerns, both families and clients report significantly improved life functioning. The trick is to operationalize the processes required to form such partnerships. This is the goal of the remainder of this chapter.

Occasionally practitioners participating in developing the collaboration process initially express sentiments that they *already* use a collaborative model in their work with families. However, when they begin to analyze their sessions, they find them lacking in certain critical features of partnership; they then appreciate opportunities to increase these skills. Similarly, practitioners may feel initially that they are not *doing* enough for clients by taking a less directive, more collaborative approach. As they experiment with ways to write goals for specific care providers and enjoy the

---

*Most of the clinical materials described in the remainder of this chapter, which are designed to increase collaboration between professionals and families, have been developed from an ongoing demonstration grant (#H133-A-980027) funded by the U.S. Department of Education as part of the Oregon Brain Injury Model System awarded by the National Institute on Disability and Rehabilitation Research.

fruits of helping people implement plans that work for their own situations, the discomfort diminishes. Many of the cognitive rehabilitation techniques discussed in other chapters are best carried out via collaborative interactions. For example, if families decide that increased attention is an important goal, they can be trained to provide attention process training (see Chapter 5). Giving families information about options and methods helps them select approaches that will best meet their needs.

Fundamental Requirements for Practitioners

An analysis of family–professional partnerships working on different goals suggests that successful collaboration depends upon the following five practitioner skills and characteristics:

1. Practitioners need to exercise excellent listening and interview skills. This is not a natural process for most practitioners and takes effortful, deliberate practice. Forming partnerships with families requires practitioners to use their interview and listening skills in order to understand these factors:

- Individual families' concerns, and their priorities among the issues they hope to address
- The daily routines and roles for relevant members in the home or community setting
- The pressures and frustrations currently experienced by the caregivers and clients
- The history of care, especially what families feel was helpful and what was not helpful about any previous services they have received
- Differences in perspective between family members
- Dreams, hopes, and goals that families hold for the clients

2. Clinical collaborations are most useful when practitioners have up-to-date knowledge about brain injury. Clients and families find it helpful to hear responses to their questions from practitioners with experience and knowledge in brain injury rehabilitation. For example, they are helped by explanations of the organic nature of problems they observe, lists of options of strategies that might be tried to help a particular problem, and stories from other cases.

3. Practitioners need to hone their observational skills. Families respond well to observations from practitioners about trends the practitioners observe, either in what families/clients report across sessions or in the clients' actual behavior. The process of "holding up a mirror" allows families to reflect on what the practitioners are observing. It also provides a means for the practitioners to verify and check out clinical perceptions.

4. Practitioners need to be flexible. Often the treatment focus will

change as issues and priorities evolve. Sometimes a plan does not work when the family members try it out in their actual day-to-day lives. It is helpful when practitioners accept that families, and individuals within families, differ in their capacities and their goals. The clinical process is more successful when practitioners can relinquish control while still providing structure and support. The clinical process is more therapeutic when practitioners view families' "failure to follow through" as a problem with the treatment plan—that is, as a poor fit, rather than noncompliance.

5. Practitioners need to structure the therapy process in ways that meet the specific needs of the families and help them implement systems or strategies to lessen challenges. Most family members (including the persons with brain injury) benefit from the opportunity to do the following:

- Tell their stories in a complete manner
- React to observations made by the practitioners
- Take data (or make systematic observations) about specific behaviors of concern and review it with the practitioners
- Ask questions
- Hear how well they are doing, given their circumstances
- "Talk to" other family members, using practitioners to help them convey their messages
- Laugh or cry with professionals who seem to understand their challenges

These five practitioner skills are implemented throughout the therapeutic process. Dividing therapy into three overlapping, cyclical phases can promote the use of these important collaborative behaviors. The three clinical phases are (1) interviewing, (2) identifying and prioritizing goals, and (3) monitoring change and revisiting goals. Interview techniques may be predominantly employed in the initial sessions, but are critical in all client meetings. They are discussed next.

Successful and Productive Interviews

The key to working collaboratively often does not lie in a therapist's having the correct answer, but in asking the correct question. As reviewed above, conducting careful interviews is critical to establishing and maintaining an effective collaboration. Unfortunately, interviewing is often not a core skill provided in the training of rehabilitation professionals. It can be helpful to think of three different types of questions.

1. *Open questions or themes.* An open question covers a broad area and may lead the discussion in a number of different directions, depending upon the response.

Example of an open question: "Can you describe a typical day?"

2. *Closed questions.* Closed questions ask for specific information; they help a family provide details to a practitioner. If they are *nonleading* questions, they do not imply a value judgment (e.g., imply that a situation is difficult, good, or bad). Occasionally, however, it makes sense to ask a *leading* question based on earlier responses. For example, a clinician may inquire about problems if respondents have already indicated they are experiencing problems.

> Example of a closed, nonleading question: "What rehabilitation services did you receive?"

> Example of a closed, leading question: "What are some of the problems you encountered with your previous therapy?"

3. *Impression questions.* Impression questions are periodically posed by a practitioner to clarify and/or verify his or her understanding of what a family has shared. Answers to these questions often facilitate an expansion on the underlying nature of what was said, as well as provide an opportunity for the practitioner to check out the accuracy of his or her perceptions.

> Example of an impression question: "Am I correct that the most troublesome problem right now is your son's inappropriate social interactions?"

An interview guide is provided in Appendix 13.2. It provides sample wording for interview questions in the following key areas: family structure, brain injury, current situation, family functioning, experiences with service providers, community supports, and goals. The interview questions were selected because of their utility in helping families reflect upon challenges and identify strategies they could successfully implement. Table 13.2 provides a list of specific interview tips. As noted above, interviewing is the first clinical phase, although interview skills are important in all phases; identifying and prioritizing goals constitute the next important clinical phase, which is also best carried out in collaboration among rehabilitation professionals, clients, and their family members or other significant caregivers.

Identifying and Prioritizing Goals

In the second clinical phase, practitioners and families/clients determine the goals they want to address. During this process, a family's members share their challenges and strengths, and reflect on what works and does not work within their family. The rehabilitation professional learns about the family's communication style and how best to relate to them. He or she also works to understand the family's priorities, and considers how best to use the family members' expertise on their situation to generate options for areas that may be useful to target. The practitioner further notes the fam-

TABLE 13.2. Interview Tips

Plan interview.
- Use an interview guide with questions highlighted that are particularly relevant to the case.
- Make sure you allow adequate time for the interview.
- Plan how you will incorporate the different perspectives of family members. Sometimes it will be most helpful to interview people separately, so that they feel more comfortable giving their honest appraisal of situations. If you do this, it is important to bring people back together and share your impressions.

Listen more, talk less.
- Sometimes the hardest work is to keep silent and listen actively. Most of us find we have to squelch our normal inclination to talk.
- Tolerate silence.

Listen on all three levels (this requires great attention and concentration—interviews should feel effortful).
- Level 1: Listen to what each person is saying; concentrate on his or her words.
- Level 2: Listen to the inner voice—what is behind the words. If the person says, "I have grown a lot from these experiences," is he or she also saying, "This has been very, very hard"? You can do this by reflecting back the emotions you believe to underlie what the person is saying.
- Level 3: Stay tuned to time constraints, how much has been covered, and how far there still is to go. Stay tuned to the progress of the interview so you can move forward as appropriate. Closed questions will help an interview move forward.

Reflect and summarize.
- After reflecting on what you have learned from the interview, share your impressions with the family. Provide a summary of what you have learned about the family's history, strengths, challenges, etc. Let the family provide additional information or correct any misperceptions.
- Periodically summarize important points that you think will lead to the identification of a therapy goal.

Verify.
- If you have theories about ideas that were implied but not stated, verify whether your theory is true. Example: "It sounds like the family expected more progress."

Validate.
- Validate that the family members have faced difficult challenges, have made progress, care about each other, etc.

Clarify.
- Look for opportunities to educate the family members about brain injury in ways that will help them better understand their situation. Example: "It is not unusual for people with brain injury to 'get stuck' on a topic. This is called *perseveration*. It is particularly common when there is damage to the region of the brain behind the forehead."
- Whenever possible, use the family's vocabulary. For example, if the family has described a problem with a client's "get up and go," it might be helpful to continue using this term rather than substituting your own vocabulary and using "initiation."

TABLE 13.2. (*continued*)

- Ask questions when you do not understand; don't just let things pass. For example, if you are confused about a sequence of events or circumstances, you can ask for clarification, using the word "again" to indicate you know that you have been told.
- If the client uses words that are vague, ask him or her to explain further. For example, you might ask, "What do you mean when you said you found work *difficult?*"

Keep people on track.
- Help to keep people focused on the interview by asking for concrete details (closed, nonleading questions) about a situation if they get off topic or stay too long on a topic.

When possible, avoid interrupting.
- If an important question occurs to you while someone is talking, you can jot it down and follow up on it later. It is helpful to people if they can complete their full thoughts.

Use appropriate attending behavior.
- Use behavior that is appropriate, given individual and cultural considerations, for demonstrating that you are genuinely listening to an individual. Examples, within a mainstream North American context: Smile; make eye contact; nod at junctures; lean toward the person.
- Stay on topics of interest to the individual.

Note. Some of these tips have been drawn from Ivey and Ivey (1999) and Seidman (1991).

ily's questions about brain injury and its consequences, and responds to these in a helpful manner.

During the process of clarifying areas of concern, families are helped to develop a system to observe or measure the contexts in which their challenges and/or successes are occurring. Table 13.3 summarizes the process of helping families identify and prioritize target areas. Some of these clinical actions will be carried out during the interview process; others will actually be implemented in the sessions following the initial interview and corresponding diagnostic sessions.

It is important that a clinician help the family members clarify *their* concerns; often these concerns are different from the therapeutic goals the practitioner might choose. For example, during the process of identifying goals, one mother realized that her biggest concern was that the aides working in the supported living facility where her son was living did not understand her son's inability to control his behavior. She felt they acted in ways that increased his difficulty with impulsivity. Hence she used content from her partnership meetings with the speech–language pathologist to develop a list of suggestions to the aides for working with her son. (This list is provided in Appendix 13.3, as it has many good suggestions for managing impulse control problems.)

Once family members (including the client) have identified and begun

TABLE 13.3. Reminders for Goal Identification and Prioritization

Check out observation from interview or previous sessions about what goals or priorities you think clients/families have communicated. Examples:
- "It is sounding to me like your husband's tendency to sit and not start any activity is of primary concern—is that correct?"
- "Am I correct that the family is most bothered by the anger outbursts?"
- "Would being able to leave your husband alone for short periods of time be one of your top priorities?"
- "Sounds like things are pretty challenging across most domains. Would figuring out what services are available be your first goal?"

Empower families to be good observers. Example:
- "We have found that families are the best experts on what is most helpful to them. Only you know your circumstances. It would be really helpful if you could make observations about [state the issue of concern] when it is occurring. We find that families often are the ones that figure out ways to deal with problems if we give them an opportunity to observe the situation. Would you be able to make observations?"

Many families need concrete examples of relevant observational factors. Asking them what factors would be important to track or notice may help them focus on the following:
- What was occurring right before/after the issue of concern arose
- How relevant people responded to the issue
- Time of day
- Level of fatigue, stress, understanding on the part of the individual with brain injury or the family member
- Setting or other environmental factors
- Medication cycle
- Other topics, as needed

Be sure to pay attention to strategies/accommodations that families/clients are already using.
- It is much easier to build on existing strategies than to try to introduce new behaviors.
- Check out your observations of "successful management" with the family members and see whether these match their perceptions.

Collaboratively design a data collection system or agree on how family members will make their observations. (You might want to have them observe successful instances rather than the problem areas, in order to identify possible strategies or environmental modifications that mitigate an issue of concern.) Examples:
- Design data collection protocols together (written charts or logs).
- Agree on the questions that you will be asking them in the next session (oral interview).
- Have them tell you everything they can about the specific situation/behavior they want to monitor.
- Have them keep a "journal" or make unconstrained written entries describing the situation/behavior of interest.
- Give them copies of calendar pages for them to document relevant information.
- Provide information by talking into a voice memo recorder.

TABLE 13.3. (*continued*)

Try out the data/information-gathering system and solicit feedback.
- Did the family members make observations? If not, what prevented them from doing so?
- Did the family members feel that the system was useful and manageable?
- Did paying more attention to issues of concern help them feel more in tune with the situation?

Make modifications based on family feedback. Examples:
- Developing a less cumbersome method (e.g., your interviewing the client/family each time, rather than the family's independently tracking information)
- Providing the family with more structure (e.g., written directions with a data form)

---

to formulate a plan to address issues of concern, the therapy process moves to the next phase, which monitors change and reevaluates goals.

Monitoring Change and Revisiting Goals

In the third therapeutic phase, the family/client and practitioner generate ideas for strategies to address issues of concern. The family provides information (through either oral reports or home data sheets) about how well strategies are working. The practitioner helps design data collection sheets when appropriate and reinforces progress. The practitioner also checks to see whether the issues of concern are improving and/or whether other ones are emerging. The practitioner makes observations across sessions and helps the family members to analyze any data they provide. Assistance with problem solving is provided by the practitioner as needed. The practitioner may point out discrepancies between stated goals and family behavior. The interview and collaboration skills discussed thus far are used in all of these interactions with families. Figure 13.1 summarizes the process involved in this stage.

Commonly, one of the goals that is identified is the need for more information about brain injury. It is helpful when the information is *requested* as part of the collaboration process; this suggests that the family is most likely to utilize it. Alternatively, practitioners can ask families if they would like more information on a specific topic especially if the practitioner feels there is a specific need. The importance and effectiveness of providing families with information are well documented in the literature (Wallace et al., 1998). The provision of effective education requires that clinicians have access to resources; that they *themselves* understand the topics of interest to their clients; and that they have the skills to adapt information so it is understandable to a wide variety of learners.

Holland and Shigaki (1998) describe a three-phase model of educa-

Begin session by asking open question about issues of concern—for example, "We were going to talk about what you noticed in terms of [state the *issue of concern*]. What did you find out?"

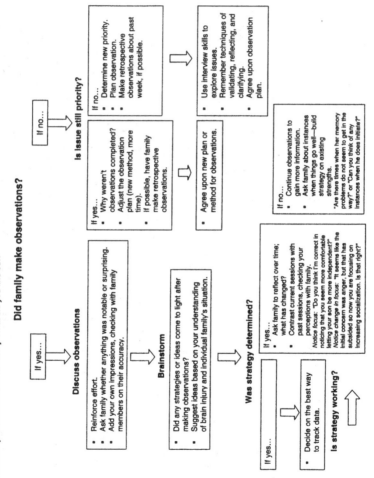

Did family make observations?

If yes...

Discuss observations

- Reinforce effort.
- Ask family whether anything was notable or surprising.
- Add your own impressions, checking with family members on their accuracy.

Brainstorm

- Did any strategies or ideas come to light after making observations?
- Suggest ideas based on your understanding of brain injury and individual family's situation.

Was strategy determined?

If yes...

- Ask family to reflect over time; what has changed?
- Contrast current sessions with past sessions, checking your perceptions with family.
  Notice focus: "Do you think I'm correct in noticing that you seem more comfortable letting your son be more independent?"
  Notice change in focus: "It seems like the initial concern was anger, but that has subsided so now you are focusing on increasing socialization. Is that right?"

- Decide on the best way to track data.

Is strategy working?

Is issue still priority?

If no...

- Determine new priority.
- Plan observation.
- Make retrospective observations about past week, if possible.

If yes...

- Why weren't observations completed?
- Adjust the observation plan (new method, more time).
- If possible, have family make retrospective observations.

- Agree upon new plan or method for observations.

- Use interview skills to explore issues.
- Remember techniques of validating, reflecting, and clarifying.
- Agree upon observation plan.

If no...

- Continue observations to gain more information.
- Ask family about instances when things go well—build strategy on existing strengths.
  "Are there times when her memory problems do not seem to get in the way?" or "Can you think of any instances when he does initiate?"

FIGURE 13.1. Components of the monitoring process.

tional needs for families: (1) an intensive care unit or acute phase, (2) an inpatient rehabilitation phase, and (3) an outpatient/community reintegration phase. These researchers also provide an extensive bibliography. Educational support may be provided in a number of formats. For example, Brown and colleagues (1999) compared education at a distance (via telephone support) and traditional on-site caregiver support groups, and showed them to be equally effective.

Forming True Partnerships: A Summary

The clinical power of using family and patient expertise to direct treatment is acknowledged in the rehabilitation community. Each family employs different coping strategies and holds a unique set of values and circumstances that affects its reaction to a member's brain injury. Recognizing families as experts in determining rehabilitation goals and how they will be achieved has direct bearing on maintaining improvements in unique family contexts.

True partnerships between rehabilitation professionals and families/clients can be promoted by dividing the therapy process into three clinical phases: interviewing, goal identification and prioritization, and ongoing monitoring. During this process, families are helped to focus on their own issues of concern and to evaluate their own functioning. In a highly collaborative mode of interaction, families learn to build on existing strengths and/or to adopt new more functional patterns of behavior or environmental modification. Examples of the implementation of this process with two families are provided in Table 13.4.

TABLE 13.4. Implementation of the Collaborative Process with Two Families

Client/family	Interview/goal identification process	Monitoring
	Family 1	
Adult son 2 years after brain injury, living with his parents. His wife has divorced him, and the plan is for him to remain in the care of his parents as long as necessary.	Parents identify son's lack of initiation as their major concern. They worry that he is not stimulated enough. They do not like to leave him, because he will "just sit on the couch." Son passively agrees that increased initiation is a good goal.	Parents and son agree to track instances of when son is and is not initiating. Mom comes to initial sessions with a notebook filled out with her documentation of a few instances when son initiated and times when he did not. Clinician helps family members note trends. For example, they note that the times when son initiated were when he had visitation with his children. Their initiation journal also leads to a discussion about how much help son needs or doesn't need. This leads to parents' setting up a plan for son to make his own breakfast. The focus of the monitoring begins to be on how much Dad helps son. Dad begins to observe that he helps son more than is necessary. The family together begins to focus on activities son can do independently and likes to do. Eventually, family members report that initiation is no longer their primary concern.
	Family 2	
High school student 1 year after severe, uncontrollable seizures that have caused brain damage. Etiology is unknown (probably encephalitis), but "illness" has occurred twice (during two separate periods) over the course of 2 years.	Daughter expresses desire to "be normal." She wants age-appropriate privileges such as driving, dating, and hanging out with friends. Mom wants to see whether there is any possibility for cognitive rehabilitation and improvement of her daughter's awareness of what she can and she cannot do.	Mom begins to track her concerns and feelings about her daughter's functioning. Because it is difficult for her to find the time to keep a structured log (she has two other young children), the clinician elicits the information via an interview format each week. This process leads to educating Mom about the effects of frontal brain injury, which seems to help Mom better understand some of daughter's behavior. Daughter begins some cognitive remediation therapy, and Mom meets with clinician alone. Clinician observes the incremental success she observes in Mom's report of what she allows daughter to do. Daughter goes on her first overnight visit with a friend since she got sick; she goes on a date; Mom helps her be evaluated to go to the community college. The process of meeting with the clinician is focused on supporting Mom in letting go and helping her understand brain injury.
Mother is the primary caregiver.	Mom also expresses living in constant fear that her daughter will become sick again and the recovery process will have to start anew. Mom describes intense anxiety about continued recovery and possible relapses.	Over time, Mom goes from requesting extra clinician time to saying she'd like to check in by phone when she has questions. Daughter increases her level of functioning and independence as she gets more freedom and practice. Awareness remains limited.

REFERENCES

Bontke, C. F. (1997). Managed care in traumatic brain injury rehabilitation: Psychiatrist's concerns and ethical dilemmas. *Journal of Head Trauma Rehabilitation, 12*, 37–43.

Brown, R., Pain, K., Berwald, C., Hirschi, P., Delehanty, R., & Miller, H. (1999). Distance education and caregiver support groups: Comparison of traditional and telephone groups. *Journal of Head Injury Rehabilitation, 14*(3), 257–268.

de Shazer, S. (1985). *Keys to solutions in brief therapy.* New York: Norton.

de Shazer, S. (1988). *Clues: Investigating solutions in brief therapy.* New York: Norton.

Holland, D., & Shigaki, C. L. (1998). Educating families and caretakers of traumatically brain injured patients in the new health care environment: A three phase model and bibliography. *Brain Injury, 12*(12), 993–1009.

Horwitz, R. C., Horwitz, S. J., Orsini, J., Antoine, R. L., & Hill, D. M. (1998). Including families in collaborative care: Impact on recovery. *Families, Systems and Health, 16*(1–2), 71–83.

Ivey, A. E., & Ivey, M. B. (1999). *Intentional interviewing and counseling: Facilitating development in a multicultural society.* Pacific Grove, CA: Brooks/Cole.

Kay, T., & Cavallo, M. M. (1991). Evolutions: Research and clinical perspectives on families. In J. M. Williams & T. Kay (Eds.), *Head injury: A family matter* (pp. 121–150). Baltimore: Paul H. Brookes.

Karpman, T., Wolfe, S., & Vargo, J. W. (1985). The psychological adjustment of adult clients and their parents following closed head injury. *Journal of Applied Rehabilitation Counseling, 17*(1), 28–33.

Karlovits, T., & McColl, M. (1999). Coping with community reintegration after severe brain injury: A description of stresses and coping strategies. *Brain Injury, 13*(11), 845–861.

Kosciulek, J. F., & Lustig, D. C. (1999). Differentiation of three brain injury family types. *Brain Injury, 13*(4), 245–254.

Kreutzer, J. S., Gervasio, A. H., & Camplair, P. S. (1994). Primary caregivers' psychological status and family functioning after traumatic brain injury. *Brain Injury, 8*(3), 197–210.

Linn, R. T., Allen, K., & Willer, B. S. (1994). Affective symptoms in the chronic stage of traumatic brain injury: A study of married couples. *Brain Injury, 8*(2), 135–157.

Lucyshyn, J. M., Albin, R., & Nixon, C. (1997). Embedding comprehensive behavioral support in family ecology: An experimental, single case analysis. *Journal of Consulting and Clinical Psychology, 65*, 241–251.

Lucyshyn, J. M., Nixon, C., Glang, A., & Cooley, E. (1996). Comprehensive family support for behavior change in children with ABI. In G. H. S. Singer, A. Glang, & J. M. Williams (Eds.), *Children with acquired brain injury: Educating and supporting families* (pp. 99–131). Baltimore: Paul H. Brookes.

Man, D. W. K. (1998). The empowering of Hong Kong Chinese families with a brain damaged member: Its investigation and measurement. *Brain Injury, 12*, 245–254.

Metcalf, L. (1998). *Solution focused group therapy.* New York: Free Press.

Mintz, M. C., Van Horn, K. R., & Levine, L. J. (1995). Developmental models of social cognition in assessing the role of family stress in relatives' predictions following traumatic brain injury. *Brain Injury, 9*(2), 173–186.

Perlesz, A., Kinsella, G., & Crowe, S. (1999). Impact of traumatic brain injury on the family: A critical review. *Rehabilitation Psychology, 44,* 6–35.

Prigatano, G. (1986). *Neuropsychological rehabilitation after brain injury.* Baltimore: Johns Hopkins University Press.

Seidman, I. E. (1991). *Interviewing as qualitative research: A guide for researchers in education and the social sciences.* New York: Teachers College Press.

Sohlberg, M. M., Glang, A., & Todis, B. (1998). Improvement during baseline: Three case studies encouraging collaborative research when evaluating caregiver training. *Brain Injury, 12*(4), 333–346.

Wallace, C. A., Bogner, J., Corrigan, J. D., Cinchot, D., Mysiw, W. J., & Fugate, L. P. (1998). Primary caregivers of persons with brain injury: Life change 1 year after injury. *Brain Injury, 12*(6), 483–493.

Ylvisaker, M. (1998). *Traumatic brain injury rehabilitation: Children and adolescents.* Boston: Butterworth–Heinemann.

Ylvisaker, M., & Feeney, T. J. (1998). *Collaborative brain injury interventions: Positive everyday routines.* San Diego, CA: Singular Press.

APPENDIX 13.1

OLDER CHILD QUESTIONNAIRE, WITH SAMPLE ANSWERS TO OPEN QUESTIONS

1. Would you say that your parent's head injury was . . .
   A. a serious injury?
   B. a medium injury?
   C. a mild injury?

2. How different does your parent seem than before the injury?
   A. Very different
   B. Somewhat different
   C. A little different
   D. No different

3. Has your parent's injury changed how you relate to him or her?
   A. Yes, a lot
   B. Sort of
   C. No

4. If your relationship is different, can you give an example?

   Response on questionnaire of a high school girl whose father had a brain injury:

   We can't sit and talk like before. I have to rely on my mom more for everything. I never go to my dad.

   Response on questionnaire of a middle school boy whose father had a brain injury:

   If I go outside to play basketball, he usually doesn't want to come. I only ask my mom stuff because my dad gets too frustrated.

5. Does your parent ever do things that embarrass you?
   A. Often
   B. Sometimes
   C. Rarely
   D. Never

6. List changes in your parent you think have been caused by your parent's head injury.

   Response on questionnaire of a high school girl whose father had a brain injury:

   He has a lot less self-confidence and is a lot slower in everything. He has a harder time controlling his temper. He apologizes every time he says something mean, but he says a lot of mean things.

He takes a long time saying things. He doesn't remember reruns or old friends a lot of times.

Response on questionnaire of a middle school boy whose father had a brain injury:

He gets mad easily. When he tells a story, he talks, but not about the point of the story.

7. List anything you think has recovered.

Response on questionnaire of a high school girl whose father had a brain injury:

When he first got out, he wouldn't let us help him, and he wouldn't even try to get better. Now he knows he has problems. He accepts that he has a disability, and that makes him less bitter.

Response on questionnaire of a middle school boy whose father had a brain injury:

He plays solitaire and doesn't get quite as mad.

8. Check anything you want to know more about the following:

_____ What happened to your parent's brain

_____ What kind of therapies your parent does here

_____ Why your parent acts certain ways or does certain things now or in the past

_____ What to do when your parent gets mad or irritated

_____ Other stuff (describe)_____

APPENDIX 13.2

INTERVIEW GUIDE

Sample introduction for interview: In order for me to be of most help to you, I want to learn as much as I can about your situation. You are the expert on your situation, and you have learned a lot from your experiences. I can contribute my knowledge and experience in rehabilitation. The first step is for me to use you as a resource to learn more about your situation. I'll begin by asking some questions.

I. *Family structure.* Tell me about your family.
   - Who lives in the home?
   - What is the nature of the extended family (children, grandparents, siblings, etc.)?
   - Who else is involved in the individual's life (friends and social institutions)?

   Sample impression question: So it sounds like you and your husband are pretty much the only visitors at the nursing home?

II. *Brain injury.* Describe the nature of the injury and its effects.
   - What caused the injury?
   - Relate the events that happened immediately after the accident/event.
   - What types of problems did the individual experience early on? Describe any medical complications.
   - (Ask for information relevant to the brain injury, such as site of damage, surgeries, length of coma, length of posttraumatic amnesia, length of hospitalization, medications.)
   - What other information about the brain injury itself might be helpful for us to know?

   Sample impression questions: Am I correct in my understanding that . . .
   the injury was relatively [severe/mild]?
   there has been much improvement, in spite of the grim prognosis by the doctors?
   you have received [a lot/not much] information about the brain injury?

III. *Current situation.* What is happening with the family now?
   - Describe [person's own/injured person's] current functioning.
   - How has the family situation changed?
   - What is it like living with a person who has a brain injury?
   - What are some of the challenges/successes/stressors for the injured person? For the family?
   - What is currently going well for the injured person? For the family?
   - What is a typical day/week like for your family? For the family member with the brain injury?

Sample impression questions:
    It sounds like one of the biggest stressors is . . .
    So days go better when . . .

IV. *Family functioning.* How does the family work together?
   - What activities or routines does your family enjoy? (What makes the injured person happiest?)
   - Which activities or routines are difficult or avoided?
   - How would you describe the way your family copes with problems or stress (e.g., humor, avoidance, stoicism, etc.)? Is it the same for each person?

Sample impression question: It sounds like one of the ways the family has adapted to the current situation is to . . .

V. *Experiences with service providers.* Describe your experiences with professional and agency supports.
   - What agencies, professionals, or care settings have you been involved with? (Examples: acute or rehab. care, transition to school or work, ongoing outpatient medical/rehab., financial.)
   - Thinking back on the people/professionals you have worked with, what was a positive experience?

Sample impression question:
    It sounds like you had an excellent experience with [fill in the type
        of service]. What did they do there that worked well for you?
   - Were there any negative experiences?

Sample impression questions:
    It sounds like you had a frustrating experience with [fill in the type
        of service]. What do you wish they had done differently there?

    So if you were to give advice to a family in your same situation, you
        might tell them to . . .

VI. *Community supports.* Tell me about support you have or have not received in your community.
   - What other supports have you sought or received? (Examples: support group, religious affiliation, Twelve-Step program.)
   - How do others *try* to help you? How *should* they help you?

VII. *Goals.* Tell me about any goals you have.
   - What would you like to work on now? Why?
   - What would need to happen in order for us to be able to work on that goal?
   - Describe improvements/changes you would expect in 6 months.

Sample impression question: So it sounds like you would like to focus on [fill in the type of strategy] in the first phase of our work together.

Is there anything that I didn't ask that you feel is important for us to know?

APPENDIX 13.3

A MOTHER'S RESPONSE TO THE GOAL
IDENTIFICATION PROCESS: A LIST FOR AIDES

List of Effective Strategies for Dealing with Issues That Are Problematic for My Son (T.)

1. Give T. positive choices, as opposed to telling him what he should do. He gets very excited and irrational when he feels he is being pushed and has no control over his life.

2. Humor—It works wonders with T.

3. Anger explosions—Stop and redirect T. firmly to a safe place (his apartment, a walk around the complex). Once T. has become angry, he has great trouble disengaging. He needs to have stimuli reduced. Often he may not even remember the explosion. This can be a dangerous time for T. Remember that direct confrontation may escalate the situation.

4. Changes—Changes are very difficult for T. Established routines are critical for his comfort. Avoid switching things around where possible, as he is not very flexible.

5. Social behavior—T. is very disinhibited and often lacks social appropriateness. This is his most significant area of impairment, and he has made very slow progress. When he gets feedback about his behavior, he becomes very defensive. I do not think he has the ability to understand why he was inappropriate. Others will need to be patient with this, as I do not think it will change. I ask you to consider the fact that often we seem to be asking people like T. to fix something they cannot even see is broken.

WORKING WITH SPECIAL POPULATIONS

14

Rehabilitation of Children with Acquired Cognitive Impairments

Traumatic brain injury (TBI) is a now well-studied area, particularly with regard to the cognitive, emotional, and behavioral sequelae of TBI in adults. The National Institutes of Health Consensus Development Panel on Rehabilitation of Persons with Traumatic Brain Injury (1999), however, concluded that there are three peaks of incidence for TBI: children aged 5 years or younger, adolescents and young adults aged 15 to 24, and seniors aged 75 and older. Therefore, a large proportion of persons with TBI are adolescents and young children. Children and adolescents also sustain brain injury secondary to other etiologies, including anoxic/hypoxic incidents, brain tumors with associated irradiation treatment, vascular episodes, and other neurological diseases and disorders. In addition, many developmental disorders—particularly those believed to involve frontal brain structures, such as Attention-Deficit/Hyperactivity Disorder (ADHD) and Fetal Alcohol Syndrome—are associated with cognitive impairments.

There is now a substantial body of clinical reports and research documenting the effectiveness of different rehabilitation techniques for improving or compensating for cognitive deficits following brain injury in adults. However, research on the effectiveness of cognitive rehabilitation for pediatric clients remains scarce. Given the high incidence of childhood/adolescent brain injury and its impact on schools, families, and vocational potential, it is an important area requiring further study.

EFFECTS OF BRAIN INJURY
IN CHILDREN VERSUS ADULTS

TBI in children most often results from vehicular accidents, falls, sports injuries, and child abuse. The pathophysiology of TBI in children is similar to that of adult TBI, and, as with adults, the frontal and temporal lobes are the most vulnerable regions to traumatic injury. Pediatric TBI is also associated with diffuse axonal injury (DAI)—the widespread injury related to the stretching and tearing of axons, which occurs when the brain is subjected to rapid acceleration, deceleration, and rotational forces. Despite the similar mechanisms of injury, children are less likely to sustain loss of consciousness, given the same level of injury as an adult. In addition, their recovery of basic motor, sensory, and language functions tends to be more rapid than adults, so that children may look better sooner after injury, despite underlying damage.

Until recently, it has been believed that the child's brain is more "plastic" or flexible than the mature brain, and therefore less susceptible to permanent damage (Kennard, 1942). This belief is amply stated in the so-called *Kennard Principle*: If you are going to have brain damage, have it early! (See Chapter 3 for a more detailed discussion of this issue.) However, many studies have demonstrated significant deficits following TBI in childhood (Knights et al., 1991; Levin et al., 1993). And, indeed, some studies showed greater deficit in the youngest age groups examined (Brink, Garrett, Hale, Woo-Sam, & Nickel, 1970; Ewing-Cobbs, Thompson, Miner, & Fletcher, 1994). Similarly, in a study of early nonfocal injury by Taylor and Alden (1997), the development of cognitive and behavioral competencies was more adversely affected the earlier in life an injury was incurred. It is likely that the capacity for functional compensation may vary across brain regions and cognitive domains, and that damage to multiple systems may interact to produce greater disability. Infants and young children may appear to recover relatively well from early focal injury, such as a localized stroke or penetrating brain wound, as there is considerable plasticity in surrounding tissues and homologous regions of the other hemisphere. Brain regions are not yet as dedicated to certain functions. With diffuse, widespread, or bilateral injury, these same mechanisms for plasticity may not be available (Kolb, 1995). Levin, Benton, and Grossman (1982) have noted that "there is no impressive evidence indicating that immaturity confers any advantage in withstanding the effects of diffuse cerebral insult" (p. 190). Finger and Almli (1985) state that there is no evidence that further development of the brain (after a TBI) proceeds in a normal manner, or that postinjury reorganization or growth in the brain's structure necessarily underlies apparent behavioral recovery.

Theoretically, there are a number of possible explanations for these findings. One explanation may be an artifact of the populations examined.

Younger children are more often injured by child abuse, and it has been suggested in particular that shaking a child violently results in considerable DAI. It is estimated that child abuse accounts for the most severe injuries in children less than 1 year of age, and that it accounts for 10% of all injuries for children less than 5 years of age (Johnson, 1992). Ewing-Cobbs, Duhaime, and Fletcher (1995) have postulated that this may account for the findings in some studies, as this group of children is likely to experience multiple episodes of injury/abuse, and may also suffer other forms of neglect or maltreatment.

Another explanation is that significant deficit associated with early brain injury is probably related to the rapid development of many important skills during childhood. Ewing-Cobbs and colleagues (1994) have suggested that these skills are more vulnerable to brain injury at different ages, because rates of skill acquisition vary with age. Thompson and colleagues (1994) have also proposed that rapidly emerging skills are most vulnerable to the effects of brain injury. Adult brain injury may disrupt established skills, which will need to be relearned. In children, if a cognitive structure has not yet developed, new learning has to take place after the brain injury with no support from old learning. Many skills develop rapidly in early childhood; hence TBI or other brain injury sustained at this time may be devastating to a child's development. In addition, for some realms of cognitive function, earlier injury may disrupt acquisition of basic competencies that provide necessary foundations for later development.

Cognitive deficits most frequently reported after TBI in children are similar to those reported in adults, and include deficits in attention and concentration, memory, and executive functions (Anderson, Fenwick, Manly, & Robertson, 1998; Donders, 1993; Kaufmann, Fletcher, Levin, & Miner, 1993). Despite similar causes, pathophysiology, and resulting cognitive deficits, there are a number of very important differences between the child and the adult who sustains a TBI. As any parent or educator is well aware, a child is not a small adult. Mateer, Kerns, and Eso (1997) state that the long-term effects of cognitive deficits, superimposed on an active developmental process, produce a very different pattern of recovery in children than in adults. The interaction of development and brain injury can produce a phenomenon known as *growing into deficit*. That is, a child who has presumably made an adequate recovery from TBI or other brain injury may not begin to demonstrate specific cognitive and/or behavioral deficits until he or she gets older.

The frontal lobes are the last brain region to develop. As noted throughout this book, they are believed to subserve the executive functions, which include such diverse abilities as planning, organization, initiation, response inhibition, self-monitoring and regulation, and cognitive flexibility. A child with a brain injury may not adequately develop many of these abilities in early adolescence, when they normally emerge and stabilize. The combination of increased complexity in the adolescent's academic and social environment, and the delayed or impaired development of executive functions, may result in the emergence of deficit in an adolescent who appeared to have made a full recovery during childhood. This phenomenon has been identified in several reports of children who sustained frontal lobe injuries in late childhood (Eslinger, Grattan, Damasio, & Damasio, 1992; Marlowe, 1992; Mateer & Williams, 1991; Price, Daffner, Stowe, & Mesulam, 1990; Williams & Mateer, 1991).

It is also plausible that different structures subserve emerging versus established skills. Classic work by Goldman (1974) showed monkeys with damage to dorsolateral prefrontal cortex exhibiting no deficit on a delayed-alternation task until they were older, whereas monkeys that received lesions to the orbitofrontal regions of the prefrontal cortex demonstrated deficits immediately. If an area is functionally immature at the time of injury, deficit may not be observable until the function assumes dependency on the damaged region. Anderson, Damasio, Tranel, and Damasio (1999) provide detailed case reports of two young adults who had sustained focal frontal injuries prior to the age of 16 months. Despite normal neurological examinations, and largely average-range neuropsychological test findings, both cases had remarkable histories of impaired decision making, behavioral dyscontrol, markedly impaired social functioning, and abnormal emotional responding. Residual frontal damage was confirmed by neuroimaging. This issue highlights the need for long-term monitoring of children with TBI, since evolution of the nature of demonstrated difficulties is very likely, particularly if the prefrontal region has been damaged.

THE IMPORTANCE OF ONGOING ASSESSMENT

The assessment of children with TBI or other brain injury is complex. It is important to distinguish between a *deficit* (a persistent impairment) and a *delay or lag in development* (which entails the supposition that a child may eventually "catch up") resultant from a brain injury. A brain injury may affect the onset of a skill (i.e., it may be delayed), the order of emergence of a skill, the rate of skill development, and/or the degree of development of a skill. The evolution of performance on standard measures of intelligence after childhood brain injury provides a good example. Immediately after injury, the child may demonstrate essentially average IQ, particularly in the verbal domain, since most of the IQ score is accounted for by abilities, knowledge, or skills that the child has already acquired (e.g., knowledge of word meanings, basic social reasoning). Measures of nonverbal performance may be somewhat more affected, since they require more problem solving and speed. The child may therefore look quite good in terms of intelligence upon return to school. If, however, there are residual problems with attention and memory, the child may fail to keep up with his or her peers, and over the years may begin to fall further and further behind on measures like IQ or achievement tests. Particularly with a child, it is important to assess abilities often, as skills change rapidly and there are important interactions between development and injury effects. A detailed discussion of assessment issues in acquired pediatric brain injury is beyond the scope of this chapter, but several good texts and treatises are available with regard to these issues.

THE REHABILITATION CONTEXT FOR CHILDREN

Traditionally, rehabilitation for adults with brain injuries involves many different modalities. There may be professionals working with an injured person to improve cognitive, speech, and motor functioning, in addition to vocational and family functioning. Often the main context for such an adult is the workplace; rehabilitative efforts are geared toward getting the person back to work or setting up some type of supported or assisted work experience. In contrast, beyond the acute stage of injury and hospital-based rehabilitation, the primary context for rehabilitation with children who have sustained TBI or other brain injury is school.

School is a complex environment requiring academic, social, and behavioral skills for success. Many children with brain injury have difficulty in all of these realms, and often fail to keep up with their peers in terms of academic skills and social–emotional development. This often results in feelings of frustration and a lowering of self-esteem, which may be accompanied by behavioral outbursts and psychosocial difficulties. After many months or years of failure, a child's downward developmental trajectory is difficult to reverse (Ylvisaker, 1998). Adequate education of teachers is essential to successful reintegration of a child with TBI or other brain injury in the classroom.

Much of the long-term rehabilitative effort will necessarily take place at school. Successful reintegration to school is an important goal for children with brain injury, and the degree of success at school is often related to later social and vocational adjustment. Crowley and Miles (1991) argue that in planning for the adult life that lies ahead for such a child, mastery of "survival levels" of academic skills must occur. Acquisition of basic academic and social competencies is crucial for eventual independence in life.

The other significant context for children with brain injury is the family. A number of studies have pinpointed the family environment as the major moderating variable for outcome for children with TBI in particular. Rivara and colleagues (1992) found preinjury level of child and family functioning to be the best predictor of behavioral outcome 1 year after injury, regardless of the severity of the injury. In a later study, they found that both academic and cognitive performance were also predicted by family functioning, as well as by severity of injury (Rivara et al., 1994). Similarly, Taylor and colleagues (1999) reported a strong relationship between child and family functioning prior to TBI and outcome 6 months after TBI. A more recent study by Taylor and colleagues examined recovery in the first year following brain injury. They found that outcome was predicted by preinjury factors, TBI severity, and measures of the postinjury family environment. In the case of severe TBI, sequelae were more marked when there were higher levels of family burden or dysfunction either prior to or following the injury.

Rehabilitation for children with brain injuries thus usually involves hospital-based treatment, the school environment, and the family, and targets cognitive, behavioral, and social issues. The specific exercises and activities that constitute the rehabilitation program for a child vary depending upon the particular needs of the child and the family, as well as the theoretical orientation and training of the rehabilitation team or teaching staff. Activities will also change as the child moves from one setting to another, and as time since the injury increases.

APPROACHES TO THE REHABILITATION OF COGNITIVE IMPAIRMENTS IN CHILDREN

Despite the need for accommodating the needs of children with brain injury and the widespread interest in this population, there are as yet very few studies examining the efficacy of specific rehabilitation procedures for children with impaired cognitive abilities (see Mateer, Kerns, & Eso, 1996, for a review). Management of acquired cognitive impairments for both children and adults can be conceptualized in a variety of ways. Most approaches fall into one of the following three categories:

- The adoption of specialized teaching strategies and academic supports
- The implementation of compensatory devices and strategies
- Retraining of underlying cognitive abilities

Adoption of Specialized Teaching Strategies and Academic Supports

Probably the most common and widespread approach to educating children with brain injury is the implementation of specialized teaching strategies and/or academic supports by special educators, teachers and/or teaching support staff within the classroom and the curricula. Students with acquired brain injury, like all students, will learn best in an educational setting that provides clear instruction, adequate practice, clear and consistent feedback, and ongoing assessment. In addition, many of the techniques found effective with other students with disabilities can also be helpful for students with brain injury. There are numerous resource books designed to provide information about working with these students in the classroom, many of which elaborate on these basic techniques (Begali, 1991; DeBoskey, 1996; Glang, Singer, & Todis, 1997; Mira, Tucker, & Tyler, 1992; Pollock, Fue, & Goldstein, 1993; Savage & Wolcott, 1995).

Instruction must take into account a child's level of academic ability. Traditional assessment in schools consists of annual group-administered standardized measures. For students with brain injury, more individualized assessment is recommended to guide instructional programming. A strong academic assessment is often supplemental to a neuropsychological examination. Such testing can help to document specific academic strengths and weaknesses. A child with an acquired brain injury is likely to have a particularly spotty and uneven profile, depending on the degree and location of injury, and the age at which it occurred. An understanding of the child's preinjury profile is also beneficial.

Once the instructor has evaluated the child's level of ability, instructional plans and curricula can be established or adapted. At this point, individualized approaches to meet the student's needs may be articulated. A list of commonly recommended strategies for working with children with impairments of attention, memory, language, and executive functions, adapted from Thomson and Kerns (2000), is provided in Appendix 14.1.

Individualized tutoring designed to provide repetition and work with a child at his or her specific level is often recommended, although there are few actual data to guide instructors in this approach. Crowley and Miles (1991) conducted a single-case study with a 14-year-old adolescent boy 18 months after injury. They targeted math skills and utilized a math test as their outcome measure. Neuropsychological measures were not found to be sensitive to this youth's difficulties. They conducted a thorough error analysis in order to guide remediation efforts. A total of 40 hour-long one-on-one sessions were conducted. The process of tutoring involved over-practicing of skills, performing careful checks, and daily charting of successes. Improvement on the math test, at the end of the remediation period, was not judged to be significant. However, accuracy on daily homework assignments increased substantially, and the authors felt that the student demonstrated improved self-monitoring during tests in other areas, suggesting some generalization of the strategies learned. The authors argued for the importance of specifically tailored, flexible intervention strategies.

Ann Glang and her colleagues (Glang, Singer, Cooley, & Tish, 1992) have promoted the use of *direct instruction* techniques in students with acquired brain injury. Direct instruction, which initially grew out of the work of Bereiter and Engelmann in the early 1960s, is regarded by many educators as the most systematic approach to the design and delivery of curricula to build and maintain basic academic skills. The visible features of direct instruction are small-group instruction, frequent responding by students, and active-participation-oriented classrooms. To teach new concepts effectively, the teacher develops daily lessons that have the following standard parts:

* *Introduction.* This involves careful modeling of any new skills or strategies by the teacher, and overt labeling of any internal (thinking) skills involved in the activity.
* *Guided and independent practice.* Research with children without learning impairments has shown the importance of providing sufficient practice on new skills to ensure mastery at each step of the learning process. For students with acquired brain injury, who may have impaired memory and learning abilities, providing adequate practice on new skills and concepts is essential.
* *Guided assistance.* At this stage the teacher gradually fades the amount of guidance or the number of prompts provided, in order to assist the student in using the strategy or skill with different examples.
* *Cumulative review.* The skill is systematically reviewed and practiced so that it is maintained. Cumulative review of material ensures integration of new skills with previously learned information.

In addition to specifying essential elements of lesson design, direct instruction identifies the most effective management and delivery techniques. During the lesson, the teacher should maintain a brisk instructional pace, require frequent student responses, provide adequate processing (thinking) time when student responses are requested, monitor student responses, and provide feedback to correct any incorrect responses. An example of a daily lesson design (from Archer et al., 1989) is provided in Table 14.1.

Glang and colleagues (1992) investigated the efficacy of direct instruction techniques with three elementary school children who had sustained severe TBI. Postinjury time for all students was at least 1 year.

* The first participant was an 8-year-old boy who was tutored twice weekly over a 6-week period. Reasoning skills, math story problems, and addition and subtraction were targeted. A multiple-baseline-across-content-area design was used, with instruction introduced sequentially once baseline performance stabilized. Probe measures were taken during each session. Improvements were noted for all areas.
* The second participant was a 6-year-old girl with severe deficits in expressive language and mild deficits in receptive language and visuomotor ability. She was tutored two to three times per week for a total of 12 ses-

TABLE 14.1. Direct Instruction: An Example of a Daily Lesson Design

	Description of component	Example wording
Opening		
Attention	Gains the student's attention	"Thank you. We are going to begin."
Review	Review prior knowledge necessary for today's lesson	"In our last lesson, we . . ."
Expectations/goals	State the expectations or goals for today's lesson	"Today we will learn . . ."
Body		
Model (teacher does it)	Demonstrate the skill or strategy for the students.	"Today you will learn . . ."
Prompt (teacher and student do it)	Assist the student in performing the skill simultaneously or by verbally prompting the students.	"Let's do this together."
Check (student does it)	Carefully observe the students as they perform the skill or strategy that was modeled or prompted.	"It's your turn to . . ."
Guided practice (teacher does it)	Set up other examples that require the same skill or strategy. Prompt and check the practice by assisting or setting up peer practice.	"Let's do these together."
Independent practice	Assign seatwork or independent assignment.	"Now it's your turn to work by yourselves."
Close		
Review	State the skill or strategy that was learned in today's session.	"Today we learned . . ."
Preview	Connect the skill or strategy to what will be learned in the next lesson.	"Tomorrow we will learn . . ."
Independent work	Assign homework that reviews skills from previous lessons	"For homework you will . . ."

Note. From Archer et al. (1989). Copyright 1989 by the Council for Exceptional Children. Reprinted by permission.

sions. An AB design was used to assess the effectiveness of the instructional program for this child. She improved on sentence repetition (accompanied by observations by her teacher of increased spontaneous verbalizations) and sound identification.

• The final case focused on behavioral rather than academic/cognitive skills. Behavioral self-management was taught by direct instruction to a

10-year-old boy who demonstrated aggressive behavior in the context of academic instruction. His cognitive deficits included a significant visuo-spatial deficit, poor fine motor control, and dysarthric speech. He received direct instruction in spelling words, math facts, and keyboarding for 12 sessions. A reward system (points) was set up for appropriate behavior and was used during the baseline phase. During the direct instruction phase, the student was taught a self-management strategy for dealing with his frustration. Results indicated that the point system alone did not alter this boy's behavior. Once he was taught the self-management strategy, there was an increase in his on-task behavior. There was also indication of gener-alization to other areas. The authors interpret their findings as support for the use of direct instruction techniques for teaching both academic and behavioral skills to children with brain injuries.

Direct instruction techniques, and other effective instructional prac-tices for students with acquired brain injury, are described in a text by Glang and colleagues (1997). They note that direct instruction provides structure and repetition, and that it reduces errors by providing cues and prompts until skills are well established. It also promotes enjoyment of learning and self-esteem. All of the factors are particularly beneficial for children with brain injury.

Implementation of Compensatory Devices and Strategies

Compensatory approaches involve developing and training the use of tools that help children with brain injury accommodate to cognitive impair-ments; they include checklists, study materials, memory books, and various organizational strategies. Regardless of the specific strategy to be trained, learning principles need to be considered. Material to be learned may need to be simplified and repeated. Errorless learning techniques, such as those embodied in direct instruction approaches, can also be very beneficial.

Kerns and Thomson (1998) described the successful use of memory compensations with a 13-year-old adolescent girl with acquired brain in-jury. She suffered from an astrocytoma in the area of the optic chiasm and hypothalamus, which extended into the third ventricle. Irradiation treat-ment resulted in very significant impairment of memory and new learning. The authors described the process of training the girl to use a memory notebook. They utilized a three-stage behavioral training approach, similar to that we have advocated elsewhere (Sohlberg & Mateer, 1989). Although the girl was able to learn to use a comprehensive system, she found it diffi-cult to adapt it to the fast pace of school. Consequently, use of the memory system was supplemented by introduction of a very detailed daily checklist designed to guide her through each day at school. Follow-up assessment carried out 2 years after the initial assessment revealed little change in her performance on neuropsychological measures of memory over time. However, she continued to use the memory notebook with positive effect. Observations by teachers and school counselors confirmed that her problems with remembering to turn in assignments and to come to class had ceased. Research has shown minimal success in restoring function to damaged memory systems, and these authors did not make any claims in that respect. However, this study illustrated the effective training and continued use of a memory notebook system with positive impact in the school environment.

Ylvisaker and Feeney (1998) promote an approach to working with children and adolescents with cognitive impairments that focuses on providing external support through the establishment of structure and routine. They promote use of advanced organizers and visual aids to support daily routines. They also emphasize the need to individualize treatment and to provide choices.

Retraining of Cognitive Abilities

Another approach to rehabilitation with children involves direct retraining. In this approach, tasks are designed to provide practice in an underlying cognitive ability such as attention. A large body of research has examined the effectiveness of attention process training in adults, and a few studies suggest the possible effectiveness of this approach in older children and adolescents with TBI (Thomson, 1995; Thomson & Kerns, 2000).

Thomson (1995) carried out direct retraining of attention abilities, using materials from the Attention Process Training (APT) program (Sohlberg & Mateer, 1987), with six high-school-age individuals who had sustained TBI at least 12 months earlier. The study utilized a multiple-baseline-across-subjects design, with three participants receiving APT after four baseline assessments, and the remaining three undergoing eight baseline assessments before participating in APT. APT was administered three times weekly in 30-minute sessions for 12 weeks. Experimental measures included the Children's Paced Auditory Serial Addition Task (CHIPASAT; Johnson, Roethig-Johnston, & Middleton, 1988), the Attention Deficit Disorder Evaluation Scale: School Version Rating Form (ADDES; McCarney, 1989), the Analytical Reading Inventory (ARI; Woods & Moe, 1995), and two mathematics worksheets. Improvements were made on the CHIPASAT, the ARI, and the math worksheets. Despite changes on these psychometric measures of attentional ability, there was no change on behavioral measures of inattention or impulsivity as rated on the ADDES. Such changes were not necessarily expected, as difficulties with the cognitive processes involved in attending are not always associated with overt behavioral manifestations of inattention. However, Thomson (1995) noted that the content of adult training materials was not interesting or engaging to adolescents.

Thomson and Kerns (2000) reported two single-case studies using attention process training materials. A 9-year-old girl with mild TBI participated in eight 1-hour weekly sessions. In addition, her parents received education about brain injury. She demonstrated considerable improvement on tests of attention. Improvement in attention and concentration abilities was also observed by her parents in her home environment. This child received treatment more than 12 months after injury, and the authors felt that the gains were probably related to the treatment tasks. A 17-year-old girl with mild TBI underwent a similar 8-week period of 1-hour weekly attention process training sessions; she also received compensation training with a memory system. In addition, the client and her mother received psychological counseling together around issues dealing with adjusting to living with her injury. At posttest, improvements on tests of attention and concentration, executive functioning, new learning, and memory were noted. The girl also demonstrated successful use of her compensatory memory system. The authors suggest that the data provide preliminary evidence for the efficacy of modified attention process training materials with younger clients.

Despite these successes, several problems have been associated with the application of adult-oriented materials to children and adolescents. Perhaps most importantly, the basic requirements of some of the tasks (such as manipulating numbers or letters) may not yet be well developed, particularly in young children. Exercises using such materials will then not work on attention skills per se. In response to these concerns, direct attention process training materials have been modified for work with younger children (Kerns, Eso, & Thomson, 1999). As in the treatment of adults, activities are hierarchically organized in different domains, with children completing tasks of increasing difficulty upon success with lower-level tasks. The content of tasks is modified, however, such that the basic cognitive skills required are within a child's repertoire, and the materials are more interesting to children. The Pay Attention materials developed for use with young children are based on pictures of members of "families" and rely on concepts familiar to children, such as age, gender, hair color, wearing of hats or glasses, and family relationships. Tasks include sorting cards by features, cancellation tasks, searching for items in "homes," listening for targets on an audiotape, and completing tasks with distraction. Kerns and colleagues (1999), studying a sample of children with ADHD, reported more improvement on a variety of measures of attention and academic functioning in children who underwent training with Pay Attention, than in children who underwent a equivalent amount of time working on nonspecific computer games. These studies lend some support to the notion of improving underlying cognitive abilities through targeted training.

Brett and Laatsch (1998) reported results of a study in which cognitive rehabilitation exercises were carried out at school as part of the students' educational programs. Ten high school students engaged in biweekly cognitive remediation sessions for 20 weeks. The cognitive remediation sessions were administered by trained schoolteachers and consisted primarily of computer tasks and some one-on-one activities. The study utilized neuropsychological tests administered before and after treatment. The program of therapy was based upon a developmental model of cognitive rehabilitation involving three levels: (1) alertness, attention, and concentration; (2) perception and memory; and (3) executive processes such as problem solving. The authors reported a "modest but significant" improvement in verbal memory skills, whereas performance on tests in the areas of attention/concentration, problem solving, executive functions, and self-esteem did not show significant change. Qualitatively, the authors reported that most of the students responded positively to the focused attention received from an adult.

Another area of functioning that has been targeted for direct training is the aspect of communication known as *pragmatics* (see Chapter 10). Wiseman-Hakes, Stewart, Wasserman, and Schuller (1998) examined the retraining of pragmatics through peer group training, using a modification of a commercially available training program, Improving Pragmatic Skills in Persons with Head Injury (Sohlberg et al., 1992). Six adolescents aged 14 to 17 years, whose postinjury time ranged from 4 months to 9 years, participated in the study. The program duration was 6 weeks, 4 days per week for 1 hour each day. The groups were facilitated by a speech–language pathologist. Outcome measures were the Rehabilitation Institute of Chicago Rating Scale of Pragmatic Communication Skills (Burns, Halper, & Mogil, 1985) and the Communication Performance Scale (Ehrlich & Sipes, 1985). The authors reported significant group changes on both measures between pretreatment and follow-up. They also noted that corresponding changes were observed clinically in natural settings. For example, positive communication behaviors were carried over into unstructured time and were observed by parents, teachers, and therapists.

REVIEW OF PEDIATRIC INTERVENTION STUDIES

Although research in pediatric cognitive rehabilitation is as yet limited, it is promising that it has begun. The articles discussed above illustrate different approaches that address a variety of communicative, academic, memory, and attention problems. It is difficult to generalize across studies because of differences in therapy and populations. The studies discussed have primarily been single-case or very small-group designs. At present, the majority of research has been carried out with early adolescents and high-school-age clients. In the future, it will be important to investigate remediation techniques for different age ranges; it is not realistic to generalize from findings of studies with adolescents to work with 6- or 7-year-olds. Similarly, there is very little to inform practice with very young children (under 5 years of age), despite the fact that this age group makes up the third highest peak in incidence for TBI. Despite the shortcomings of our current research base in the area of rehabilitation for pediatric acquired brain injury, what has been demonstrated is positive. Findings are generally encouraging: The majority of studies demonstrate some gains in cognitive function, with targeted remediation leading to corresponding improvement in naturalistic settings—which is the ultimate rehabilitative goal.

SUPPORTS FOR FAMILIES AND SCHOOLS

Effects on Families

As noted earlier, families play a critical role in the rehabilitation process for children with brain injury. There has been a transition in recent years from viewing brain injury as a medical problem to viewing it as a challenge to families (Conolley & Sheridan, 1997). The entire family system is disrupted when one member is seriously injured. The family goes through phases of adjustment to injury, as does the injured individual. Initial reactions of shock and fear give way to relief and happiness when a child comes out of coma and is stabilized. Bewilderment may follow during the initial postinjury adjustment phase, when the parent or parents are overwhelmed by dealing with their still vulnerable injured child. This is often followed by anger and discouragement when it becomes apparent that the child has difficulties in thinking and behavior and is not perhaps the "same" as prior to the injury. Mourning of losses may follow. Parents may mourn losses of skills and/or losses of significant milestones in the child's life (such as learning to drive). There may also be mourning of the loss of the "old" person (Waaland, 1998). Conolley and Sheridan (1997) state that the hoped-for endpoint of this adjustment process is family reorganization.

TBI in particular places significant burdens on caregivers. Wade, Taylor, Drotar, Stancin, and Yeates (1998) compared reported levels of stress and burden for families of children with TBI and families of children with orthopedic injuries. They found that caregivers of children with severe TBI reported significantly higher levels of family burden, injury-related stress, and parental psychological symptoms. They suggest that TBI is a source of considerable caregiver stress, even when compared with other traumatic injuries in children. Similarly, Conolley and Sheridan (1997) reported that subjective burden is more positively related to social aggression and cognitive disability than to physical disability. In addition to the emotional stresses involved with adjusting to living with a child with a brain injury, families often incur financial stresses associated with the cost of rehabilitation, time taken off work, and medical and legal costs. Waaland (1998) has stated that vulnerability for poor outcome is affected by family developmental stage, the extent of the child's disabilities, and additional adversities and stressors affecting the family. Alternatively, positive outcome or resilience is influenced by multiple factors, such as family access to resources that support rehabilitation, personal characteristics that enhance role flexibility, problem solving, and healthy communication.

Professional Support

Professionals working with children who have brain injuries can help families' adjustment to the new circumstances in a number of ways. Initially, families benefit from education about their children's injury and recovery. It has been reported that parents are typically more satisfied with their children's acute medical care than they are with the care that is received after the acute stage (Conolley & Sheridan, 1997). Information should be presented to families in easily understandable terms. Families should also be given multiple opportunities to receive this information, because they may not be able to absorb it all at once. In addition to information about the injury and about the behaviors and difficulties they may observe in the months ahead, parents benefit from information about educational and community resources. Mental health professionals may find themselves in the role of advocates, helping families to access services. Being well informed about what services and support groups are available in one's community is essential to working with families of children with brain injury. Consultation to schools is an important part of the successful rehabilitation process. Providing information to schools and helping to foster strong links between the family and the school are essential. Table 14.2 provides a

---

TABLE 14.2. Arming Parents of Children with Brain Injury with Effective Tools

- Teaching parents about brain injury and its effects
- Helping parents learn where to find out more about brain injury
- Facilitating connections with local and national support agencies
- Teaching and monitoring behavior management strategies
- Educating parents about advocacy in the schools
- Teaching coping techniques for stress and anxiety reduction
- Referral to formal psychological services as needed
- Encouraging use of respite as needed

list of tools and strategies clinicians can use to assist parents in coping and in becoming effective advocates for their children.

In addition to providing information and helping families to navigate complex educational and legal systems, mental health professionals may also be called upon to provide therapeutic interventions to families. This may be done as a preventative measure before family life has deteriorated, or may be instituted to help to remediate problems that have become difficult for a family to manage itself. Family counseling can have a number of different foci. Teaching parents strategies for managing their children's difficult behaviors is often very useful. Similarly, behavior management may need to be implemented if the family system includes siblings. Siblings often experience distress when another child in the family is injured, particularly in the case of brain injury (Orsillo, McCaffrey, & Fisher, 1993). Out of necessity, parents may be overfocused on the injured child, and siblings may act out as a way of drawing attention away from the injured child and toward themselves. Counseling can also teach valuable coping skills to parents, who may be experiencing burnout, depression, and other adverse psychological reactions. Therapists can assist parents in learning positive coping skills and in dealing with their own unique reactions to their child's injury. Sometimes marital/couple issues require attention. Two parents may have very different ideas about how to deal with their injured child. One may take an overprotective stance, while the other continues to maintain preinjury expectations for behavior and scholastic performance. This can result in parental disagreements and difficulty in supporting each other. Family or marital/couple counseling can assist parents in learning to appreciate each other's viewpoint and to develop open communication patterns.

Recently, there has been a movement toward involving parents more actively in their children's rehabilitation. Ylvisaker and Feeney (1998) argue that rehabilitation should be delivered by "everyday people" in a child's life. Hostler (1999) describes *family-centered care*, a philosophy that espouses the facilitation of family members becoming full partners in the design, delivery, and evaluation of rehabilitation services for their children and adolescents with traumatic head injury. This philosophy fosters family–professional collaboration, and views the family as the "constant" in a child's life, whereas the health care system and professionals working within that system are transient. This model respects families' individuality, unique strengths, and coping mechanisms. Unbiased information sharing between professionals and families is advocated. The family is viewed as the "expert" on the child, and the professional health care team is regarded as the "expert" on brain injury. The goal is that the merging of these two different types of expertise will result in the best possible rehabilitation program for the child. (For further discussion of working collaboratively with family members, see Chapter 13 of this volume.)

Sohlberg, Glang, and Todis (1997) have developed a program entitled

Student Centered Education Management and Advocacy (SCEMA) as a systematic, student-centered team approach to identifying the needs of secondary students with brain injury. The program involves a student, the teachers, and the parents. An example of the SCEMA materials is a Homework Monitoring Form, designed to assist parents in identifying some of the difficulties their child may be having with completing homework.

As discussed earlier, school is a very important place for any child, and an important context for consideration in planning a rehabilitation program for a child with brain injury. Rehabilitation efforts may take place at school, with exercises and activities being facilitated by teachers or teachers' assistants, or they may take place at a specialized center. Whatever the case, rehabilitation is focused on preparing the child for school and optimizing the child's chances for success at school in the academic, social–emotional, and behavioral realms. Success in school is a very important metric of the success of rehabilitation interventions.

Like families, schools require education about brain injury and about each student's unique circumstances and needs. Ylvisaker (1998) outlines how a child with brain injury is different from a child with congenital learning disabilities in a number of ways. First, the child with brain injury may show more variability than the child with learning disabilities. Second, performance on tests of academic achievement may be misleading if the information tested is based on previously learned material. The child with brain injury may appear to be doing better cognitively than is actually the case. Third, the student with brain injury may display acute psychosocial difficulties that are not observed in students with learning disabilities. Behaviors may be surprising or may seem out of character for the former student. Finally, children with brain injury may also display unpredicted and unexpected difficulties years after injury, due to delayed onset of deficits. Each child with brain injury may have a unique pattern of cognitive strengths and weaknesses, and the diagnosis of brain injury alone is not enough to describe an appropriate educational plan. It is important for schools to understand each and every one of these factors.

Just as parents are incited to be more and more involved in the rehabilitation process, school personnel are often being recruited to carry out the recommendations of neuropsychological assessment reports. Parents and teachers often find themselves in the role of therapists for students with brain injuries. Brett and Laatsch (1998), as noted earlier, described an outreach study where rehabilitation activities were carried out in a public high school and were delivered by specially trained teachers with backgrounds in special education. Although they reported some success, they also described a number of barriers to carrying out rehabilitation within the students' school environment. Primarily, these problems included the ever-present difficulty of not enough teachers to justify one-on-one hours for students with special needs. The physical layout of the school was another barrier, in that there were not enough private rooms for testing or for carrying out the rehabilitation activities without interruption or distractions. Brett and Laatsch also described a lack of environmental support for achievement, which they characterized as sample-specific. Flexibility and sensitivity to the restrictions and economic realities of schools are required for a successful and realistic plan that can be implemented at school.

SUMMARY

Empirical support for the efficacy of interventions aimed at improving cognitive functioning in children with brain injury is growing. However, many questions still remain to be answered. Studies still need to address issues of generalizability of gains made on experimental tasks. The question of whether these translate into gains in the real world is of paramount importance, because the ultimate goal of rehabilitation is improved functioning on daily activities. Another important issue is the maintenance of treatment effects. Studies with long-term follow-up periods should begin to answer the question of whether gains made during rehabilitation persist over time. Research addressing the cognitive sequelae and remediation of cognitive problems in adults with TBI and other forms of brain injury is well underway. However, there is much less available to guide the rehabilitation specialist who is working with children. Can we, for example, improve or repair "foundation" skills, upon which future skills are built?

The research base examining the efficacy of cognitive rehabilitation techniques specifically designed for a pediatric population is currently small, as noted previously. However, the available research has shown consistently positive results. For those interested in exploring this issue further, there are numerous unanswered questions to address. In addition to the issues of maintenance and generalizability discussed above, there are issues that are unique to the pediatric context. We need further exploration of the nature of recovery for children at different ages; do they show a recovery curve similar to adults, and when is the best time to intervene? Many rehabilitation materials are modified extensions of materials developed for adults. How applicable are these materials, and to what age ranges? Does school-based rehabilitation work, and what supports are required for this to take place? The importance of family functioning for a child's postinjury functioning has been demonstrated. What interventions and supports best serve families? What combination of rehabilitation activities and family interventions is most efficacious in producing a favorable outcome? These and many other questions remain to be answered in providing empirically sound guidance for practicing rehabilitation clinicians. Children are our most challenging clients in some ways, because they present with the complexity of a brain injury superimposed on a continuing developmental process. The effects of their brain injury may be lifelong and affect all aspects of functioning. Pediatric rehabilitation is therefore one of the most important areas of research in neuropsychology as we enter the 21st century. We will be able to offer more to our pediatric clients and their families than we have in the past, with the beginning of a solid research base.

REFERENCES

Anderson, S. W., Damasio, H., Tranel, D., & Damasio, A. R. (1999). Impairment of social and moral behavior related to early damage in human prefrontal cortex. *Nature-Neuroscience, 2*, 1032–1037.

Anderson, V., Fenwick, T., Manly, T., & Robertson, I. (1998). Attentional skills following traumatic brain injury in childhood: A componential analysis. *Brain Injury, 12*(11), 937–949.

Archer, A., Isaacson, S., Adams, A., Ellis, E., Morehead, J. K., & Schiller, E. P. (1989). *Academy for effective instruction: Working with mildly handicapped students.* Reston, VA: Council for Exceptional Children.

Begali, V. (1991). *Head injury in children and adolescents: A resource and review for school and allied professionals.* Brandon, VT: Clinical Psychology.

Brett, A. W., & Laatsch, L. (1998). Cognitive rehabilitation therapy of brain-injured students in a public high school setting. *Pediatric Rehabilitation, 2*(1), 27–31.

Brink, J. D., Garrett, A. L., Hale, W. R., Woo-Sam, J., & Nickel, V. L. (1970). Recovery of motor and intellectual function in children sustaining severe head injuries. *Developmental Medicine and Child Neurology, 12*, 565–571.

Burns, M., Halper, A. S., & Mogil, S. I. (1985). *Clinical management of right hemisphere dysfunction.* Rockville, MD: Aspen.

Conolley, J. C., & Sheridan, S. M. (1997). Pediatric traumatic brain injury: Challenges and interventions for families. In E. D. Bigler, E. Clark, & J. E. Farmer (Eds.), *Childhood traumatic brain injury: Diagnosis, assessment, and intervention* (pp. 177–189). Austin, TX: Pro-Ed.

Crowley, J. A., & Miles, M. A. (1991). Cognitive remediation in pediatric head injury: A case study. *Journal of Pediatric Psychology, 16*(5), 611–627.

DeBoskey, D. S. (1996). *An educational challenge: Meeting the needs of students with brain injury.* Houston, TX: HDI.

Donders, J. (1993). Memory functioning after traumatic brain injury in children. *Brain Injury, 7*, 431–437.

Ehrlich, J. S., & Sipes, A. L. (1985). Group treatment of communication skills for head trauma patients. *Cognitive Rehabilitation, 3*(1), 32–38.

Eslinger, P. J., Grattan, L. M., Damasio, H., & Damasio, A. R. (1992). Developmental consequences of childhood frontal lobe damage. *Archives of Neurology, 49*, 764–769.

Ewing-Cobbs, L., Duhaime, A. C., & Fletcher, J. M. (1995). Inflicted and noninflicted traumatic brain injury in infants and preschoolers. *Journal of Head Trauma Rehabilitation, 10*, 13.

Ewing-Cobbs, L., Thompson, N. M., Miner, M. E., & Fletcher, J. M. (1994). Gunshot wounds to the brain in children and adolescents: Age and neurobehavioral development. *Neurosurgery, 35*, 225–233.

Finger, S., & Almli, C. R. (1985). Brain damage and neuroplasticity: Mechanisms of recovery or development? *Brain Research Reviews, 10*, 177–186.

Glang, A., Singer, G., Cooley, E., & Tish, N. (1992). Tailoring direct instruction techniques for use with elementary students with traumatic brain injury. *Journal of Head Trauma Rehabilitation, 7*(4), 93–108.

Glang, A., Singer, G. H., & Todis, B. (1997). *Students with acquired brain injury: The school's response.* Baltimore: Paul H. Brookes.

Goldman, P. S. (1974). An alternative to developmental plasticity: Heterology of CNS structures in infants and adults. In D. G. Stein, J. R. Rosen & N. Butters (Eds.), *Plasticity and recovery of function in the central nervous system* (pp. 149–174). New York: Academic Press.

Hostler, S. L. (1999). Pediatric family-centered rehabilitation. *Journal of Head Trauma Rehabilitation; 14*(4), 384–393.

Johnson, D. A. (1992). Head injured children and education: A need for greater delineation and understanding. *British Journal of Educational Psychology, 62*, 404–409.

Johnson, D. A., Roethig-Johnston, K., & Middleton, J. (1988). Development and evaluation of an attentional test for head injured children: I. Information processing capacity in a normal sample. *Journal of Child Psychology and Psychiatry, 29*(2), 199–208.

Kaufmann, P. M., Fletcher, J. M., Levin, H. S., & Miner, M. E. (1993). Attentional disturbance after pediatric closed head injury. *Journal of Child Neurology, 8*, 348–353.

Kennard, M. A. (1942). Cortical reorganization of motor function. *Archives of Neurology and Psychiatry, 48*, 227–240.

Kerns, K. A., Eso, K., & Thomson, J. (1999). Investigation of a direct intervention for improving attention in young children with ADHD. *Developmental Neuropsychology, 16*(2), 273–295.

Kerns, K. A., & Thomson, J. (1998). Implementation of a compensatory memory system in a school age child with severe memory impairment. *Pediatric Rehabilitation, 2*(2), 77–87.

Knights, R. M., Ivan, L. P., Ventureyra, E. C. G., Bentivoglio, C., Stoddardt, C., Winogron, W., & Bawden, H. M. (1991). The effects of head injury in children on neuropsychological and behavioral functioning. *Brain Injury, 5*, 339–351.

Kolb, B. (1995). *Brain plasticity and behavior.* Mahwah, NJ: Erlbaum.

Levin, H. S., Benton, A. L., & Grossman, R. G. (1982). *Neurobehavioral consequences of closed head injury.* New York: Oxford University Press.

Levin, H. S., Cuihane, K. A., Mendelsohn, D., Lilly, M. A., Bruce, D., Fletcher, J. M., Chapman, S. B., Harward, H., & Eisenberg, H. M. (1993). Cognition in relation to magnetic resonance imaging in head-injured children and adolescents. *Archives of Neurology, 50*, 897–905.

Marlowe, W. B. (1992). The impact of a right prefrontal lesion on the developing brain. *Brain and Cognition, 20*, 205–213.

Mateer, C. A., Kerns, K. A., & Eso, K. L. (1996). Management of attention and memory disorders following traumatic brain injury. *Journal of Learning Disabilities, 29*(6), 618–632.

Mateer, C. A., Kerns, K. A., & Eso, K. L. (1997). Management of attention and memory disorders following traumatic brain injury. In E. D. Bigler, E. Clark, & J. E. Farmer (Eds.), *Childhood traumatic brain injury: Diagnosis, assessment, and intervention* (pp. 153–175). Austin, TX: Pro-Ed.

Mateer, C. A., & Williams, D. (1991). Effects of frontal lobe injury in childhood. *Developmental Neuropsychology, 7,* 359–376.

McCarney, S. B. (1989). *Attention Deficit Disorder Evaluation Scale: School Version Rating Form.* Columbia, MO: Hawthorne Educational Services.

Mira, M. P., Tucker, B. F., & Tyler, J. S. (1992). *Traumatic brain injury in children and adolescents: A sourcebook for teachers and other school personnel.* Austin, TX: Pro-Ed.

National Institutes of Health (NIH) Consensus Development Panel on Rehabilitation of Persons with Traumatic Brain Injury. (1998, October). *Consensus conference: Rehabilitation of persons with traumatic brain injury.* [Online]. Available: http://www.odp.od.nih.gov/consensus/

Orsillo, S. M., McCaffrey, R. J., & Fisher, J. M. (1993). Siblings of head-injured individuals: A population at risk. *Journal of Head Trauma Rehabilitation, 8,* 102–115.

Pollock, E., Fue, L. D., & Goldstein, S. (1993). *A teacher's guide: Managing children with brain injury in the classroom.* Salt Lake City, UT: Neurology, Learning and Behavior Center.

Price, B. H., Daffner, R. R., Stowe, R. M., & Mesulam, M. M. (1990). The compartmental learning disabilities of early frontal lobe damage. *Brain, 113,* 1383–1393.

Rivara, J. B., Fay, G. C., Jaffe, K. M., Polissar, N. L., Shurtleff, H. A., & Martin, K. M. (1992). Predictors of family functioning one year following traumatic brain injury in children. *Archives of Physical Medicine and Rehabilitation, 73,* 899–910.

Rivara, J. B., Jaffe, K. M., Polissar, N. L., Fay, G. C., Martin, K. M., Shurtleff, H. A., & Llao, S. (1994). Family functioning and children's academic performance and behavior problems in the year following traumatic brain injury. *Archives of Physical Medicine and Rehabilitation, 75,* 369–379.

Savage, R. C., & Wolcott, G. F. (1995). *An educator's manual: What educators need to know about students with traumatic brain injury.* Alexandra, VA: Brain Injury Association.

Sohlberg, M. M., Glang, A., & Todis, B. (1997). *Student Centered Education Management and Advocacy (SCEMA) project.* Eugene, OR: Teaching Research.

Sohlberg, M. M., & Mateer, C. A. (1987). Effectiveness of an attention-training program. *Journal of Clinical and Experimental Neuropsychology, 9,* 117–130.

Sohlberg, M. M., & Mateer, C. A. (1989). Training use of compensatory memory books: A three stage behavioral approach. *Journal of Clinical and Experimental Neuropsychology, 11,* 871–891.

Sohlberg, M. M., Perlewitz, P. G., Johansen, A., Schultz, J., Johnson, L., & Hartry, A. (1992). *Improving pragmatic skills in persons with head injury.* Tuscon, AZ: Communication Skill Builders.

Taylor, H. G., & Alden, J. (1997). Age-related differences in outcomes following childhood brain insults. *Journal of the International Neuropsychological Society, 3,* 555–567.

Taylor, H. G., Yeates, K. O., Wade, S. L., Drotar, D., Klein, S. K., & Stancin, T. (1999). Influences on first-year recovery from traumatic brain injury in children. *Neuropsychology, 13*(1), 76–89.

Thomson, J. B. (1995). Rehabilitation of high school-aged individuals with traumatic brain injury through utilization of an attention training program. *Journal of the International Neuropsychological Society, 1*(2), 149.

Thomson, J. B., & Kerns, K. A. (1999). Mild traumatic brain injury in children. In S. A. Raskin & C. A. Mateer (Eds.), *Neuropsychological management of mild traumatic brain injury* (pp. 233–251). New York: Oxford University Press.

Thompson, N. M., Francis, D. J., Stuebing, K. K., Fletcher, J. M., Ewing-Cobbs, L., Miner, M. E., Levin, H. S., & Eisenberg, H. M., (1994). Motor, visual–spatial, and somatosensory skills after closed head injury in children and adolescents: A study of change. *Neuropsychology, 8*(3), 333–342.

Waaland, P. K. (1998). Families of children with traumatic brain injury. In M. Ylvisaker (Ed.), *Traumatic brain injury rehabilitation: Children and adolescents* (pp. 345–368). Newton, MA: Butterworth–Heinemann.

Wade, S. L., Taylor, H. G., Drotar, D., Stancin, T., & Yeates, K. O. (1998). Family burden and adaptation during the initial year after traumatic brain injury in children. *Pediatrics, 102*(1, Pt. 1), 110–116.

Williams, D., & Mateer, C. A. (1991). Developmental impact of frontal lobe injury in middle childhood. *Brain and Cognition, 20*, 196–204.

Wiseman-Hakes, C., Stewart, M. L., Wasserman, R., & Schuller, R. (1998). Peer group training of pragmatic skills in adolescents with acquired brain injury. *Journal of Head Trauma Rehabilitation, 13*, 23–36.

Woods, M. L., & Moe, A. J. (1995). *Analytical Reading Inventory: Assessing reading strategies for literature/story, science, and social studies* (5th ed.). Old Tappan, NJ: Simon & Schuster.

Ylvisaker, M. (Ed.). (1998). *Traumatic brain injury: Children and adolescents*. Newton, MA: Butterworth–Heinemann.

Ylvisaker, M., & Feeney, T. J. (1998). Everyday people as supports: Developing competencies through collaboration. In M. Ylvisaker (Ed.), *Traumatic brain injury rehabilitation: Children and adolescents* (pp. 369–384). Boston: Butterworth–Heinemann.

APPENDIX 14.1

CLASSROOM STRATEGIES FOR EDUCATING CHILDREN WITH ACQUIRED COGNITIVE IMPAIRMENTS

A. Inattentiveness
- Cue the child to pay attention to important information.
- Allow the child to take frequent breaks.
- Present information in a short and concise format.
- Provide several repetitions of information, in order to allow for fluctuations in attention.
- Speak slowly and distinctly, and face the child when speaking.
- Stop periodically to summarize important points.
- Seat the child in an area free of distractions, such as near the front of the classroom, or away from noises such as heating vents, clocks, or fans, and away from windows and doors.
- Allow the child to use earplugs or a headset during independent work time.
- Keep the child's desk or other work area free from clutter.
- Work with the child in small groups whenever possible, in order to minimize distractions from other students.
- Prepare the child for new situations in advance.
- Allow sufficient time between tasks.
- Require the child to attend to only one activity at a time.

B. Motor Restlessness
- Allow the child to stand while working.
- Assign the child active jobs, such as erasing the blackboard or handing out papers.

C. Speech and Language Processing Problems
- Utilize paraphrasing, repetition, and summarizing.
- Provide concrete and concise verbal information.
- Encourage nonverbal communication, such as gesturing or signing.
- Allow the student time to formulate a response.
- Provide opportunities for verbal expression in a small group.
- Provide alternative options for responding.
- Supplement oral instructions with written instructions and/or visual information such as pictures or maps.

D. Difficulties with Memory and Learning
- Utilize the "three R's": repetition, review, and rehearsal.
- Ensure that previously learned information can be recalled over time before presenting new information.
- Use mental imagery or other mnemonics when appropriate.
- "Anchor" new learning to previous experience.

- Use scaffolding and overlearning.
- Use errorless learning techniques (i.e., have the child avoid "guessing" at words, spellings, or math facts).
- Avoid the use of multistep instructions, or provide written instructions.
- Have the child immediately repeat information to check accuracy.
- "Reteach" material, such as including a few old spelling words on new spelling lists or reintroducing facts in another context.
- Teach use of a memory notebook, organizer, or checklist system.
- Post information to be remembered, such as schedules of assignments.
- Utilize a peer note taker.
- Provide a tape recorder to record assignments and lectures.

E. Executive Functioning and Problem-Solving Skills
- Provide a highly structured and consistent, routine environment.
- Use well-defined goals and objectives.
- Provide meaningful choices.
- Provide assistance with identification of appropriate solutions.
- Provide assistance with shifting solutions.
- Shorten or simplify tasks when necessary.
- Help the child break down assignments, and estimate how much time he or she will need to complete each part.
- Assign a classroom "buddy" who can assist the student when confused or experiencing problems.

Note. From Thomson and Kerns (1999). From *Neuropsychological Management of Mild Traumatic Brain Injury* by Sarah Reskin and Catherine Mateer. Copyright 1999 by Oxford University Press. Used by permission of Oxford University Press, Inc.

15

Management Strategies for Mild Traumatic Brain Injury

As indicated in Chapter 2 of this volume, the severity of traumatic brain injury (TBI) occurs on a broad continuum, from very mild concussions to severe, life-threatening injuries. The largest proportion of TBI occurs within the mild to moderate spectrum. Indeed, it has been estimated that approximately 75% of all cases can be categorized as mild TBI (MTBI). In addition to TBI, various other neurological and psychiatric diagnoses can be associated with mild to moderate cognitive impairments. These include multiple sclerosis, brain tumor, electric shock injuries, mild hypoxic episodes, some limited cerebrovascular episodes, and schizophrenia, to name a few. The approaches to working with mild cognitive impairments and associated behavioral, emotional, and social consequences outlined in this chapter may be appropriate for use with a wide variety of clients who have differing etiologies. Most of the literature on mechanisms, consequences, and treatment, however, is based on MTBI, so discussion of this area will be the major focus of this chapter.

The classification of TBI severity is a large problem within both clinical and research settings (for recent reviews, see Binder, 1997; Kibby & Long, 1996). Alexander (1995) has argued the importance of defining the severity of TBI by acute injury characteristics, rather than by the severity of symptoms at random points after trauma. The rationale behind this is that early physical, behavioral, and cognitive features are the best indications of severity of the trauma, whereas later-stage symptomatology reflects a broader spectrum of factors—including not only direct injury effects, but emotional responses and adjustment to injury-related factors.

The definition of MTBI has generated considerable controversy. All agree that some kind of traumatic insult to the head, in the form of a blow and/or subjection to acceleration/deceleration forces, is necessary for the diagnosis. Rimel, Giordani, Barth, Boll, and Jane (1981) defined characteristics of MTBI as a loss of consciousness (LOC) of 20 minutes or less, a Glasgow Coma Scale (GCS) score of 13 or greater, no evidence of intracerebral hematoma, no subsequent deterioration of neurological status, and hospitalization of less than 48 hours. Although it was one of the first attempts to quantify MTBI, this definition did not incorporate an estimate of posttraumatic amnesia (PTA), which has been shown to be a sensitive indicator of long-term recovery in more severe injuries. In addition, some researchers have argued that LOC is not a necessary condition for MTBI, as absence of unconsciousness does not preclude significant effects, particularly when cortical structures such as the frontal lobes are injured (Alexander, 1995; Berrol, 1992).

The Mild Traumatic Brain Injury Committee of the Head Injury Special Interest Group of the American Congress of Rehabilitation Medicine (Kay, Newman, Cavallo, Ezrachi, & Resnick, 1992) defined MTBI as a traumatically induced physiological disruption of brain function manifested by *at least one* of the following:

1. A period of LOC.
2. Any loss of memory for events immediately before or after the accident.
3. Any alteration in mental state at the time of the accident (e.g., feeling dazed, disoriented, or confused).
4. Focal neurological deficits that may or may not be transient.

In addition, LOC, when it occurs, may not exceed 30 minutes; GCS score must be at least 13 by 30 minutes after the injury; and PTA must be less than 24 hours. Also, standard radiological studies—including computed tomography (CT) and magnetic resonance imaging (MRI) scans, if they are done—must be interpreted as normal.

Although this definition has gained fair acceptance, some disagreements remain (e.g., the necessity of LOC), and it is widely recognized that both the GCS score and PTA have limitations in the way they are employed to classify mild head injuries. The GCS not only has limited sensitivity in discriminating less severe head injuries (Jennett, 1998), but may be administered at different times after injury (e.g., at the scene of an accident, during emergency transportation, on arrival at the emergency department, or during hospital admission), making reliance on this measure for clinical or research purposes problematic. PTA is also formally assessed quite inconsistently, if at all, and its duration is often difficult to determine with any precision from retrospective reports of what the person remembers following the injury. PTA can be underestimated due to *islands of memory,* which are isolated recollections that do not occur within continuous memory for events. It is also misleading if the resolution of PTA is defined solely on the basis of orientation to time and place. Indeed, there is little correlation in the acute postinjury period between correctly responding to orientation questions and subsequently remembering that such questions were asked. Conversely, PTA can be overestimated by the inclusion of impaired orientation or arousal due to medication, alcohol, or drugs that are ingested prior to or after injury. Nevertheless, PTA is widely considered to be the best severity index of MTBI, because it typically lasts beyond the resumption of a normal GCS score and allows for a finer gradation of mental status.

Many, though certainly not all, individuals with MTBI are seen in an emergency care setting or in a doctor's office immediately after or within a few days of injury. Typically, a constellation of early postconcussion symptoms is reported in the days and weeks following injury (Binder, 1986; Evans, 1992, 1994). These often include physical symptoms, such as headache, dizziness, tinnitus, blurred or double vision, sensitivity to noise or light, fatigue, and/or sleep disturbance. Also prevalent are cognitive symptoms—including difficulty with concentration and attention, memory difficulties, and slowed mental processing—although these may not be fully recognized or reported until the individual attempts to resume preinjury activities such as returning to work. Some emotional changes, especially irritability and other forms of emotional lability, are also often seen quite early after injury. Other emotional changes, including depression and anxiety, are typically not seen until some time after injury, particularly if the individual has not been able to return successfully to all aspects of his or her preinjury functioning. Thus the emotional lability and irritability are usually seen as more biologically based, whereas depression and anxiety are more often interpreted as reflecting a reaction to dealing with physical and cognitive consequences of the injury.

It is important to recognize that the majority of individuals with MTBI appear to make excellent recoveries. Longitudinal studies of unselected samples of individuals seen with MTBI suggest that about 70% report resolution of symptoms by 3–6 months after injury (Kraus & Nourjah, 1998); by 12 months after injury, about 85% are typically asymptomatic (Alves, Macciocchi, & Barth, 1993; Mateer, 1992). Nevertheless, a substantial minority, in the range of 8–15%, continues to report symptoms and to experience difficulties a year or more following MTBI. In addition, there is evidence that various factors, including age and the occurrence of a prior brain injury, are negative prognostic factors for persisting deficits (Binder, 1986; Evans, 1992). Richards (2000) found that elderly subjects with MTBI performed more poorly on neuropsychological tests than either young adults with MTBI or elderly controls, and that age and the occurrence of a MTBI exerted additive versus interactive effects on cognitive performance decrements. Even when individuals who have had MTBI are asymptomatic or appear to have had very good recoveries, they may continue to show subtle cognitive impairments (Stuss et al., 1985), and their cognitive abilities continue to be more vulnerable under adverse conditions.

When symptoms persist for more than a year following MTBI, the term *postconcussive syndrome* (PCS) is often applied. There has been a long-standing disagreement about the fundamental nature of PCS. Some clinicians and researchers believe that persistent symptoms reflect, at least in part, underlying neurological abnormality or inefficiency secondary to the injury. Others are skeptical of any persisting organic abnormalities; they view the maintenance of symptoms as a reflection of premorbid problems, and/or as a consequence of emotional factors such as depression or anxiety. Still others have expressed beliefs that persisting symptoms are perpetuated by health care professionals who have convinced clients that they are "brain-injured" and have suffered permanent damage, and/or that complaints and poor neuropsychological performances are exaggerated or malingered for the purpose of secondary gain.

Although PCS is often considered as a single-entity syndrome, several investigators have argued that the sequelae of MTBI fall into multifactorial groupings that form distinct symptom clusters (Bohnen, Twijnstra, & Jolles, 1992b; Levin et al., 1987; Lishman, 1988). Cicerone and Kalmar (1995), for example, identified, through discriminant analysis of symptoms in 37 patients with MTBI and subsequent PCS, four factors (cognitive, somatic, affective, and sensory). Based on these factors, they identified four patient clusters: (1) those with minimal symptoms, (2) those with primarily cognitive–affective symptoms, (3) those with primarily somatic symptoms, and (4) those with global symptoms. Cicerone and Kalmar suggested that different mechanisms may underlie these different symptom clusters, and that both psychological and organic factors need to be considered in a comprehensive model of MTBI.

Indeed, a biopsychosocial model for understanding MTBI and PCS that acknowledges both physiogenic and psychogenic factors and their interaction in the development of symptoms is probably the most useful and productive approach (Alexander, 1995; Karzmark, Hall, & Englander, 1995; Lishman, 1988; McClelland, 1996). The following section outlines evidence for both physiogenic (i.e., neurological or physiological) factors and psychogenic (i.e., psychosocial and emotional) factors in the development and expression of MTBI and PCS.

EVIDENCE FOR PHYSIOGENIC VERSUS PSYCHOGENIC FACTORS IN MTBI

Evidence for Physiogenic Factors

It used to be thought that temporary LOC or concussion was a purely transient event, akin to "short-circuiting," which left no permanent damage to nerve cells. However, modern imaging has provided some evidence of potentially longer-lasting effects (Newberg & Alavi, 1996). MRI has revealed focal brain lesions in MTBI that are undetected by CT. They appear in the grey matter, the white matter, or at grey–white matter junctions (Yodoto, Kurokawa, & Otsuka, 1991; Zasler, 1993). In a series of 50 patients with TBI, 40 of whom were categorized as having MTBI, 80% of the subjects had lesions detected by MRI compared to 20% of subjects who had lesions detected on CT (Levin, Williams, Eisenberg, High, & Guinto, 1992). There has also been some evidence of diffuse axonal injury in MTBI. Mittl and colleagues (1994) found MRI evidence of diffuse axonal injury in approximately 30% of patients with MTBI who had normal CT findings.

Even when CT and MRI suggest normal structural integrity, more sensitive indicators of functional integrity have demonstrated abnormalities. Ruff, Crouch, and Troster (1994) reported abnormalities on positron emission tomography (PET), a measure of glucose metabolism, in nine individuals with PCS, all of whom had normal CT and MRI findings. Abnormalities were observed in the anterior temporal and frontal lobes, the same brain regions that have been extensively implicated in more severe TBI. Similarly, Humayan, Presty, and Lafrance (1989) reported that in comparison to control participants, MTBI patients had decreased metabolism in medial temporal, posterior temporal, and posterior frontal regions. Varney, Bushnell, Nathan, and Kahn (1995) also reported significant anterior mesial temporal hypoperfusion and orbitofrontal hypoperfusion in a series in subjects with MTBI who had poor social and vocational outcomes, but who demonstrated no CT or MRI abnormalities. In addition, Strich (1961) and Gennarelli (1993) described neuronal changes after MTBI on postmortem examinations of individuals who died of other causes. Thus the notion that concussion is a purely transient event does not appear to hold in all circumstances.

Evidence for Psychogenic Factors

There is also considerable support for emotional and psychosocial contributors to persistent problems following MTBI. Several investigators have found a significant association between the frequency, intensity, and duration of postconcussion symptoms and daily stress levels (Gouvier, Cubic, Jones, Brantley, & Cutlip, 1992; Radanov, Stefano, Schnidrig, & Ballinari, 1991). Similarly, Cicerone (1991) found little relationship between objective assessment and magnitude of complaint. Rather, subjective awareness and report of limitations are closely related to other indicators of subjective distress. On the other hand, there is no clear preinjury pattern of personality or social functioning that predicts outcome from MTBI (Fenton, McClelland, Montgomery, MacFlynn, & Rutherford, 1993).

It has also been suggested that involvement in litigation plays a large role in symptom severity and duration, although formal studies have suggested that individuals who are not in litigation have similar symptoms, and that symptoms do not necessarily resolve when litigation is over (Fee & Rutherford, 1988). Nevertheless, there is little doubt that litigation can sometimes play a role, particularly in the context of rehabilitation, in that the injured person, his or her family, or an attorney may perceive that symptoms must remain if there is to be compensation for damages. In addition, there is no doubt that litigation of any kind is stressful, and that it tends to focus an individual on problems and limitations rather than on progress, successes, and achievements.

Possible Interactions of Physiogenic and Psychogenic Factors

In attempting to specify the interaction between biological and social–emotional factors, a number of authors have discussed long-term effects of MTBI in terms of a stress and coping hypothesis (Kay et al., 1992; Kay, 1993; Marsh & Smith, 1995; Raskin & Mateer, 2000). Most variations of this hypothesis suggest that persisting symptoms are primarily caused by patients' unsuccessful coping with reduced cognitive efficiency following injury. Symptoms such as anxiety and depression are seen as the result of the chronic effort by patients with MTBI to overcome and compensate for their deficits. Problems are often exacerbated secondary to increased stress that occurs when an individual attempts to resume normal family and work responsibilities. From this perspective, cognitive difficulties as well as persisting pain and fatigue result in feelings of frustration and loss of control, which fuel depression and anxiety.

An alternative hypothesis is that individuals who are depressed or anxious cope poorly with the injury and its effects, resulting in poor cognitive performance. Research supporting the causal direction of these effects has yielded mixed results. Barth and colleagues (1983) found that level of depression in patients with MTBI, as measured on the Depression scale of the Minnesota Multiphasic Personality Inventory, was significantly related to the Halstead Impairment Index. Atteberry-Nennet, Barth, Loyd, and Lawrence (1986) reported a significant association between level of depression (Beck Depression Inventory) and verbal intellect, verbal learning, and Trail Making Test (TMT) performance. In contrast, Raskin, Mateer, and Tweeten (1998) found no correlation between depression and cognitive performance in patients with MTBI, and Ruttan (1998) reported that depression was largely independent of cognitive performance in patients with MTBI a year or more following injury. Reitan and Wolfson (1997) reviewed the literature in this area and concluded that emotional disturbance, considered alone, is not a reliable basis for predicting or producing poor neuropsychological test scores. It is always important to recognize that correlation does not imply causality, and that causal influences can be bidirectional.

In general, there appears to be a growing consensus that causes of and vulnerability to the development of PCS arise at both the physical and psychological levels, and that these interact with social expectancies. There are many observed and measured interrelationships among injury variables, demographic variables, cognitive variables, and emotional/personality variables. Causal or contributory mechanisms are complicated and probably vary significantly from case to case. At this point, the biopsychosocial model seems to be the most comprehensive and best supported.

NEUROPSYCHOLOGICAL PATTERNS

In this section we review research findings pertaining to the cognitive effects of MTBI. Descriptions of and references to particular neuropsychological tests are provided in Chapter 4, which deals with assessment in general. As with more severe injuries, the most common areas of neuropsychological difficulty for individuals with MTBI involve attention, speed of processing, learning efficiency, and executive functions.

Attention Deficits

Performance on tasks involving simple focused attention, such as forward digit span, cancellation tasks, digit–symbol substitution, and Part A of the TMT, may be impaired in the first few months after MTBI but typically returns to normal (Cicerone, 1996; Dikmen, Machamer, Winn, & Temkin, 1995; Leininger, Gramling, Farrell, Kreutzer, & Peck, 1990; Raskin et al., 1998).

In contrast, subjects with MTBI often demonstrate difficulty, relative to controls, on externally paced tasks that require them to sustain attention to multiple pieces of information over time, in response to a continuous rate of stimulation (Cicerone, 1997; Gronwall & Wrightson, 1974; Raskin et al., 1998). Part B of the TMT requires an individual to alternate searching for and responding to letters and numbers. Raskin and colleagues (1998) found impaired performance on this task in 28% of a group of subjects with MTBI who continued to be symptomatic more than 1 year after injury. Similarly, Ogden and Wolfe (1998) found a significant difference between participants with MTBI and controls on TMT Part B 2 years after injury.

Consistent with frequent complaints of not being able "to do more than one thing at once," studies using dual-task paradigms have demonstrated that subjects with MTBI do relatively worse than controls on such tasks. Cicerone (1996), for example, required participants to complete a cancellation task while simultaneously solving simple math problems presented every 5 seconds. Dual-task demands slowed both controls and subjects with MTBI, but the proportion of decline was much greater for the latter. Similarly, many researchers have replicated the sensitivity of the Paced Auditory Serial Addition Task (PASAT) to MTBI (Cicerone, 1997; Leininger et al., 1990; Ponsford & Kinsella, 1992).

Memory Deficits

Verbal learning following MTBI has been understudied. Some studies have shown poor initial learning of word lists (Leininger et al., 1990), but the duration of dysfunction remains controversial. Some researchers have argued that memory difficulties resolve between 1 and 3 months after injury (Dikmen et al., 1995; Levin et al., 1992), whereas other studies demonstrate persistent problems even 1 year after injury (Bohnen, Jolles, & Twijnstra, 1992a; Ruff et al., 1994). This discrepancy is probably largely accounted for by the use of unselected samples (consecutive cases seen in the emergency room and followed over time) versus selected samples (individuals seen clinically with complaints of persistent symptoms). Given that 85–90% of individuals recover by 1 year, the unselected samples should show much higher performance than the selected samples. This is a continuing problem when researchers are studying a relatively low-base-rate phenomenon such as PCS.

Differences may also relate to the specific aspect of learning that is addressed. For example, Raskin and colleagues (1998) found recall of a word list after a single presentation (recall on Trial 1 of the California Verbal Learning Test [CVLT]) to be impaired in subjects with MTBI, although recall improved substantially by Trial 5, and learning was maintained over time. Similarly, Mateer (1992) reported that subjects with MTBI performed more poorly on Trial 1 of the Rey Auditory Verbal Learning Test than either controls or subjects with moderate to severe TBI, but did not differ from controls on Trial 5 of the learning trials or on short- or long-term delayed recalls; these results suggested that the problem is one with attention to or with self-initiated strategic encoding of information to be learned, not with retention of material.

Impairments in Executive Functions

Executive functions (discussed at length in Chapter 8) include cognitive abilities involved in the initiation, planning, and regulation of complex behavior, and those that govern efficiency and appropriateness of task performance. Performance on the Wisconsin Card Sorting Test (WCST), a widely used measure of executive functions, is commonly impaired after moderate to severe TBI. Mateer (1992) reported that subjects with MTBI achieved a comparable number of categories to controls, but had significantly more losses of set. She argued that such problems are not related to the conceptual aspects of the task, but to the attentional and/or working memory demands. The Consonant Trigrams Test (CTT), another commonly used measure of executive functions, requires an individual to retain three letters in mind during various periods of distraction (counting backward). Stuss, Stethem, Hugenholtz, and Richard (1989) found that CTT performance distinguished patients with TBI from controls, and that the longer the duration of PTA or coma, the worse the performance on the CTT. Of relevance to this discussion, however, is that CTT performance was sufficiently sensitive to differentiate mildly concussed patients from control participants.

Verbal fluency tasks demand retrieval from long-term memory, sustained attention, and the executive control of retrieval processes. Functional neuroimaging investigations have implicated bilateral frontal and temporal regions in verbal fluency. Raskin and Rearick (1996) compared subjects with MTBI and controls on phonemic (F, A, and S) and semantic (animals) verbal fluency tasks. Subjects in the MTBI group produced significantly fewer words on both tasks, although, like the control group, they employed both phonemic and semantic retrieval strategies. The subjects with MTBI also made more errors than controls, suggesting problems in executive self-monitoring.

Summary of Neuropsychological Findings

Results in the literature on the cognitive effects of MTBI have been complicated by use of different measures and by the use of selected versus unselected samples. Although investigations of unselected samples, like those of Dikmen and colleagues (1995) are extremely valuable in determining the natural history of the effects of MTBI, they are limited in what they can tell us about cognitive patterns in symptomatic individuals. Raskin and colleagues (1998) provided information from a large sample of individuals who were still reporting symptoms and functional problems more than a year after injury, but comparisons were only made with test-based norms rather than a matched sample. In a recent study, Richards (2000) undertook a comparison of young and elderly individuals with MTBI (with symptoms lasting longer than 1 year) and both young and elderly controls on a wide range of attention, memory, and executive function tasks. MTBI effects were seen on backward digit span, letter cancellation, TMT Parts A and B (sequencing and switching errors), a Digit–Symbol test (omission and commission errors), the CVLT (total words recalled across five trials), verbal fluency, the CTT (omissions and commissions), and the percentage of perseverative responses on the WCST. Consistent with other studies, Richards reported age effects but not MTBI effects, on the percentage of information retained on the CVLT after a delay, and on the number of categories achieved on the WCST.

On the whole, the literature suggests that MTBI may have long-term effects in some individuals on complex attention, working memory, efficiency of new learning, speed of processing, generative fluency, and self-monitoring of responses. Negative effects on simple attention, retention of learned information, linguistic skills, and conceptual abilities are far less common.

INTERVENTION APPROACHES FOR DIFFERENT PHASES AND CIRCUMSTANCES

Despite the level of interest in causes and effects of MTBI, and in the associated short- and long-term symptoms, few studies have focused on effective interventions for these individuals (Raskin & Mateer, 2000). In this section we focus first on early interventions in the immediate postinjury period, and then discuss strategies and approaches for individuals with persistent symptomatology. The need to consider special circumstances is also discussed.

The Role of Early Intervention/Education

Perhaps the most common experience for individuals who sustain a concussion or MTBI is to be seen in an emergency room or doctor's office immediately after or within a day or two of the injury. They usually undergo a standard neurological examination, and are reassured that nothing is seriously wrong and that they can expect a complete recovery. Physicians have traditionally been reluctant to suggest to individuals with such injuries that they may experience adverse symptoms for some period of time—presumably because they do not want to suggest or prompt symptoms that might not otherwise emerge, and because the usual expectation is for full recovery. Indeed, there has been concern that providing information about the common symptoms of MTBI will result in iatrogenic symptom development and/or maintenance. But what is the evidence for such beliefs and for the effects of early intervention in general?

In one of the first studies to look at this issue, Kelly (1975) reported that postconcussive symptom rates were actually higher when measured some months later in patients who had been given no explanation for their symptoms. Similarly, Minderhoud, Boelens, Huizenga, and Saan (1980) reported that subjects who received a printed manual about the nature, causes, and expected course of recovery actually reported significantly fewer postconcussive symptoms at 6 months after injury than did control subjects who did not receive such information. Gronwall (1986) also looked at the effectiveness of providing early information in reducing postconcussive symptoms. Subjects in one group were given reassurance that various postconcussive symptoms are ordinary, transient effects of head injury, and they were given a booklet providing suggestions for how to cope with them. They were encouraged to resume preinjury activities gradually, and they were given instructions for stress management techniques. Three months after injury, the untreated (i.e., uninformed) patients were nine times more likely to be symptomatic than were those who received the "intervention." Alves and colleagues (1993) also reported that information lowered risk for persistence of PCS at a 6-month follow-up.

Mittenberg, Tremont, Zielinski, Fichera, and Rayls (1996) also looked at the effect of early educationally oriented interventions. Subjects in this study included 29 subjects with MTBI, who had a mean GCS score of 14.86. The treated group was given a 10-page manual entitled "Recovery from Mild Head Injury: A Treatment Manual for Patients" (Mittenberg, Zielinski, & Fichera, 1993), whereas the control subjects were provided with only standard treatment and discharge information. The treated patients showed significantly shorter symptom duration than untreated patients, fewer symptoms at 6 months, fewer symptomatic days, and lower average symptom severity levels. Table 15.1 lists the percentage of initially symptomatic patients who continued to report specific symptoms 6 months after injury. It was clear that informed subjects fared significantly better after injury across a broad range of common symptoms than did those who were treated in the standard fashion.

Effective and important early messages appear to include information that normalizes postconcussion symptoms and provides a realistic explanation of their bases (Lawler & Terregino, 1996). Without this information,

TABLE 15.1. Percentage of Patients with MTBI
Who Remained Symptomatic at 6 Months after
Injury, with and without Early Information

Symptom	Group	
	Control	Treatment (informed)
Headache	86%	44%
Fatigue	82%	47%
Memory	80%	38%
Concentration	80%	29%
Anxiety	58%	38%
Depression	56%	27%
Dizziness	50%	36%

Note. From Mittenberg, Tremont, Zielinski, Fichera, and Rayls (1996). Copyright 1996 by Elsevier Science, Inc. Adapted by permission.

or with information suggesting that significant symptoms are extremely unlikely, individuals are more apt to attribute the MTBI effects to other causes and/or to worry that they are "doing something wrong," are "lazy," or are "going crazy." Also important is information that helps these individuals to regulate their lifestyle and environment to reduce or avoid problems. Simple strategies such as taking an extra few weeks away from work, returning to work part-time, declining some other responsibilities for a period, or simply getting rest and reducing distraction can be very helpful. Individuals with MTBI should also be educated to recognize early signs of stress and to take steps to reduce or control such feelings. Finally, the individuals should be encouraged to develop a variety of compensations, such as using a diary or other memory aid during the period of recovery. Table 15.2 summarizes the various messages.

Strategies to Use When Symptoms Persist

Several variables, some not yet fully identified, appear to put some individuals at risk for and/or contribute to persistent problems (Conboy, Barth, & Boll, 1986; Ho & Bennett, 1997). These include injury-related variables; variables related to an individual's age; and the person's premorbid cognitive, emotional, social, personality, and behavioral functioning. Also important are variables related to the individual's postinjury experiences, including any consequences for work, family, and/or social functioning. Another important variable may be the interpretations that the person makes with regard to the injury.

　　When a clinician is working with an individual who demonstrates persisting effects of MTBI, we recommend a number of steps. First, it is important to conduct a thorough neuropsychological assessment to identify both preinjury and current cognitive strengths and weaknesses, and to determine their fit with the commonly recognized effects of MTBI. The evaluation should also include a thorough evaluation of the person's background, and a history related to the injury and early effects of clinical course after the injury. Assessment of emotional status and of current functional adaptation is also crucial. With this information in place, the

---

TABLE 15.2. Important Messages in the Acute/Early Stage of MTBI

- Normalize early physical, cognitive, and emotional postconcussion symptoms
- Provide a realistic explanation as to their cause
- Suggest ways to regulate lifestyle and environment to reduce or avoid problems
- Educate about signs of stress and suggest ways to reduce it
- Encourage interim use of compensations during the period of recovery
- Reinforce strong likelihood of full recovery

clinician can explore alternative explanations for persisting symptoms or reduced function. The first step in treatment is usually to provide some information about the common effects of MTBI. This often results in validating the person's own experience and provides reassurance. Without focusing on emotional or personality factors as causal, the therapist can then begin to explain how emotional responses to cognitive failures or inefficiency can affect functional adaptation. Treatment focusing on improving underlying cognitive skills (such as attention), and on assisting the person to develop and use effective compensations (e.g., a compensatory memory system), should then be considered. Although it has been suggested that there is "no role" for cognitive rehabilitation in individuals with MTBI (Alexander, 1995), our experience does not support this. Indeed, many individuals with MTBI have responded very well to cognitively oriented interventions and have made very significant improvements in their functioning (Mateer, Sohlberg, & Youngman, 1990; Raskin & Mateer, 2000). Another important goal of intervention should be to promote self-regulation of emotional response due to frustration and cognitive failure. Many individuals with MTBI feel that their cognitive difficulties occur "out of the blue" and are out of their control. It is important to foster and reestablish a sense of mastery over the environment and oneself. Table 15.3 sets forth some general clinical guidelines for managing persistent MTBI.

The Need to Consider Special Circumstances

In some individuals with MTBI, there may be causes for symptoms and behaviors that, though consequences of the injury, suggest alternative, noncognitive approaches to intervention. In such cases, intervening at the level of improving or compensating for cognitive inefficiency may not be effective or fruitful. Alternative explanations for symptoms may include a primary pain disorder (e.g., posttraumatic migraine), a sleep disturbance, or other comorbid medical or psychiatric problems. The following case study illustrates one such situation.

TABLE 15.3. General Clinical Guidelines for Managing Persistent MTBI

- Validate the experience of the person
- Do not prematurely confront emotional factors as primary
- Reestablish the shaken sense of self
- Involve the family
- Focus on emotional adjustment along with the cognitive problems
- Sort out the primary from the secondary deficits

Case Example of Sleep Disturbance Following MTBI

Carl was a 43-year-old man who worked as an accountant with a mortgage company. He had been married for 16 years and had two young children. He was involved in a motor vehicle accident in which his vehicle was struck on the driver's side by a truck; he was belted and his airbag deployed. He reported no retrograde amnesia and only a brief period of anterograde amnesia; his GCS score was 15. Carl's injuries included a broken clavicle, a wound at the base of his skull on the left side, two broken ribs, and a minor knee injury. He returned to work 2 weeks later, but upon return to work reported concerns with his attention and memory. He also reported very significant sleep disturbance, to the degree that he had his wife call him at his office several times a day to make sure that he was not sleeping. Neuropsychological testing indicated that his IQ was in the superior range (97th percentile), but that his verbal memory was only average (Wechsler Memory Scale—III General Memory Index, 45th percentile), and his nonverbal memory was significantly below expectations for his background and IQ (Rey Figure Recall, 15th percentile; Rey Visual Design Learning, 18th percentile). Because of his significant sleep disorder, a sleep disorder evaluation was recommended. This included a 2-night sleep study with electroencephalogram, electro-oculogram, electromyogram, and a multiple sleep latency test. The study indicated that Carl demonstrated more than the expected number of periodic limb movements, as well as disturbed distribution of alpha–delta brain wave activity during sleep. Hypersomnolence secondary to sleep interruption and low sleep efficiency was diagnosed. It was recommended that he undergo a trial period of treatment with trazodone, following which Carl experienced substantial resolution of not only his sleep difficulties, but his problems with attention and concentration. Although not feeling fully "back to normal," he was able to resume a full range of work and home activities, with some accommodations.

In this example, focusing on the predominant sleep disturbance had a very positive effect on this man's everyday functioning. Indeed, sleep difficulties/disorders are extremely common after MTBI, and comprehensive sleep studies can often help to pinpoint problems and identify appropriate interventions. Other noncognitive factors affecting performance and adjustment after MTBI may include associated pain problems or psychiatric disorders. In another case seen by one of us, an unexpected psychiatric abnormality emerged over a year following the injury.

Case Example of a Psychiatric Disturbance Following MTBI

Daniel, a college literature instructor, suffered an MTBI in a motor vehicle accident in the summer. Upon return to work in the fall, he experienced fatigue, as well as some memory and organizational difficulties that affected his lecturing. He had a reduced teaching load in the fall, but resumed his full duties in the winter. All seemed to be going well until he was brought into the college president's office, threatened with dismissal, and shown examples of terribly rude and hurtful remarks he had written on students' papers. Daniel had always received very positive teaching ratings and few complaints, and was frankly shocked that he had made the comments. Upon further inquiry, his wife acknowledged a period (beginning about 16 months after the injury) during which her husband began talking very quickly, sleeping little, and expressing grandiose or unrealistic plans. A Manic Episode was suspected, and a review of the literature revealed definite reports of Manic Episodes occurring many months after TBI (Taylor & Jung, 1998). Episodes were unrelated to family history, previous psychiatric functioning, or severity of injury, and were most commonly associated with posterior frontal and anterior temporal damage.

SPECIFIC TECHNIQUES FOR WORKING WITH INDIVIDUALS WITH MTBI

Specific techniques for working with cognitive impairments following MTBI are, in many cases, similar to or the same as those indicated in prior chapters in this text that address management of attention, memory, and executive function disorders. For example, approaches to working with attention problems include environmental modifications and strategies; attention process training; and psychosocial support to achieve a higher level of adjustment to changes, self-regulation, and self-control. Before beginning the actual interventions, we find it useful to have the individual complete the self-report Attention Rating Scale (Ponsford & Kinsella, 1991), as well as an individualized list of cognitively based problems that are interfering with everyday function. The individual may report having difficulty driving, problems with meal preparation, slowness or errors in the workplace, difficulty dealing with distraction, and/or fatigue. The problem list yields insight into the person's awareness, the extent and nature of functional problems, and the person's current way of dealing with or responding to the problems. Goals, framed in functional terms, are mutually discussed and agreed upon. Table 15.4 lists several useful techniques for working with individuals with MTBI, which are discussed in more detail in the following sections.

Environmental Modifications

Clients are provided with information about ways in which environmental factors can influence cognitive performance. Together with their therapists, they can explore ways in which the environment may be altered. These may include such things as turning off the radio or TV when preparing

TABLE 15.4. Useful Techniques for Working with Individuals with MTBI

* Environmental modifications
* Improving, and fostering generalization of, attention skills
* Increasing metacognitive awareness of attention and memory functioning
* Time pressure management (TPM) training
* Specific memory interventions/compensations
* Improving memory self-efficacy
* Fostering self-management and self-regulation of cognitive and emotional functioning
* Cognitive-behavioral interventions
* Coping effectiveness training and preparation for lapses

dinner or doing homework, or undertaking more limited shopping trips in smaller stores or at quieter hours.

Improving Underlying Attention Skills

A number of studies have shown positive effects on attention skills in individuals with MTBI following attention process training. Repeated practice on tasks requiring a high degree of working memory and self-monitoring appears to be beneficial in improving performance on unpracticed tasks requiring similar and/or related abilities. Elsewhere, we (Mateer et al., 1990) reported on the results of a comprehensive treatment program involving attention process training, use of external memory aids, and psychosocial adjustment. Five participants with MTBI demonstrated significant improvements on several cognitive measures. There were significantly decreased times to completion on TMT A and B; improved recall over five learning trials, and better delayed recall, on the Auditory–Verbal Learning Test; and improved Acquisition and Recall scores on the Randt Memory Test. Although improvements were well beyond those expected from practice effects alone, these individuals were all involved in a multidisciplinary program involving cognitive rehabilitation, psychosocial support, and vocational interventions, with an emphasis on developing effective coping skills. This made it difficult to know to what factors the change should be attributed. However, in one report, an individual who did only the cognitive exercises (because of distance constraints) made substantial gains on TMT Part B, on the Stroop Test, and on verbal fluency (Mateer, 1992). This gentleman, who did not start the training until 16 months after his injury, was able to return to full-time work as a university professor of economics. Indeed, gains in return to work and in vocational productivity were reported in the great majority of subjects with MTBI who completed a program designed particularly to address this population (Mateer et al., 1990).

Fostering Generalization of Attention Skills and Strategies

In 1994, we (Sohlberg, Johnson, Paule, Raskin, & Mateer) developed the Attention Process Training II (APT-II) program, a set of training materials designed for work with individuals with less severe injuries. Along with a large set of exercises involving sustained, selective, alternating, and divided attention (described in Chapter 5), the APT-II incorporates more formal ways of addressing the generalization of training. Specific, individualized generalization exercises are created and carried out at home or at work. Specific parameters are set with regard to the nature of the activity, the setting, the time of day or duration of the activity, level of difficulty, and measure of success. The client completes information about his or her performance on the activity, and activity sheets are discussed and modified as part of the therapy. Examples of generalization activities for sustained attention include reading for various amounts of time, persisting on a telephone calling activity, or (for a student) working on a homework exercise. For generalization activities in the selective attention domain, various kinds of distraction or interference are introduced in association with specific activities. Within the divided attention domain, simpler functional tasks are combined, and measures of performance/success are obtained for each. Since emotional responses to cognitively demanding tasks are common, scoring/rating criteria often incorporate subjective ratings of stress, irritability, or frustration. Comments also include information about coping strategies, such as taking a break or turning off the distraction briefly. An example of the use of generalization exercises focusing on divided attention is provided below.

Case Example of Using Attention Generalization Exercises

Jill was a 35-year-old parts clerk for a large automotive distribution company serving a large metropolitan region. She was involved in a motor vehicle accident in which she sustained brief loss of consciousness and a PTA of about 5 hours. Upon return to work a couple of months later, she had difficulty with headaches, felt "overwhelmed," made many mistakes, and often left work early. Jill received training in divided attention tasks (APT-II). In conjunction with a representative of her union, she then engaged in generalization exercises at the workplace. Much of her work involved working with invoices and packing orders, and with looking up parts numbers and prices from catalogues in a busy office. Jill began with a series of exercises in which she practiced finding specific information within a set time limit. She then worked on identifying whether there was any missing information on the invoices, a more difficult task. The next step was to work on looking up and transferring parts numbers and price codes—first in a quiet room, then while on the phone with a confederate who provided some distraction, and then while on the phone at a busy counter. Throughout the training she monitored her level of stress, and learned to take regular breaks and to use breathing techniques for relaxation. Over subsequent sessions, she was able to increase her time on task and to reduce the number of times she needed to take a break. Once successful, she independently initiated using the strategies while at home preparing dinner and while driving. She successfully returned to full-time work in her preinjury capacity, although initially she had been ready to quit.

Metacognitive Interventions

One APT-II component is a metacognitive intervention, which involves the use of attention lapse logs and attention success logs. These logs are kept by the client at home or at work. The first type of log is initially used to help both the client and therapist to monitor the frequency of attention lapses. The log form also asks the client to identify what he or she did in response to each lapse and what he or she might have done to avoid the problem or improve performance. This allows the therapist to look for patterns associated with attention lapses (e.g., time of day or setting), as well as to look for generalized effects of treatment. For the client, it also begins reinforcing the notion that some control over the occurrence of lapses is possible, and that the responses to lapses can be more or less effective. The treatment attempts to build awareness of the interplay between lapses and emotional responses, and to facilitate enhanced feelings of self-control. The attention success log is then introduced in order to reduce the focus on failures, to highlight successes, and to build on feelings of success and control. Clients record situations or events in which they might have had difficulty, but were successful, and then speculate about what it is they did to facilitate that success. The goal of this process is to build insight, self-confidence, and an understanding that clients can, to a large extent, exert influence and control over situations and themselves so as to increase success. Examples of completed attention success and failure logs are provided in Appendices 15.1 and 15.2.

Training in Time Pressure Management

A common source of frustration after MTBI is difficulty managing tasks under time pressure. Slow information processing and difficulties with organization are common consequences of brain injury at all levels of severity. Many clients with MTBI experience a feeling of "information overload" in daily tasks that once were relatively easy. Fasotti, Kovacs, Eling, and Brouwer (2000) have described a technique called *time pressure management* (TPM), a set of cognitive exercises designed to help subjects learn to give themselves enough time to deal with the task at hand. These strategies may entail the enhancement of awareness, the optimalization of planning and organization, the rehearsal of task requirements, and/or the modification of the task environment. The main cognitive strategies encouraged in TPM training are listed in Table 15.5. One group received TPM training, with a focus on dealing with time-limited tasks. Another group received concentration training consisting of reminders to "focus," and not to get distracted by "irrelevant sounds" or by "your own irrelevant thoughts." Although both groups improved on a pair of complex tasks under time pressure, subjects who participated in TPM training made more "managing steps" after training than they had before, or than did the control group. However, they did not appear to use more "prevention strategies."

Specific Memory Interventions

Effective memory interventions for clients with MTBI include facilitating the use of memory aids and both external and internal organizational strategies (e.g., key finders, notebooks/organizers, minicomputer devices, sophisticated watches, voice recorders, and pagers). Although the training and use of internal mnemonic strategies is not usually recommended in individuals with moderate to severe injury, due to the heavy demands on abstraction, initiation, and awareness, individuals with less severe impairments often use such strategies with more success. For example, a nurse we worked with, who was unable to return to her previous work in a cognitively demanding emergency room following MTBI, decided to take an opportunity to do hospice nursing. In order to do so, she needed to take a written test pertaining to common cancer medications and side effects. She learned the information by using a set of mnemonic strategies, similar to those commonly used to remember such sets of information as the cranial nerves. These techniques can be helpful in remembering small-domain, specific bodies of information that are relatively unchanging. Many indi-

---

TABLE 15.5. The Cognitive Strategies in Time Pressure Management—Objectives

1. To *recognize* the time pressure in the task at hand
   - Are there two or more things to be done at the same time?
   - Is there enough time available to tackle both?

2. To *prevent* as much time pressure as possible
   - Make a short plan of which things can be done before the actual task begins
   - Eliminate distractions or actions which do not need to be done

3. To *deal* with time pressure as quickly and effectively as possible
   - Identify the steps that will be taken to complete the tasks
   - Look regularly at the plan
   - Make an emergency plan in case of overwhelming time pressure

Note. From Fasotti, Kovacs, Eling, and Brouwer (2000). Copyright 2000 by Psychology Press, Ltd. Reprinted by permission.

viduals with MTBI, perhaps because they tend to have good awareness of their difficulties, are usually very open and receptive to the introduction of external memory aids and strategies. Because they have retained many cognitive skills, they can often learn to use quite sophisticated and powerful external systems, as well as internal strategies, readily and effectively.

Improving Memory Self-Efficacy

Another area we have found useful to address with individuals who have had MTBI is the area of metamemory and memory self-efficacy. This is similar to the attention self-efficacy work described earlier. *Self-efficacy* refers in this context to individuals' beliefs about their own memory capacity, the degree to which their memory has changed, and the degree to which their memory performance is under their personal control. Self-efficacy beliefs are important because they have been shown to influence the level of effort an individual is willing to put forth on a task, and higher processing effort is known to produce better performance (Lachman, Steinberg, & Trotter, 1987; Lachman, Weaver, Bandura, Elliott, & Lewkowicz, 1992). Research has shown that self-efficacy beliefs can influence behavior in a variety of ways. Beliefs about memory predict not only memory performance, but also how much subjects are willing to wager on their performance. Beliefs about the likelihood that one will experience cognitive difficulty have also been shown to covary with stress. Even neurologically normal subjects who judge themselves inefficacious on memory tasks, and who believe they lack control over their memory, show poorer memory performance than subjects who have higher estimates of memory self-efficacy. Overall, these findings suggest that the belief that one has a poor memory may lead to increased dependence on others, avoidance of memory challenges, and a pattern of helplessness and demoralization in the face of memory difficulties. Thus a more positive sense of cognitive self-efficacy should improve overall level of cognitive functioning and emotional adjustment. We have found that working toward more positive memory self-statements is valuable in increasing adjustment, confidence, and willingness to try new activities.

Fostering Self-Management and Self-Regulation of Emotional Functioning

Although it is important to address cognitive inefficiencies and/or impairments directly, it is also important to consider social, behavioral, and emotional issues that affect cognitive functioning. MTBI often results in a variety of negative emotions and beliefs that can significantly influence a person's performance and functional adjustment. Many individuals with MTBI and their families report significant problems with irritability and quickness to anger. These feelings often appear secondary to frustration, and are exacerbated by stress. Individuals with MTBI, depending on the circumstances of their injury, may also have feelings of victimization, mistreatment, and unfairness. These feelings seem to be most common when they see the injury as no fault of their own, and can be exacerbated by protracted litigation or by changes in their work or relationships following the injury. Anxiety is also common, and frequently relates to feelings of losing control and of uncertainty. Many individuals with MTBI are particularly frustrated by their inability to predict how they will function, and, in general, feel more sensitive and irritable. Other common emotions include feelings of loss and/or depression. These feelings are most commonly related to postinjury perceptions of inadequacy, failure, and inability to achieve or maintain internal goals and expectancies. All of these emotions can contribute to increased stress. Interestingly, it has been suggested that stress itself not only can lead to changes in memory performance, but may result in physiological changes in the hippocampus (Bremner, 1999; Gould & Tanapat, 1999).

Many factors affect emotional compensation following MTBI. As indicated above, self-esteem is often undermined or shattered, in part secondary to cognitive difficulties, and in part due to disturbed regulation of affect and a fragile sense of control. There may also be a magnification of premorbid tendencies. For example, questioning and dismissal by health care professionals with regard to MTBI symptoms may trigger prior feelings of invalidation, abuse, and/or rejection in someone with a history of abuse or neglect, or in someone with a fragile sense of self prior to injury. In an interesting and disturbing recent report, Reeves, Beltzman, and Killu (2000) describe two patients with a history of sexual abuse who, following mild to moderate brain injuries, reported experiencing the reemergence of intrusive sequelae associated with their past abuse. Symptomatology was similar to that commonly seen in association with Posttraumatic Stress Disorder and included intense, vivid, and intrusive flashbacks of the past sexual trauma; behavioral and affective disturbances; nightmares; and hypervigilance. This occurred after years of not experiencing these types of intense recollections. The authors suggest possible explanations for the phenomena, particularly in relation to the notion of decreased inhibitory control as a consequence of the injury. They suggest that sensitive inquiry regarding abuse history should be considered part of the clinical interview with patients who have sustained neurological trauma.

Other premorbid psychological styles may also respond "catastrophically" to the seemingly relatively mild effects of an injury. An individual who has a strong need for control and/or perfectionistic tendencies is likely to react strongly to even subtle changes in ability, compared to someone with a more relaxed attitude about his or her performance. Someone with a very dependent personality may feel "paralyzed" by even subtle cognitive symptoms, and may dip below a critical threshold for coping, resulting in increased fear and anxiety. These reactions can further exacerbate the cognitive impairment, such that mental processing is affected to a degree that goes well beyond that predicted by the apparent injury severity. It is this interplay among subtle cognitive deficits, significant current social stressors, and underlying emotional needs and conflicts that can result in degrees of withdrawal and decompensation that appear excessive in light of apparent potential for better functioning. Ruff, Camenzuli, and Mueller (1996) provide an excellent description and discussion of some of the ways in which preexisting personality features may affect recovery patterns and response to rehabilitation (a more lengthy discussion of this issue is provided in Chapter 12).

We concur with Cicerone, Kay, and others who have worked extensively with individuals experiencing persistent effects of MTBI (Cicerone, Smith, Ellmo, & Mangle, 1996; Kay et al., 1992; Kay, 1993; Raskin & Mateer, 2000) that a major goal of psychosocial therapy is to reconcile discrepancies among patients' own assessment of their functioning and their performance-based competencies; their sense of preinjury identity and ability; and their subjective expectations for future successful functioning. It is important to validate the *experience* of persons with MTBI, but it is also vital to encourage alternative *interpretations* of symptoms as appropriate. Although emotional factors are important, it is not wise to confront emotional factors prematurely. Among the primary goals of treatment should be reestablishing the shaken sense of self, and building and reinforcing self-efficacy and self-regulation.

Approaches to working with individuals with the emotional sequelae of MTBI include educationally oriented approaches, cognitive-behavioral interventions, stress and coping interventions, time management training, and other traditional forms of psychotherapy. (We discuss cognitive-behavioral interventions and coping interventions in more detail below.) Examples of educational approaches include suggesting and teaching approaches to dealing with various problems such as frustration and irritability. For example, in assisting clients to deal better with frustration, clients may be told that although too much frustration is problematic, a little frustration may be a good thing because the individual is stretching to make gains. They may also be told that it is all right to back off, calm down, and try again; helped to learn when they should take a break; assisted in learning signs of fatigue or frustration; and encouraged to select their challenges (Judd, 1999).

Cognitive-Behavioral Interventions

Cognitive-behavioral treatments, which are discussed in more detail in Chapter 12, are based on the premise that cognitions, thoughts, and beliefs affect emotion and behavior, and that self-talk is a powerful mediator of feeling and action (Dobson, 2000). Individuals who harbor feelings of guilt, low self-esteem, avoidance, denial, or entitlement often hold a variety of extreme, negative, and/or dysfunctional beliefs that perpetuate negative affect and a sense of helplessness. These distortions take a variety of forms, including dichotomous thinking, overgeneralization, selective abstraction, arbitrary inference, personalization, and catastrophization, all of which have been defined earlier. The goal of cognitive-behavioral interventions is to help a person identify and modify dysfunctional beliefs. This is done through identification of the person's beliefs and the content of self-talk in response to different situations, and then assisting the person to assess the situation and his or her performance in a more rational and positive manner. The treatment typically involves understanding the person's belief system by having him or her keep a daily record of dysfunctional thoughts, and then facilitating self-statements that are more positive. Cognitive-behavioral interventions for depression and social isolation/withdrawal are often helpful, but should be supplemented by efforts to increase activity and social involvement. Identifying and scheduling pleasurable events and planning social activities are valuable adjuncts to treatment.

Coping Effectiveness Training and Preparation for Lapses

Another approach is known as *coping effectiveness training*. King and Kennedy (1999) have described the use of a coping effectiveness training model in individuals with spinal cord injury, and have demonstrated significant decreases in such individuals' depression and anxiety. The program is administered in seven 75-minute sessions; it involves appraisal training, problem solving, coping skills, and fostering social support. We have recently used this approach in a group of individuals with MTBI, who demonstrated gains in reported self-efficacy and subjective stress. A key component of the intervention involves fostering positive self-control statements. Examples of statements generated by subjects include "I intend to be in control—not my emotions or cognitive problems," "I can and will learn and use strategies to regain control," and "I will teach my body and brain not to respond to my emotions first."

Although many of these techniques are useful in increasing confidence, we have also found that it is important to prepare for lapses. Following a period of increased coping, an unexpected or feared lapse or perceived failure can result in a cascade of negative self-statements, increased cognitive distortions, and decreased use of coping skills, all of which can contribute to an increased probability of further lapses. Indeed, there is a substantial literature on relapse prevention in cognitive-behavioral therapy (see, e.g., Dobson, 2000). Preparing clients for such lapses, and emphasizing that they do not mean progress is not being made, have become essential parts of our discussions.

SUMMARY

A biopsychosocial model incorporating physiogenic and both premorbid and current psychogenic factors is best suited for understanding the long-term outcome following MTBI. Cognitive inefficiencies often set the stage for negative emotional reactions of frustration, anger, irritability, and depression. Therefore, it is important to address the cognitive component in interventions through education, direct training, and work on accommodations and compensations. Attention to the role of emotional responses in mediating cognitive difficulties is an important adjunct to treatment. It is also valuable to identify individuals' beliefs about their cognitive abilities, and to foster balanced and rational perspectives about their functioning. Treatment should foster self-understanding and a sense of personal efficacy and empowerment. It is likewise important to understand pre- and postinjury emotional vulnerabilities and personality factors that can interact with the deficits, the postinjury circumstances and experiences, and the treatment.

REFERENCES

Alexander, M. P. (1995). Mild traumatic brain injury: Pathophysiology, natural history, and clinical management. *Neurology, 45,* 1253–1260.

Alves, W. M., Macciocchi, S. N., & Barth, J. T. (1993). Postconcussive symptoms after uncomplicated mild head injury. *Journal of Head Trauma Rehabilitation, 8,* 48–59.

Atteberry-Bennett, J., Barth, J. T., Loyd, B. H., & Lawrence, E. C. (1986). The relationship between behavioral and cognitive deficits, demographics, and depression in patients with minor head injuries. *International Journal of Clinical Neuropsychology, 8,* 114–117.

Barth, J. T., Macciocchi, S. N., Girodani, B., Rimel, R., Jane, J. A., & Boll, T. J. (1983). Neuropsychological sequelae of minor head injury. *Neurosurgery, 13,* 529–533.

Berrol, S. (1992). Terminology of post-concussive syndrome. In L. J. Horn & N. D. Zasler (Eds.), *Rehabilitation of post-concussive disorders: State of the art reviews* (pp. 1–8). Philadelphia: Henley & Belfus.

Binder, L. M. (1986). Persisting symptoms after mild head injury: A review of the postconcussive syndrome. *Journal of Clinical and Experimental Neuropsychology, 8,* 323–346.

Binder, L. M. (1997). A review of mild head trauma: II. Clinical implications. *Journal of Clinical and Experimental Neuropsychology, 19,* 432–457.

Bohnen, N., Jolles, J., & Twijnstra, A. (1992a). Neuropsychological deficits in patients with persistent symptoms six months after mild head injury. *Neurosurgery, 30,* 692–695.

Bohnen, N., Twijnstra, A., & Jolles, J. (1992b). Post-traumatic and emotional symptoms in different subgroups of patients with mild head injury. *Brain Injury, 6,* 481–487.

Bremner, J. D. (1999). Does stress damage the brain? *Biological Psychiatry, 45,* 797–805.

Cicerone, K. D. (1991). Psychotherapy after mild traumatic brain injury: Relation to the nature and severity of subjective complaints. *Journal of Head Trauma Rehabilitation, 4,* 30–43.

Cicerone, K. D. (1996). Attention deficits and dual task demands after mild traumatic brain injury. *Brain Injury, 10,* 79–89.

Cicerone, K. D. (1997). Clinical sensitivity of four measures of attention to mild traumatic brain injury. *Clinical Neuropsychologist, 11,* 266–272.

Cicerone, K. D., & Kalmar, K. (1995). Persistent postconcussion syndrome: The structure of subjective complaints after mild traumatic injury. *Journal of Head Trauma Rehabilitation, 10,* 1–17.

Cicerone, K. D., Smith, L. C., Ellmo, W., & Mangle, H. R. (1996). The neuropsychological rehabilitation of mild traumatic brain injury. *Brain Injury, 10*(4), 277–286.

Conboy, T. J., Barth, J., & Boll, T. J. (1986). Treatment and rehabilitation of mild and moderate head trauma. *Rehabilitation Psychology, 31*(4), 203–215.

Dikmen, S. S., Machamer, J. E., Winn, H. R., & Temkin, N. R. (1995). Neuropsychological outcome at 1-year post head injury. *Neuropsychology, 9,* 80–90.

Dobson, K. S. (2000). (Ed.). *Handbook of cognitive-behavioral therapies* (2nd ed.). New York: Guilford Press.

Evans, R. W. (1992). The postconcussion syndrome and the sequelae of mild head injury. *Neurologic Clinics, 10,* 815–847.

Evans, R. W. (1994). The postconcussion syndrome: 130 years of controversy. *Seminars in Neurology, 14,* 32–39.

Fasotti, L., Kovacs, F., Eling, P., & Brouwer, W. H. (2000). Time pressure management as a compensatory strategy training after closed head injury. *Neuropsychological Rehabilitation, 10,* 47–65.

Fee, C. R. A., & Rutherford, W. H. (1988). A study of the effect of legal settlement on postconcussion symptoms. *Archives of Emergency Medicine, 5,* 12–17.

Fenton, G., McClelland, R., Montgomery, A., MacFlynn, G., & Rutherford, W. (1993). The postconcussional syndrome: Social antecedents and psychological sequelae. *British Journal of Psychiatry, 162,* 493–497.

Gennarelli, T. A. (1993). Mechanisms of brain injury. *Journal of Emergency Medicine, 11,* 5–11.

Gould, E., & Tanapat, P. (1999). Stress and hippocampal neurogenesis. *Biological Psychiatry, 46,* 1472–1479.

Gouvier, D. W., Cubic, B., Jones, G., Brantley, P., & Cutlip, Q. (1992). Postconcussional symptoms and daily stress in normal and head-injured college populations. *Archives of Clinical Neuropsychology, 7,* 193–212.

Gronwall, D. (1986). Rehabilitation programs for patients with mild head injury:

Components, problems and evaluation. *Journal of Head Trauma Rehabilitation, 1*(2), 53–62.

Gronwall, D., & Wrightson, P. (1974). Delayed recovery of intellectual function after minor head injury. *Lancet, ii,* 605–609.

Ho, M. R., & Bennett, T. L. (1997). Efficacy of neuropsychological rehabilitation for mild–moderate traumatic brain injury. *Archives of Clinical Neuropsychology, 12*(1), 1–11.

Humayan, M. S., Presty, S. K., & Lafrance, N. D. (1989). Local cerebral glucose metabolism in mild closed head injured patients with cognitive impairments. *Nuclear Medicine Communications, 10,* 335–344.

Jennett, B. (1998). Some international comparisons. In H. S. Levin, H. M. Eisenberg, & A. L. Benton (Eds.), *Mild head injury* (pp. 22–34). New York: Oxford University Press.

Judd, T. (1999). *Neuropsychotherapy and community integration: Brain illness, emotion and behavior.* New York: Kluwer Academic/Plenum.

Karzmark, P., Hall, K., & Englander, J. (1995). Late-onset post-concussion symptoms after mild brain injury: The role of premorbid, injury-related, environmental, and personality factors. *Brain Injury, 9,* 21–26.

Kay, T. (1993). Neuropsychological treatment of mild traumatic brain injury. *Journal of Head Trauma Rehabilitation, 8,* 74–85.

Kay, T., Newman, B., Cavallo, M., Ezrachi, O., & Resnick, M. (1992). Toward a neuropsychological model of functional disability after mild traumatic brain injury. *Neuropsychology, 6,* 371–384.

Kelly, R. E. (1975). The post-traumatic syndrome: An iatrogenic disease. *Forensic Science, 6,* 17–24.

Kibby, M. Y., & Long, C. J. (1996). Minor head injury: Attempts at clarifying the confusion. *Brain Injury, 10,* 159–186.

King, C., & Kennedy, P. (1999) Coping effectiveness training for people with spinal cord injury: Preliminary results of a controlled trial. *British Journal of Clinical Psychology, 38*(1), 5–14.

Kraus, J. F., & Nourjah, P. (1998). The epidemiology of mild uncomplicated head injury. *Trauma, 28,* 1637–1643.

Lachman, M. E., Steinberg, E. S., & Trotter, S. D. (1987). The effects of control beliefs and attributions on memory self-assessments and performance. *Psychology and Aging, 2,* 127–271.

Lachman, M. E., Weaver, S. L., Bandura, M., Elliott, E., & Lewkowicz, C. J. (1992). Improving memory and control beliefs through cognitive restructuring and self-generated strategies. *Journal of Gerontology, 47,* 293–299.

Lawler, K. A., & Terregino, C. A. (1996). Guidelines for evaluation and education of adult patients with mild traumatic brain injuries in an acute care setting. *Journal of Head Trauma Rehabilitation, 11*(6), 18–28.

Leininger, B. E., Gramling, S. E., Farrell, A. D., Kreuzer, J. S., & Peck, E. A. (1990). Neuropsychological deficits in symptomatic minor head injury patients after concussion and mild concussion. *Journal of Neurology, Neurosurgery and Psychiatry, 53,* 293–296.

Levin, H. S., Mattis, S., Ruff, R. M., Eisenberg, H. M., Marshall, L. F., & Tabaddor, K. (1987). Neurobehavioral outcome following minor head injury: A three-center study. *Journal of Neurosurgery, 66,* 234–243.

Levin, H. S., Williams, D. H., Eisenberg, H. M., High, W. M., & Guinto, F. (1992). Serial MRI and neurobehavioral findings after mild to moderate closed head injury. *Journal of Neurology, Neurosurgery and Psychiatry, 55*, 255–262.

Lishman, W. A. (1988). Physiogenesis and psychogenesis in the "post-concussional syndrome." *British Journal of Psychiatry, 153*, 460–469.

Marsh, N. V., & Smith, M. D. (1995). Post-concussion syndrome and the coping hypothesis. *Brain Injury, 9*, 553–562.

Mateer, C. A. (1992). Systems of care for post-concussive syndrome. In L. J. Horn & N. D. Zasler (Eds.), *Rehabilitation of post-concussive disorders: State of the art reviews* (pp. 143–155). Philadelphia: Henley & Belfus.

Mateer, C. A., Sohlberg, M. M., & Youngman, P. K. (1990). The management of acquired attention and memory deficits following mild closed head injury. In R. Wood (Ed.), *Cognitive rehabilitation in perspective* (pp. 68–95). London: Taylor & Francis.

McClelland, R. J. (1996). The post-concussional syndrome: A rose by any other name. *Journal of Psychosomatic Research, 40*, 563–568.

Minderhoud, J. M., Boelens, M. E., Huizenga, J., & Saan, R. J. (1980). Treatment of minor head injuries. *Clinical Neurology and Neurosurgery, 82*, 127–140.

Mittenberg, W., Tremont, G., Zielinski, R. E., Fichera, S., & Rayls, K. R. (1996). Cognitive-behavioral prevention of postconcussive syndrome. *Archives of Clinical Neuropsychology, 11*(2), 139–146.

Mittenberg, W., Zielinski, R. E., & Fichera, S. (1993). Recovery from mild head injury: A treatment manual for patients. *Psychotherapy in Private Practice, 12*, 37–52.

Mittl, R., Grossman, R. I., Hiehle, J. F., Hurst, R. W., Kauder, D. R., & Gennarelli, T. A. (1994). Prevalence of MRI evidence of diffuse axonal injury in patients with mild head injury and normal head CT findings. *American Journal of Neuroradiology, 15*, 583–589.

Newberg, A. B., & Alavi, A. (1996). Neuroimaging in patients with traumatic brain injury. *Journal of Head Trauma Rehabilitation, 17*, 65–79.

Ogden, J. A., & Wolfe, M. (1998). Recovery from the post-concussion syndrome: A preliminary study comparing young and middle-aged adults. *Neuropsychological Rehabilitation, 8*, 413–431.

Ponsford, J., & Kinsella, G. (1991). The use of a rating scale of attentional behavior. *Neuropsychological Rehabilitation, 1*, 241–257.

Ponsford, J., & Kinsella, G. (1992). Attentional deficits following closed-head injury. *Journal of Clinical and Experimental Neuropsychology, 14*, 822–838.

Radanov, B. P., Stefano, G. D., Schnidrig, A., & Ballinari, P. (1991). Role of psychosocial stress in recovery from common whiplash. *Lancet, 338*, 712–715.

Raskin, S. A., & Mateer, C. A. (Eds.). (2000). *Neuropsychological management of mild traumatic brain injury*. New York: Oxford University Press.

Raskin, S. A., Mateer, C. A., & Tweeten, R. (1998). Neuropsychological assessment of individuals with mild traumatic brain injury. *The Clinical Neuropsychologist, 12*, 21–30.

Raskin, S. A., & Rearick, E. (1996). Verbal fluency in individuals with mild traumatic brain injury. *Neuropsychology, 10*, 416–422.

Reeves, R. H., Beltzman, D., & Killu, K. (2000). Implications of traumatic brain injury for survivors of sexual abuse: A preliminary report of findings. *Rehabilitation Psychology, 45*, 205–211.

Reitan, R. M., & Wolfson, D. (1997). Emotional disturbances and their interaction with neuropsychological deficits. *Neuropsychology Review, 7*, 221–228.

Richards, B. (2000). *The effects of aging and mild traumatic brain injury on neuropsychological performance.* Unpublished doctoral dissertation, York University, Toronto, Ontario, Canada.

Rimel, R. W., Giordani, B., Barth, J. T., Boll, T. J., & Jane, J. A. (1981). Disability caused by minor head injury. *Neurosurgery, 9*, 221–228.

Ruff, R. M., Camenzuli, L., & Mueller, J. (1996). Miserable minority: Emotional risk factors that influence the outcome of a mild traumatic brain injury. *Brain Injury, 10*(8), 551–565.

Ruff, R. M., Crouch, J., & Troster, A. (1994). Selected cases of poor outcome following minor brain trauma: Comparing neuropsychological and positron emission tomography assessment. *Brain Injury, 8*, 297–304.

Ruttan, L. A. (1998). *Depression and neuropsychological functioning in mild traumatic brain injury.* Unpublished doctoral dissertation, York University, Toronto, Ontario, Canada.

Sohlberg, M. M., Johnson, L., Paule, L., Raskin, S. A., & Mateer, C. A. (1994). *Attention Process Training II: A program to address attentional deficits for persons with mild cognitive dysfunction.* Puyallup, WA: Association for Neuropsychological Research and Development.

Strich, S. J. (1961). Shearing of nerve fibers as a cause of brain damage due to head injury. *Lancet, ii*, 443–448.

Stuss, D. T., Ely, P., Hugenholtz, H., Richard, M. T., LaRochelle, S., & Poirier, C. A. (1985). Subtle neuropsychological deficits in patients with good recovery after closed head injury. *Neurosurgery, 17*, 41–47.

Stuss, D. T., Stethem, L. L., Hugenholtz, H., & Richard, M. T. (1989). Traumatic brain injury: A comparison of three clinical tests and analysis of recovery. *The Clinical Neuropsychologist, 3*, 145–156.

Taylor, C. A., & Jung, H. Y. (1998). Disorders of mood after traumatic brain injury. *Seminars in Clinical Neuropsychiatry, 3*(3), 224–231.

Varney, N. R., Bushnell, D. L., Nathan, M., & Kahn, M. D. (1995). NeuroSPECT correlates of disabling mild head injury: Preliminary findings. *Journal of Head Trauma Rehabilitation, 10*, 18–28.

Yodoto, H., Kurokawa, A., & Otsuka, T. (1991). Significance of magnetic resonance imaging in acute head injury. *Journal of Trauma, 31*, 351–357.

Zasler, N. D. (1993). Mild traumatic brain injury: Medical assessment and intervention. *Journal of Head Trauma Rehabilitation, 8*, 13–29.

APPENDIX 15.1

EXAMPLE OF A COMPLETED APT-II ATTENTION LAPSE LOG

Name _____DB_____

Instructions from therapist ___Record mistakes or lapses of attention___
___at home or on the road.___

Date/Time	Describe lapse in attention	What did you do (or could you have done) to manage lapse?
3-4 9:00	Put teapot on stove, forgot to put stove on	Don't leave the kitchen without checking
3-5 9:30	Burned pancakes—smoke! Lost coffee cup, found it in microwave	Don't leave kitchen Wait or check for coffee in microwave
3-6 7:30	What am I doing in the basement? What tool did I want?	Repeat to myself what I'm after
3-7 10:00	Forgot to write mileage down in truck	Keep Post-It Note on dash
3-7 3:00	Dropped phone	Watch where I place things
3-7 9:00	Found the bathtub full of cold water	Throw towel over my shoulder when I'm running a bath
3-8 8:00	Forgot to take medication	Keep my medicine on counter
3-8 2:30	Attempted taxes, overload, had to stop	Tackle a smaller piece for a shorter length of time
3-8 6:00	Smoke alarm special for dinner!	Set the oven alarm!

Note. The log form is from Sohlberg, Johnson, Paule, Raskin, and Mateer (1994). Copyright 1994 by the Association for Neuropsychological Research and Development. Materials now available from Lash & Associates, 708 Young Forest Drive, Wake Forest, NC 27587. Reprinted by permission.

EXAMPLE OF A COMPLETED APT-II ATTENTION SUCCESS LOG

Name _____DB_____

Instructions from therapist ___Record instances when you felt successful
doing something that demanded attention at home or on the road.___

Date/Time	Describe attention success	Why do you think you were successful? (list strategies or management techniques)
3-10 10:00	Cleaned my chainsaw and put it back together again	Stuck with one task; no distractions, not even radio
3-11 9:30	Managed to pay all of my bills—as far as I know	I gathered and then opened every envelope I could find
3-12 7:30	Made toast, eggs, and juice	Made a plan and got all the ingredients out and ready
3-13 10:00	Remembered to make phone calls and didn't quit when I wanted to	Set aside time early in the day; made and kept a list of who I needed to call with numbers; kept notepad handy and wrote down when numbers were busy
3-14 12:00	Cleaned the house on autopilot	It was raining and I had to stay inside anyway, but I promised myself a movie if I finished

Note. The log form is from Sohlberg, Johnson, Paule, Raskin, and Mateer (1994). Copyright 1994 by the Association for Neuropsychological Research and Development. Materials now available from Lash & Associates, 708 Young Forest Drive, Wake Forest, NC 27587. Reprinted by permission.

Index